£70-00

SJAmyes

This is the first book to deal comprehensively with endocrine toxicology. It covers the whole spectrum of known toxicant effects on the endocrine system ranging from small disturbances in hormonal secretion to full endocrine neoplasia. In each chapter, internationally recognized authorities have addressed basic endocrine physiology, current techniques for studying endocrine toxicity *in vivo* and *in vitro*, known xenobiotic-induced toxicity phenomena and the latest scientific advances in understanding the underlying molecular and cellular events. Consideration is given to important issues such as dietary factors which influence endocrine toxicity, species differences in sensitivity to toxicants, and the toxicity of hormones as drugs.

The volume provides a sound basis for understanding the scientific aspects of this complex and important area of toxicology and will be a valuable source of information for all those working in this field including: regulatory and investigative toxicologists, reproductive toxicologists, pathologists and pharmacologists in industry, medicine, contract laboratories and academia.

# ENDOCRINE TOXICOLOGY

# ENDOCRINE TOXICOLOGY

*Edited by*

**Christopher K. Atterwill**
*Celltox Centre, Hatfield Polytechnic, Hatfield, Herts, UK*
*and*

**John D. Flack**
*SmithKline Beecham Pharmaceuticals, Harlow, Essex, UK*

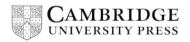

CAMBRIDGE
UNIVERSITY PRESS

Published by the Press Syndicate of the University of Cambridge
The Pitt Building, Trumpington Street, Cambridge CB2 1RP
40 West 20th Street, New York, NY 10011–4211, USA
10 Stamford Road, Oakleigh, Victoria 3166, Australia

First published 1992

Printed in Great Britain at the University Press, Cambridge

*A catalogue record for this book is available from the British Library*

*Library of Congress cataloguing in publication data*

Endocrine toxicology/edited by Christopher K. Atterwill and John D. Flack.
   p. cm.
   ISBN 0 521 40225 5 (hardback)
   1. Endocrine toxicology. I. Atterwill, C. K. II. Flack, John D.
   [DNLM: 1. Endocrine Glands—drug effects. 2. Endocrine Glands—
physiopathology. 3. Toxicology. WK 100 E5273]
   RC649.E524 1992
   616.4—dc20   91—23113   CIP

ISBN 0 521 40225 5 hardback

To: Our families and secretaries, for their patience, tolerance, and support.

# Contents

# Contributors

C.K. ATTERWILL
Celltox Centre, Hatfield Polytechnic, College Lane, Hatfield, Herts AL10 9AB, UK.

G.R. BETTON
Safety of Medicines Dept, ICI Pharmaceuticals, Mereside, Alderley Park, Macclesfield, Cheshire SK10 4TG, UK.

C.G. BROWN
SmithKline Beecham Pharmaceuticals, The Frythe, Welwyn, Herts AL6 9AR, UK.

J.C. BUCKINGHAM
Dept of Pharmacology, Charing Cross and Westminster Medical School, University of London, Charing Cross Hospital, Fulham Palace Road, London W6 8RF, UK.

C.C. CAPEN
Dept of Veterinary Pathobiology, The Ohio State University, 1925 Coffey Road, Columbus, OH 4321-1093, USA.

H.D. COLBY
Dept of Pharmacology and Toxicology, Philadelphia College of Pharmacy and Science, Woodland Avenue at 43rd Street, Philadelphia, PA 19104, USA.

R.A. COOPER
Reproductive Toxicology Branch, HERL, US Environmental Protection Agency, Research Triangle Park, NC 27711, USA.

A.D. DAYAN
DHSS Dept of Toxicology, St Bartholomew's Hospital Medical College, University of London, Dominion House, 59 Bartholomew Close, London EC1 7ED, UK.

J.D. FLACK
SmithKline Beecham Pharmaceuticals, Coldharbour Road, The Pinnacles, Harlow, Essex CM19 5AD, UK.

D. GARSIDE
Animal Research Station, Animal Biotechnology Cambridge Ltd, University of Cambridge, 307 Huntingdon Road, Cambridge CB3 0JQ, UK.

D. GILLIES
Dept of Pharmacology, Charing Cross and Westminster Medical School, University of London, Fulham Palace Road, London W6 8RF, UK.

R.W. GREENHILL
SmithKline Beecham Pharmaceuticals, The Frythe, Welwyn, Herts AL6 9AR, UK.

P. HARVEY
Safety Evaluation Department, Schering Agrochemicals Ltd, Chesterford Park Research Station, Saffron Walden, Essex CB10 1XL, UK.

C. JONES
Dept Biological Sciences, The University of Sheffield, Sheffield, Yorks S10 2TN, UK.

A.J. LEIGH
Dept of Obstetrics and Gynaecology, St George's Hospital, Medical School, University of London, Cranmer Terrace, London SW17 0RE, UK.

P.A. LONGHURST
Division of Urology, University of Pennsylvania, School of Medicine, Philadelphia, PA 19104, USA.

F.J.C. ROE
19 Marryat Road, Wimbledon Common, London SW19 5BB, UK.

G. THOMAS
Dept of Pathology, University of Wales College of Medicine, Heath Park, Cardiff CF4 4XN, UK.

M.J. TUCKER
ICI Pharmaceuticals, Mereside, Macclesfield, Cheshire SK10 4TG, UK.

R.F. WALKER
University of South Florida College of Medicine, Department of Paediatrics, Division of Endocrinology, All Children's Hospital, 801 Sixth Street South, St Petersburg, FL 3371–8920, USA.

E.D. WILLIAMS
Dept of Pathology, University of Wales College of Medicine, Heath Park, Cardiff CF4 4XN, UK.

C. WILSON
Dept of Obstetrics and Gynaecology, St George's Hospital Medical School, University of London, Cranmer Terrace, London SW17 0RE, UK.

# Preface

Studies of the effects of drugs on the endocrine system in animals and humans had largely been an area occupied by endocrinologists and pharmacologists until the late 1970s. Some pharmacological agents had even helped to progress knowledge of endocrine control mechanisms, such as the use of dopamine agonists and antagonists for delineating dopamine receptor subtypes on pituitary lactotrophs. There were exceptions to this where reproductive toxicologists had long studied the effects, for example, of heavy metals on testicular function.

An explosion of toxicological interest in the endocrine system occurred in the late 1970s and 1980s. This was in part due to enigmas such as the prevalence of species-specific rodent endocrine tumours, the effects of dietary factors on endocrine tumours, and the whole area of hormone and growth-factor related epigenetic carcinogenesis. All of these started to be of great concern to practising toxicologists and pathologists as problems in regulatory studies continued to expand.

This was mirrored by a number of prestige scientific meetings to discuss the various issues in the hope of conveying positive understanding, mechanistic suggestions, and new methods for investigative studies to regulatory authorities such as the EPA and the FDA. For example, the Pharmaceutical Manufacturers Association, the Society for Endocrinologic Pathologists and the Society for Drug Research together with the British Toxicological Society all held scientific symposia. Indeed it was the latter which largely prompted the idea for this book.

Alongside these developments the area of *in vitro* toxicology was growing fast and it is fair to say that much of the advance in this area was made *in vitro* endocrine toxicology. There are now many culture and cellular models of, for example, the thyroid, adrenal pituitary, and gonads, available for both prescreening toxicology and mechanistic work. For the thyroid in particular much of the knowledge on the role of thyroid stimulating hormone (TSH) in epigenetic thyroid tumourigenesis came from work in culture.

It is hoped this book, which we anticipate to be the first of many, will be a useful reference source to all toxicologists and pathologists in both industry and academia. Since each chapter also attempts to give a full background of endocrine physiology to each system described, the book should also be a valuable aid to students of toxicology. Although protocols for endocrine toxicological studies are not provided, as the field is not that far advanced as yet, the book should form a useful adjunct to standard toxicology textbooks in formulating investigative strategies.

# I     Introduction

C.K. ATTERWILL AND J.D. FLACK

# 1    Introduction to endocrine toxicology

The word *endocrinology* is derived from two Greek words meaning 'separated within' which recognizes, albeit rather obliquely, the mechanism by which hormones circulate within the body to stimulate specific target organs and tissues. It is this unique characteristic of the endocrine system (the ductless glands) that was the focus of the attention of the French physiologist Claude Bernard in the middle of the nineteenth century. He put forward the concept of the *milieu intérieur*, the stable internal environment of the body, regulated by a multitude of interacting control mechanisms geared to maintain the body's chemical and physical *status quo*.

Bernard postulated the theory (without knowing anything of the way endocrine glands operate) that internal secretions maintain equilibrium in response to a range of altering conditions imposed on the body. This mechanism, called homeostasis, is essentially that which is still accepted today and forms the basis of endocrine toxicology and of this book. Major, or more subtle perturbations of this complex system of homeostatic control mechanisms can lead to endocrine toxicity.

Major alterations in endocrine status have been recognized by clinical endocrinologists and physiologists for decades as resulting in disease conditions with characteristic clinical syndromes. Thus the names of Harvey Cushing (the American neurological surgeon), Robert Graves (one of a group of Irish doctors in Dublin), and Thomas Addison (a physician at Guy's Hospital in London) are associated with severe abnormalities of the pituitary, thyroid, and adrenal cortex glands, respectively, which give rise to clinical endocrine diseases described by the enduring clinical eponyms of Cushing's Syndrome, Grave's Disease, and Addison's Disease.

More subtle abnormalities of the endocrine system have had to await the isolation, extraction, characterization and measurement of the endogenous hormones. With this knowledge synthetic and medicinal chemists have been able to make highly potent and metabolically stable analogues and antagonists of the endogenous endocrine hormones. Many of these synthetically derived hormones or analogues of them were introduced as therapeutic agents before the advent of regulatory authorities and the subsequent growth in pre-clinical toxicological testing for defining toxicity in animals as an attempt to predict clinical safety.

The clinical benefits derived from these advances are absolutely staggering in their magnitude. One only has to consider the natural and synthetic glucocorticoids to realize how much impact corticosteroid therapy has had on the quality of life since the isolation and identification of cortisone in 1949 by Edward Kendall at the Mayo Clinic. Similar examples could be forwarded for oestrogens, androgens, progestogens, mineralocorticoids, insulin, and the thyroid hormones. Therapy with these hormones, their enantiomers and analogues has led in turn to detailed knowledge of their inherent target organ toxicity and activated removal mechanisms from the body enabling clinical doses to be 'fine-tuned' and less toxic analogues introduced (Atterwill *et al.*, 1988).

It is a sobering thought for the toxicologist (and the regulatory authorities concerned with protecting the public from unacceptable clinical toxicity of medicines) as to how they would cope with this situation in today's climate. The argument is frequently advanced by toxicologists that were aspirin to be tested by today's conventional toxicology protocols there would be little chance of 'clearing' the compound for clinical use and little to no chance of any regulatory authority giving aspirin a product licence. Because of the physiological potency and central role of endogenous endocrine hormones in controlling homeostasis, conventional toxicology pre-clinical testing in animals of the natural or synthetically derived hormone and analogues thereof is only appropriate if the data derived from such studies is properly interpreted by both toxicologists and regulators. Unfortunately there is a significant risk of throwing the baby out with the bathwater with this approach. It would seem more appropriate for the toxicologist to design animal studies which are targeted more specifically to the compounds under study and for the regulatory authorities to be flexible in their requests for specific types and designs of studies (Flack, 1986; Roe, 1989). This is not simply an issue of historic interest. Toxicologists and regulatory authorities face similar issues today with the new generation of neuroendocrine hormones such as hypothalamic releasing factors and other endogenous local hormones which can now be produced by biotechnology techniques on such a large scale that allows their therapeutic use for clinical conditions which will often require long term administration. Potential examples of this would be the use of nerve growth factor and growth hormone. The dangers of continual use of corticosteroids in rheumatoid arthritis were learnt from clinical practice and experimental (investigational) endocrinology not conventional toxicology. Predicting the clinical safety and how to effectively and safely use the new generation of 'natural' or chemically modified endogenous hormones, whether biotechnologically or chemically synthetically derived, will require a similar approach.

Relative to the multiple actions of exogenously administered hormones and their synthetic analogues on the complex homeostatic mechanisms of the whole body, there are comparatively few examples of xenobiotics which give rise to endocrine toxicity (Baylis & Tunbridge, 1985). The thioureas have been known for several decades to cause thyroid toxicity and indeed this knowledge has been exploited by medicinal chemists to discover effective antithyroid compounds which are of benefit for patients with symptoms of an over-active thyroid gland. Aminoglutethimide, etomidate, and ketoconazole can inhibit corticosteroid secretion by interfering with steroid hydroxylations (P450 mediated) and again this side effect, once recognized, has been utilized with clinical benefit in patients with hypercortisol secretion. On the other hand, the use of aminoglutethimide for the treatment of breast cancer has led to an appreciation of the fine titration of clinical dose to avoid adrenal toxicity. Clinical life-threatening endocrine toxicity or even toxicity leading to a loss of quality of life by xenobiotics appears to be relatively rare. In particular it is worth noting that in humans the incidence of endocrine tumours relative to all other sites is very low (Table 1.1) and there appears to be no evidence that xenobiotics are increasing this incidence. Multiple endocrine tumours in humans are very rare.

In contrast to the relatively low incidence of spontaneous and drug induced toxicity in humans the situation in the rodent and most particularly the rat is quite different. The rat has a very high spontaneous incidence of usually benign multiple endocrine tumours and yet the rat has an extremely important position in assessing the toxicological potential and safety assessment (including carcinogenic potential) of xenobiotics.

Classifications of different types of endocrine toxicity have been proposed in previous publications on this subject. Capen & Martin (1989) proposed a detailed classification based on clinical endocrine function and pathology. On the other hand Baylis & Tunbridge (1985) proposed a simpler classification based on the adverse endocrine reactions of xenobiotics which are observed clinically. From a toxicological or pre-clinical safety testing point of view we favour classifying endocrine toxicology of xenobiotics in a manner which is similar in concept to that for classifying other toxicological phenomena (CIOMS, 1983) but which we have modified to take account of the unique nature of the endocrine system.

Table 1.1. *Proportion of human cancers in the UK of hormonal origin*

| Cancer site | Rate per 100,000 living-all ages | |
| --- | --- | --- |
| | Male | Female |
| All sites | 305.6 | 281.3 |
| Endocrine/hormone sensitive sites | | |
| Breast | 0.5 | 69.1 |
| Endometrium | | 12.4 |
| Ovary | | 14.3 |
| Prostate | 21.5 | |
| Testes | 2.3 | |
| Endocrine | | |
| (excluding pancreas and gonads) | 1.4 | 2.7 |
| % Endocrine/hormonal | 8.4 | 35.0 |

(Based on Cancer Registry data – Waterhouse, 1974).

Class 1: Effects which can be predicted from the endocrine pharmacology of compounds. An example would be the oestrogens and progestogens which have a plethora of effects on metabolic parameters in addition to their actions on oestrogen sensitive target sites when administered at pharmacological doses (the therapeutic dose levels).

Class 2: Effects which again can be predicted from the endocrine pharmacology of the compound when administered at doses well in excess of the therapeutic dose level. An example would be adrenal steroid suppression and general excessive catabolism observed with high dose and prolonged use of glucocorticoids.

Class 3: Effects which could not have been predicted from the pharmacology of the compound. This group can be subclassified into: 3a. Effects which are direct or primary actions on an endocrine gland. Examples of this might be the action of ketoconazoles on adrenal and testicular function and the action of alloxan and streptozocin on the β-cell of the pancreas; and 3b. Effects on endocrine glands which are indirect or secondary to changes in other organs or control mechanisms (homeostasis). Examples here would be the actions of phenobarbitone on the rat thyroid and the effects of lactose and polyols on the rat adrenal medulla.

Class 4: Effects which cannot be predicted from pre-clinical studies because of idiosyncratic effects on the endocrine system.

As indicated by Baylis & Tunbridge (1985) the adverse effects of drugs on the endocrine system are nearly all due to normal or exaggerated pharmacological responses, that is Classes 1 and 2. Furthermore, it appears that endocrine toxicity can be detected reliably in pre-clinical studies. What is essential is that Class 3 toxic endocrine effects are classified appropriately. Class 3a effects would be expected to be seen across species whereas there are numerous examples where Class 3b effects appear to be species-specific. There seems to be no clear cut example to quote for Class 4 effects which is in contrast to several examples of compounds which have idiosyncratic effects on the immune system of susceptible humans which cannot be predicted from pre-clinical studies.

Data from Ribelin (1984) suggests that the endocrine system of the rats is sensitive to toxicity from xenobiotics. This is also supported by Hey wood (1984) in which he examined the target organ toxicity for 42 pharmaceutical compounds in the rat and dog. The endocrine system of the rat was only second to the liver as the most frequently affected target organ (38% liver, 31% endocrine). Ribelin (1984) reported that the most frequent endocrine lesion occurs in the adrenals followed by the testes but this analysis was conducted on chemicals and pharmaceuticals, and the data indicated that it was the cortical layers of the adrenal that were being predominantly effected, suggesting that the adrenal changes may be reflecting general stress responses rather than direct adrenal gland toxicity.

In another analysis conducted in conjunction with the Centre of Medicines Research this area was further explored (Tables 1.2 and 1.3). Toxicology data on 124 compounds (all pharmaceuticals) were analysed. Just under 50 per cent (61/124) of these compounds have effects on one or more endocrine glands. Similar to Ribelin (1984) the adrenals were the most frequently affected, followed by the testes and the thyroid. Where there was an effect it is of interest that about half were only weight changes, with no pathological changes observed. This confirms the suggestion that a general stress response is probably responsible. It is also of interest that 27 of the 61 compounds where endocrine changes were observed are on the market. Furthermore, it was established that of the remaining 34 compounds, the endocrine effects alone did not cause termination of development of any of the compounds. These data suggest that abnormal endocrine effects in animals caused by new pharmaceuticals do not provide insurmountable problems when considering their safety in humans.

Table 1.2. *Frequency of toxicity to endocrine glands (CMR database)*

| Organ | No. of compounds with an effect | Weight change only | Species |
|---|---|---|---|
| Adrenals | 44 | 27 | rat, dog, primate |
| Testes | 24 | 10 | rat, dog |
| Thyroid | 17 | 9 | rat, dog |
| Ovary | 14 | 7 | rat, dog |
| Pituitary | 11 | 6 | rat, dog, primate |
| Pancreas | 4 | 0 | rat, dog, primate |

61/124 compounds have effects on one or or more endocrine glands.
27/61 compounds are marketed. Endocrine effects have *not* caused termination of development for any of the remaining 34 compounds.
CMR = Centre for Medicines Research.

Table 1.3. *Frequency of toxicity to endocrine glands (CMR database) Species distribution analysis*

| Organ | No. of studies where an effect seen (wt. change only) | | |
|---|---|---|---|
| | Rat | Dog | Primate |
| Adrenals | 33(22) | 14(8) | 5(3) |
| Testes | 18(10) | 13(7) | 0 |
| Thyroid | Data not available | | |
| Ovary | 9(6) | 8(3) | 0 |
| Pituitary | 6(2) | 5(1) | 3(1) |
| Pancreas | 1(0) | 2(0) | 1(0) |
| Parathyroid | Data not available | | |

Total no. of studies. Rat = 101; dog = 87; primate = 32.
CMR = Centre for Medicine Research.

When the endocrine effects are broken down according to species it can be seen that the rat shows a greater frequency of effects than the dog or primate (Table 1.2). There are a larger number of rat studies relative to the dog and primate, nevertheless it is clear that the rat is more sensitive in picking up endocrine toxicity than the dog or primate.

In a survey of rodent carcinogenicity studies conducted by the Pharmaceutical Manufacturers Association for USA pharmaceutical companies in 1989, the tumour type by target organ cited by the highest percentage of companies was the liver (rat 47%, mouse 43%). However, individual endocrine tumours were cited by almost as many respondents. Interestingly in the case of the endocrine tumours, their occurrence as a problem in rats was cited by a much higher percentage than for mice. The endocrine tumours cited by the largest percentage of companies were mammary (43% rat, 3% mouse) followed by thyroid (27% rat, 3% mouse), pituitary (23% rat, 0% mouse), adrenal (20% rat, 0% mouse), testicular (20% rat, 0% mouse), uterine (20% rat, 6% mouse) and ovarian (13% rat, 10% mouse). It should be noted that the percentages cited do not indicate the frequency with which tumours are observed but to the respondents to the survey that cite a particular tumour type. The data provided by Tucker (Chapter 11) is consistent with and supportive of the rat being particularly susceptible to spontaneous endocrine tumours.

The reason for the marked difference between the rat and mouse is not known and emphasizes the importance of understanding species differences in endocrine physiology so that toxicological response to xenobiotics can be better appreciated. Until we have a thorough understanding of comparative endocrinology of the common species used in toxicology studies (rodents, dogs, and primates) with respect to toxic response, it will not be possible to make rational choices of species to use or exercise informed judgement and perspective with response to endocrine safety assessment. Unfortunately experimental endocrinologists have a predilection to use rats in their studies with relatively little work being done on the mouse, dog, or primate. However, it is clear that the rat has important physiological differences from humans and other species, particularly with respect to the transport of hormone from endocrine gland to target tissue, the binding and uptake of the hormone by target tissues and their receptors, and the metabolism and clearance of hormones. The validity of animal models of toxicity in assessing endocrine toxicology has indeed been the subject of considerable controversy (Flack & Swann, 1989). This is exemplified most clearly in the area of thyroid hormones.

Hormonal measurements can define the mechanisms behind morphological changes in animal studies and fortunately similar measurements can be made in clinical studies. It is, therefore, possible to make extrapolations of the potential hazards and the possible risks for humans. Detailed experimental and clinical investigations are required for the endocrine changes frequently seen in rat toxicology and carcinogenicity studies to be placed in their proper perspective.

A book of this type must inevitably include recognition of new testing strategies in investigative endocrine toxicology. Here the rise and acceptance of *in vitro* technology has made a big impact not only because of resource and ethical issues but because of a particular need in endocrine investigations to be able to dissect direct from indirect effects on a particular endocrine organ, that is Class 3a from 3b. Thus the reader will find descriptions of the use of isolated pituitary glands and hypothalami, cultured thyroid cells, and cultured adrenal cells in elucidating xenobiotic toxicity. Recent important advances in this area include the work of Thomas and Williams (Chapter 5) in defining the molecular growth control systems of thyroid epithelial cells. Furthermore, with the advent of new and important types of drugs, such as immunosuppressants, *in vitro* studies have started to help define the mechanism, species sensitivity and risk of, for example, cyclosporin on adrenal cortical function.

In the chapters that follow we have attempted to provide the reader with a comprehensive description of the anatomy and physiology of the major endocrine glands so that a toxicologic response to xenobiotics can be defined in mechanistic terms. We have not sought to provide an exhaustive catalogue of endocrine toxins. For example, the paucity of current information on the endocrine pancreas (except perhaps for the experimentally-induced diabetes, induced by alloxan and streptozocin) has led to its omission from the current text. Similarly the full spectrum of regulatory requirements or toxicity study design features could not be given worthy coverage here. However, we have attempted to bring together the expertise of experimental endocrinologists, physiologists, and toxicologists which we hope will help the reader to distil their own views and hopefully solutions to their own particular endocrine toxicity problem.

### Acknowledgement

We are grateful to Dr Cyndy Lumley at the Centre for Medicines Research, Woodmansterne Road, Carshalton, Surrey SM5 4DS, England, for supplying the previously unpublished information from the CMR toxicity database.

### References

Atterwill, C.K., Kennedy, S., Jones, C.A., Lee, D.M., Davies, S. & Poole, A. (1988). Comparison of the toxicity of orally administered L-triiodothyronine ($T_3$) in rat and cynomolgus monkey. *Toxicology*, **52**, 89–105.

Baylis, P.H. & Tunbridge, W.M.G. (1985). Endocrine disorders. In *Textbook of Adverse Drug Reactions*, 3rd edn. ed. D. M. Davies, pp. 335–51. Oxford: Oxford Medical Publications.

Capen, C.C. & Martin, S.L. (1989). The effects of xenobiotics on the structure and function of thyroid follicular and C-cells. *Toxicologic Pathology*, **17**(2), 266–93.

CIOMS (1983). *Safety Requirements for The First Use of New Drugs and Diagnostic Agents in Man. A Review of Safety Issues in Early Clinical Trials of Drugs.* Geneva: Council for International Organisations of Medical Sciences.

Flack, J.D. (1986). Toxicity: ritual, rationale and regulatory requirements in prediction and assessment of antibiotic clinical efficacy. In *Prediction and Assessment of Antibiotic Clinical Efficacy*, ed. F. O'Grady & A. Percival, pp. 141–57. London: Academic Press.

Flack, J.D. & Swann, P. (1989). Validity of animal models in endocrine pathology. *Trends in Pharmacological Sciences*, **10**, 301–3.

Heywood, R. (1984). Prediction of adverse drug reactions from animal safety studies. In *Detection and Prevention of Adverse Drug Reactions*, ed. H. Bostrun & N. Ljungstedt, pp. 173–89. Sweden: Almquist and Wiksell Int.

Ribelin, W.E. (1984). The effects of drugs and chemicals upon the structure of the adrenal gland. *Fundamentals of Applied Toxicology*, **4**, 105–19.

Roe, F.J.C. (1989). Non-genotoxic carcinogenesis: implications for testing and extrapolation to man. *Mutagenesis*, **4**, 407–11.

# II     *Hypothalamic and pituitary toxicology*

ROBERT W. GREENHILL

## 2 Anatomy, morphology and pathology of the pituitary gland in different species – implications in toxicology

### Introduction

The pituitary is both structurally and functionally the most complex of the endocrine glands. The many hormones it secretes have important roles in the maintenance of the normal structure and function of various mammalian tissues. It is not unexpected then that control of pituitary hormone production and secretion involves input from many areas of the brain through links, as yet not fully characterized, between the pituitary and the hypothalamus. In this way, the pituitary is an important conduit through which the central nervous system is able to influence body function.

In this review the gross and microscopic anatomy of the pituitary gland will be described, with particular emphasis on those species used routinely in toxicology laboratories, and current understanding of pituitary function and its control will be outlined. The extensive literature on comparative cellular morphology and spontaneous pathology will be reviewed, and may serve as a reference source for toxicologists embarking on investigative studies of endocrine toxicity.

### Development and gross anatomy

The embryological development and the gross anatomy of the pituitary gland have been well described by Holmes & Ball (1974) and Ham (1974). In the adult of all laboratory species the pituitary is divided into two main lobes separated by a cleft (Fig. 2.1), which is a remnant of its embryological development. Anterior to the cleft is the main body of the gland, the pars distalis (pars anterior). Posterior to the cleft is a narrow band of glandular tissue, the pars intermedia. Posterior to the pars intermedia and adherent to it is the pars nervosa (pars posterior, infundibular lobe). The pars nervosa is an extension of the base of the brain and is linked to it by the pituitary stalk (infundibular stalk). A projection from the pars distalis, called the pars tuberalis, extends up along the anterior

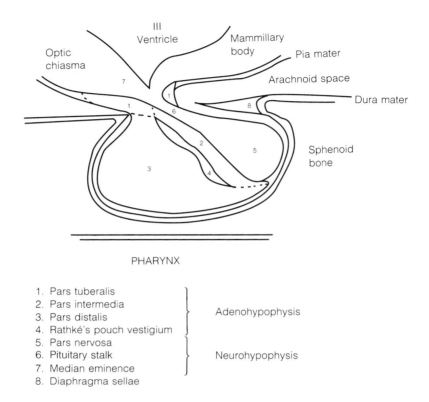

Fig. 2.1. General anatomy of the pituitary gland. (Modified from Ham, 1974.)

and lateral aspects of the pituitary stalk. The pars distalis, pars intermedia and pars tuberalis resemble endocrine tissue and constitute the adeno-hypophysis. The pars nervosa, pituitary stalk and adjoining median eminence constitute the neurohypophysis.

The pituitary lies in a depression of the sphenoid bone at the base of the skull called the fossa or sella turcica. A fold in the dura mater of the meninges, called the diaphragma sellae, forms a roof over the fossa which is pierced by the pituitary stalk. The dura mater continues onto line the fossa. The remaining layers of the meninges, the arachnoid space and the pia mater, blend with the capsule of the pituitary gland and so cannot be identified as separate layers in the fossa.

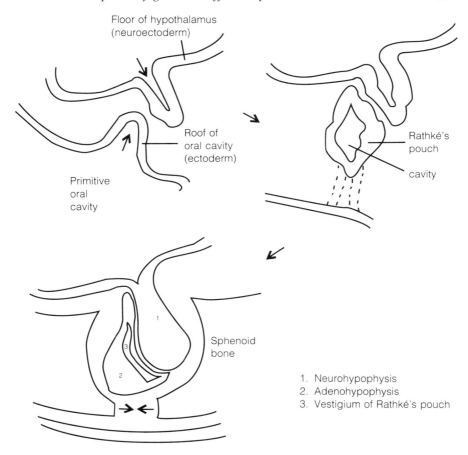

Fig. 2.2. Embryological development of the pituitary gland.

Embryologically, both the neurohypophysis and adenohypophysis are of ectodermal origin (Fig. 2.2). The neuroectoderm of the floor of the developing hypothalamus migrates ventrally to form the pituitary stalk and the pars nervosa. The ectodermal tissue in the roof of the developing oral cavity grows dorsally, towards the hypothalamus, to form a sac called Rathké's pouch. The pouch breaks away from the oral ectoderm to form a hollow island of epithelium. The cells of the anterior wall of Rathké's pouch multiply to form the pars distalis and those of the posterior wall to form the pars intermedia which becomes adherent to the lower surface of the developing pars nervosa. Lateral outgrowths of the upper part of

Rathké's pouch extend forwards and towards the midline, usually join-
ing, and becoming closely applied to the presumptive median eminence;
these form the pars tuberalis. During its development, the neural growth
carries with it an extension of the central cavity of the neural tube. In
most species this cavity later becomes obliterated.

## Comparative anatomy

In all the vertebrate classes, the pituitary gland shows remarkable
similarities in its overall morphology, for example, the pars distalis is
always the largest of the epithelial components. However, the level of
development and the extent of association between the different areas of
the pituitary vary considerably within mammalian species. Detailed
studies of the anatomy of the pituitary of a wide range of mammals were
made by Hanstrom between 1944 and 1953 and were reviewed by that
author in 1966, and cited by Holmes & Ball in 1974. The following
comparison will be restricted to the laboratory species of rodent, dog and
primate.

Pituitary anatomy most similar to that of humans is seen in the
chimpanzee and the gorilla. The orientation of the pars nervosa in relation to the hypothalamus varies from almost vertical in these primates to
almost horizontal in the dog and rodents; in the rhesus macaque (*Macaca
mulatta*) it lies at an intermediate angle. The horizontal axis tends to give
the rodent pituitary a flattened appearance, the pars distalis lies entirely
inferiorly (Fig. 2.3) in contrast to the rhesus monkey, where the pars
distalis lies in front of the pars nervosa.

In the dog, the fossa is quite shallow. The pars distalis and pars intermedia surround the pars nervosa (Fig. 2.3) and the Rathké's pouch
vestigium is usually quite spacious. The pars tuberalis forms a collar at the
junction of the median eminence and pituitary stalk, and folds can be
seen in the pars intermedia.

The rodents also show a collar-like tuberalis around the stalk up to the
hypothalamus and the pars intermedia is well developed. The pars distalis
and pars tuberalis are larger in the rat than in the mouse whilst the pars
intermedia and pars nervosa are smaller.

In the rhesus macaque, an Old World monkey, the pars distalis may
extend dorsally and caudally around the pituitary stalk. The medium-
sized pars intermedia forms a collar at the base of the stalk below the pars
tuberalis, which also has a collar-like structure. The pars intermedia is
well developed in comparison with that of the baboon (*Papio*), which is
only rudimentary, and that of humans which is present during foetal life
but largely disappears in the adult.

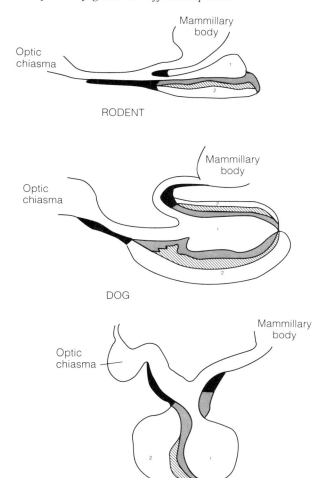

PRIMATE (Rhesus macaque: *Macaca mulatta*)

1 – Pars nervosa
2 – Pars distalis
▨ – Rathké's pouch vestigium
▦ – Pars intermedia
■ – Pars tuberalis

Fig. 2.3. Comparative anatomy of the pituitary gland. (After Hanstrom, 1966.)

New World monkeys are represented in the laboratory by the marmosets (*Callithrix*) which characteristically possess remnants of a pars tuberalis interna, an area of the pars distalis which is thought to have developed from the lateral lobes of Rathké's pouch but has a cytology distinct from that of the pars tuberalis.

## Vascular supply

The arterial and venous system of the pituitary has three vital functions: supply of blood for maintenance of endocrine metabolism; delivery of the gland's secretions to target organs and tissues; and a system through which secretory activity of the pars distalis can be controlled by feedback mechanisms and the central nervous system (CNS). The arterial supply to the pituitary is from branches of the carotid artery. However, the capillaries between the glandular elements of the pars distalis receive no direct arterial supply. Instead they form a secondary capillary bed which receives blood from specialized vessels which originate in a primary capillary bed in the median eminence. This system, by which two capillary beds are linked by veins or venules, constitutes a portal system – the hypothalamic hypophyseal portal system – which plays a central role in hypothalamic control of the pituitary. Blood reaching the pars distalis will have lost some nutrients and oxygen and gained metabolic waste products and regulatory products from the neurohypophysis.

The blood vascular system of the rat pituitary has been studied in detail by Murakami *et al.* (1987). In summary (see Fig. 2.4), the pituitary is served by the anterior, middle, accessory middle, and posterior hypophyseal arteries. The anterior and middle hypophyseal arteries extend to the median eminence to supply its mesh-like capillary bed and that of the infundibular stalk, which together form the primary capillary plexus. This plexus can be subdivided into an external and internal plexus (Page, 1988). The former is a superficial network, the morphology of which varies little between species. Its architecture is compatible with rapid exchange of materials between blood and tissue. The internal plexus arises from the external plexus and shows considerable variability between species (Page, 1988).

In addition to serving the primary plexus, the anterior and middle arteries also give off branches to the capillary plexus of the pars tuberalis which then drain into the secondary capillary plexus in the pars distalis. Branches from the middle and accessory middle arteries serve the upper third of the pars nervosa and the pars intermedia. The lower two-thirds of the pars nervosa and the pars intermedia are served by the posterior

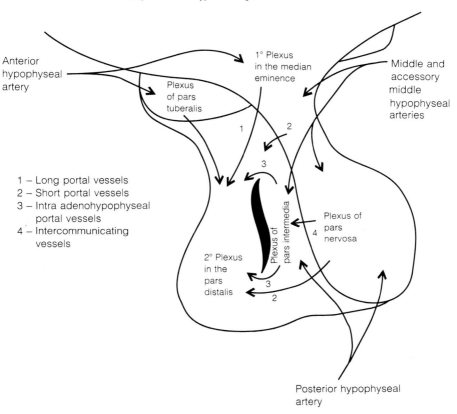

Anterior
hypophyseal
artery

1° Plexus
in the median
eminence

Middle and
accessory
middle
hypophyseal
arteries

Plexus
of pars
tuberalis

1

2

3

1 – Long portal vessels
2 – Short portal vessels
3 – Intra adenohypophyseal
    portal vessels
4 – Intercommunicating
    vessels

Plexus of
pars intermedia

Plexus of
pars
nervosa

4

2° Plexus
in the
pars
distalis

3

2

Posterior hypophyseal
artery

Fig. 2.4. Arterial supply of the rat pituitary gland.

hypophyseal artery. The capillary bed of the pars nervosa is continuous
with the primary capillary plexus and is the origin of the short portal
vessels which run into the pars distalis. The capillary bed of the pars
intermedia sends off intra-adenohypophyseal portal vessels which also
drain into the pars distalis. In addition, this capillary bed has many vessels
communicating with the capillary bed of the pars nervosa throughout the
junctional area.

It has always been assumed that blood flow in the long, short, and
intra-adenohypophyseal portal vessels is towards the pars distalis and in
the intercommunicating vessels is towards the pars intermedia. However,
Murakami's work supports earlier evidence from the mouse, rat, dog and

monkey that there may be a countercurrent between the hypophysis and median eminence which may serve as an ultrashort feedback control system for the pars distalis.

The venous system of the pituitary comprises the ventral and dorsal adenohypophyseal and neurohypophyseal veins. The latter arise deep in the pars nervosa, the former in the pars distalis; all three drain into the cavernous sinuses or basioccipital sinuses which eventually feed into the internal maxillary veins and internal jugular and vertebral veins or the external jugular, respectively.

## Hypothalamic control and function of the pituitary hormones

The adenohypophysis is the source of at least seven peptide hormones: growth hormone (or somatotrophin; GH), prolactin (PRL), thyroid stimulating hormone (TSH), the gonadotrophins: luteinizing hormone (LH) and follicle stimulating hormone (FSH), adrenocorticotrophic hormone (ACTH) and melanocyte-stimulating hormone (MSH). In addition, the neurohypophysis releases two hormones: antidiuretic hormone (ADH or vasopressin) and oxytocin. The major functions of the pituitary hormones are summarized in Table 2.1.

The release of the hormones of the adenohypophysis is controlled, in part, by the central nervous system via releasing or release inhibiting hormones from the hypothalamus. Feedback to the adenohypophysis and/or hypothalamus by hormones from the target tissues also have a regulatory role (Table 2.2). In the absence of direct innervation of the pars distalis the hypothalamic release controlling factors are synthesized by neurones and transported down unmyelinated neuronal axons of the hypothalamo-hypophyseal tract to be released into the primary capillary bed of the median eminence. The portal system, as described earlier, carries the hormones to the secondary capillary plexus which perfuses the glandular elements of the pars distalis, thus enhancing communication by delivering the chemical messengers directly to the interstitium. The neurosecretory cells of the hypothalamus are influenced by impulses received from the thalamus, limbic system and reticular activating system, and have hypothalamic autonomic regulatory functions in, for example, the cardiovascular and gastrointestinal systems (Kaufman, 1987). The secretory neurones are also responsive to circulating hormone levels from peripheral target tissues. In this way the hypothalamus plays a central role in integrating the endocrine and central nervous systems.

The neuroendocrinology of pituitary hormone regulation has recently been described in detail by Lechan (1987) and outlined by Reichlin

Table 2.1. *Major functions of the pituitary hormones*

| Hormones | Function |
|---|---|
| *Adenohypophysis* | |
| Growth hormone (GH, Somatotrophin) | Accelerates tissue growth. |
| Thyroid stimulating hormone (TSH) | Hypertrophy of thyroid epithelial cells and increased thyroid hormone synthesis and secretion. |
| Prolactin (PRL) | Promotes mammary gland development and lactation in the female. Regulates Leydig cell function in males? |
| Luteinising hormone (LH) | Induces maturation of the follicle, oestrogen secretion, ovulation and corpus luteum formation in the female. Increases synthesis and secretion of androgens in the male. |
| Follicle stimulating hormone (FSH) | Stimulates ovarian follicle growth in the female. Activates spermatogenesis in the male. |
| Adrenocorticotrophic hormone (ACTH) | Stimulates production of glucocorticoids by cells of the adrenal cortex. |
| Melanocyte stimulating hormone (MSH) | Expands melanophores and induces melanin synthesis. |
| *Neurohypophysis* | |
| Antidiuretic hormone (ADH, vasopressin) | Promotes water retention. |
| Oxytocin | Causes milk release, also uterine contraction in parturition. |

(1989). Most of the hypothalamic factors have been identified within the last 20 years, whilst the existence of others (e.g. MSH) remains speculative (Kaufman, 1987). In some cases specific groups of neurones responsible for their production have been pinpointed, whilst others are found in diverse areas of the CNS. For example the paraventricular and periventricular nuclei secrete corticotrophin releasing hormone (CRH) and other factors which seem to have a positive effect on ACTH release including vasopressin, angiotensin II and cholecystokinin.

ACTH is a polypeptide of 39 amino-acids, one of several derived from the precursor molecule pro-opiomelanocortin (POMC) which is syn-

Table 2.2. *Regulation of adenohypophyseal hormone release*

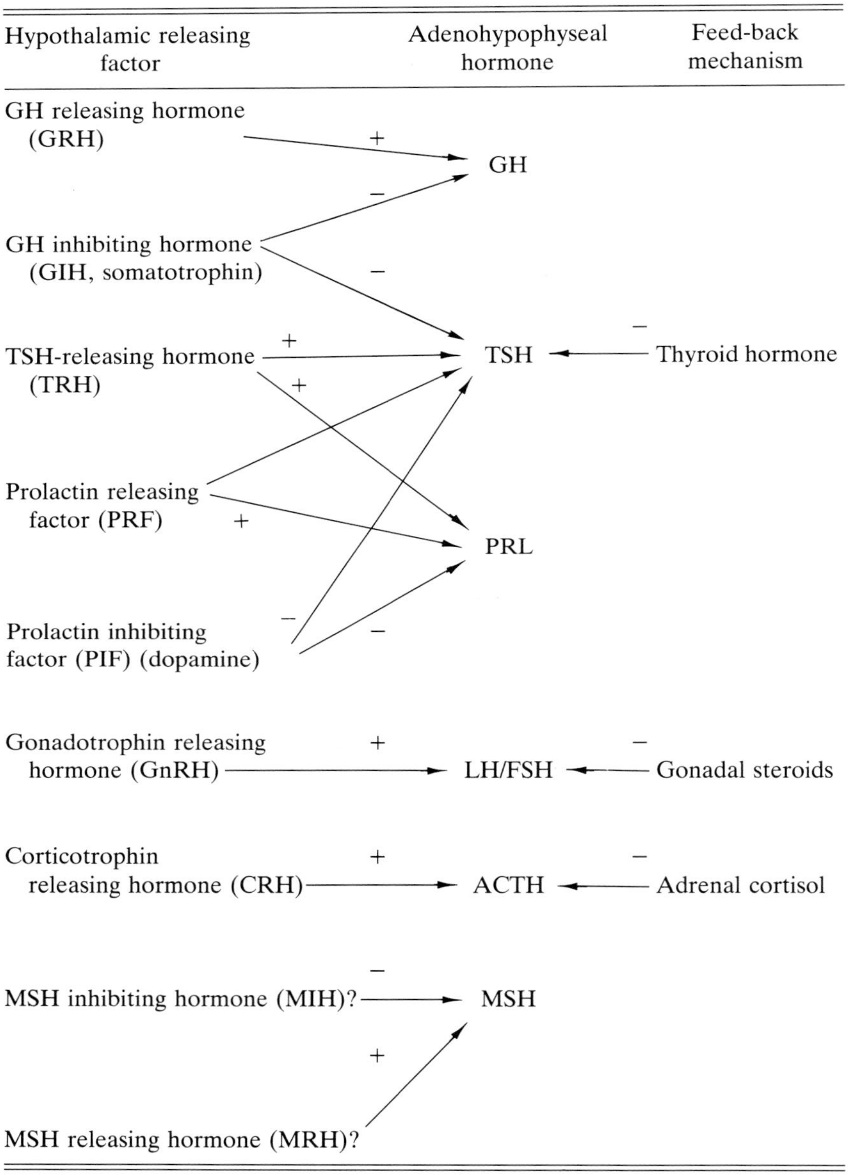

| Hypothalamic releasing factor | Adenohypophyseal hormone | Feed-back mechanism |
| --- | --- | --- |

GH releasing hormone
(GRH)     +

GH

−

GH inhibiting hormone
(GIH, somatotrophin)   −

TSH-releasing hormone  +       TSH ◄────── Thyroid hormone   −
(TRH)   +

Prolactin releasing
factor (PRF)   +

PRL

Prolactin inhibiting
factor (PIF) (dopamine)  −   −

Gonadotrophin releasing  +              −
hormone (GnRH) ────────► LH/FSH ◄──── Gonadal steroids

Corticotrophin        +             −
releasing hormone (CRH) ────► ACTH ◄──── Adrenal cortisol

−
MSH inhibiting hormone (MIH)? ──► MSH

+

MSH releasing hormone (MRH)?

GH = growth hormone; TSH = thyroid stimulating hormone; MSH = melanocyte-stimulating hormone; PRL = prolactin; LH = luteinizing hormone; FSH = follicle stimulating hormone; ACTH = adrecorticotrophic hormone.

thesized in both the pars distalis and pars intermedia of mammals. The control and the processing of POMC are different at the two sites of production; in the pars distalis the precursor is predominantly converted to ACTH (1–39) and β-lipotrophic hormone (βLPH). This is controlled mainly by the negative feedback of plasma cortisol directly on the pars distalis, but also by CRH and other hypothalamic factors, and adrenalin, which releases ACTH (Riechlin, 1989). In the pars intermedia ACTH (1–39) is further processed to α-melanocyte-stimulating hormone (α-MSH), leaving ACTH (18–39) (or corticotrophin-like intermediate lobe peptide, CLIP). Beta-LPH is further metabolized to β-endorphin and α-LPH (which in turn can be processed to β-MSH). Secretion from the pars intermedia is regulated predominantly by dopaminergic inhibition and β-adrenergic or serotoninergic stimulation (Middleton *et al.*, 1987).

The paraventricular and periventricular nuclei associated with the third ventricle also secrete growth hormone inhibiting hormone (GIH) which interacts with growth hormone releasing hormone (GRH) from the arcuate nucleus to produce a rhythmic pattern of GH release. In addition, vasoactive intestinal polypeptide (VIP) is thought to inhibit GIH secretion, thereby releasing GH, whereas catecholamines probably stimulate GH release by releasing GRH. Thyroid stimulating hormone is primarily regulated by a negative feedback suppression by thyroid hormone but secretion is controlled by thyroid hormone releasing hormone (TRH) synthesized in the paraventricular nucleus and is inhibited by dopamine and GIH. The control of gonadotrophin release is by positive and negative feedback regulation by gonadal steroids under the permissive influence of gonadotrophin releasing hormone (GnRH) (or LHRH) from neurones in the preoptic area and basal hypothalamus.

In contrast to most of the other hormones of the pars distalis, the secretion of which is dependent on the presence of a hypothalamic releasing factor (HRF), prolactin secretion is tonically inhibited by dopamine from the arcuate nucleus. Consequently it is the only hormone of the pars distalis for which destruction of the pituitary stalk results in an elevation of serum hormone level. However, several prolactin releasing factors (PRF) have been described; VIP and peptide histidine isoleucine (PHI) from the paraventricular nucleus are probably the most important. Serotonin has a dual role in increasing prolactin release by suppressing dopamine release and stimulating PRF. Other possible releasing factors for prolactin are TRH, oxytocin, vasopressin, enkephalin, cholecystokinin and angiotensin II.

In addition to secretion of controlling factors for the pars distalis, the paraventricular nuclei and the supraoptic nucleus are also responsible for producing the two hormones released by the pars nervosa; antidiuretic hormone and oxytocin. Both are derived from precursor molecules, propressophysin and pro-oxyphysin, respectively, and packaged into secretion granules. Following axonal transport to the pars nervosa, via the hypothalamo-hypophyseal system, the prehormones are stored in the axon terminals and then cleaved to release ADH and oxytocin, their carrier proteins, neurophysin II and neurophysin I, respectively, and a glycoprotein.

## Microscopic anatomy of the pituitary gland

Before morphological changes in the pituitary can be assessed a knowledge of the normal structure and cellular distribution is essential. There follows a review of the microscopic anatomy of the major regions of the pituitary, at the light and ultrastructural level, in the various laboratory animals.

### Pars distalis

The endocrine cells of the pars distalis are arranged in branching cords or nests separated by abundant capillaries that are lined by a fenestrated endothelium. The endothelium and the secretory cells are each supported by a basement membrane with a perivascular space between. This arrangement allows rapid removal of secreted hormones, but also ready access of glandular elements to regulatory factors and possible communication between cells (Page, 1988). The capillaries are also supported by the cytoplasmic processes of the stellate cells. Recent work by Soji & Herbert (1989) suggests that the stellate cells form a meshwork which may compose an information conducting system which transmits its data through gap junctions, thus allowing cell to cell communication in a gland which is lacking direct innervation.

The staining reactivity of the cells of the parenchyma, with the routine histological stain, haematoxylin and eosin, divides them into those which take up stain, the chromophils, and those which do not, the chromophobes. The chromophils can be further divided into basophils and acidophils. The basophils are those which produce the glycoprotein hormones: FSH, LH and TSH and therefore also stain with periodic acid Schiff reagent (PAS). The peptide hormones GH and PRL are produced by the acidophils. The chromophobes are smaller and lack obvious granules and may represent ACTH or MSH cells, stellate cells and undifferentiated stem cells (Capen, 1983). Chromophils may also appear chromophobic following hormone release when the cytoplasm contains no storage granules but abundant endoplasmic reticulum and Golgi apparatus actively synthesizing hormone.

In recent years the use of immunocytochemical techniques and electron microscopy have extended our knowledge of the morphological characteristics of the cells of the pituitary gland, particularly those of the pars distalis. An excellent account of the development of these techniques in their laboratory is given by Childs, Unabia & Ellison (1986). Many of the immunocytochemical studies have concentrated on the rat and are based on the early work of Baker *et al.* (1969) and Nakane (1970) and have been reviewed by Petrusz & Ordronneau (1983) and Pelletier (1984). Nakane (1975) also produced early work using the electron microscope, this area has recently been reviewed by Horvath & Kovacs (1988).

Less work, particularly ultrastructural, has been done in other laboratory species but important contributions have been made to our knowledge of the mouse by Baker & Gross (1978) and Sasaki & Iwama (1988); of the dog by El Etreby, Richter & Gunzel (1973), El Etreby & Fath El Bab (1977a,b, 1978), El Etreby *et al.* (1977), El Etreby & Dubois (1980), and El Etreby *et al.* (1980); and the non-human primate by Herbert & Hayashida (1974) and Herbert & Silverman (1983).

Classification of the cells of the pars distalis has always been controversial; typing by size and ultrastructural appearance of secretory granules was based on the theory that one cell could produce only one hormone. However, with the emergence of immunocytochemical techniques it was shown that FSH and LH (Nakane, 1970), and later PRL and GH, could be produced by the same cell; indeed it is thought that monohormonal and bihormonal cell types could have specific distributions and be subject to different regulatory influences (Horvath & Kovacs, 1988). Recent work in the rat by Losinski, Horvath & Kovacs (1989) has shown that some cells may contain GH and TSH or PRL and TSH positive granules, and in fact some granules may show dual staining. They also suggest that there may be intermediary cell types allowing transformation between GH and PRL production. The one cell–one hormone theory is then, generally accepted as obsolete for rat and humans (Horvath & Korvacs, 1988). However, Kurosumi (1986), who has done much work in this field, still denies the existence of PRL–GH cells in the rat. This author also prefers to classify morphological variants staining for the same hormone as subtypes of the same cell thus: Type I – the classical type, usually with large granules; Type II – with medium-sized or mixed large and small granules; Type III – immature forms with small granules. Yoshimura (1986) introduces the dimension of time in suggesting that a whole range of morphological subtypes of one class of cell are continuously shifting and overlapping with time.

In the rat, GH cells (somatotrophs) are the most abundant, seen throughout the lobe but showing reduced numbers in the anterior ventral region and adjacent to the pars intermedia. The cells are round to oval or polyhedral with a slightly eccentric nucleus often with a fairly prominent nucleolus (Fig. 2.5). They are often found in close association with ACTH cells, less frequently with LH or PRL cells. With the electron microscope, ovoid or round dense-cored secretory granules measuring 300–400 nm are seen throughout the cytoplasm. In some somatotrophs small granules of around 150 nm are intermingled with the larger ones.

Difficulties with the identification of GH cells by ultrastructural morphology alone have also been experienced in the mouse; Sasaki & Iwama (1988), described Type I (350 nm granules) and Type II (100–200 nm). Immunoelectron microscopy was required to distinguish the rarely seen GH Type II cells from PRL Type II and other cell types such as TSH, gonadotrophs and ACTH cells. Using the light microscope, GH cells show a similar shape and distribution to those in the rat but are reduced in numbers in the dorsocephalic region ('sex zone').

In the dog, somatotrophs are small and round to oval, and are seen singly in palisades along capillaries and most frequently in the dorsal region near the pars intermedia (El Etreby & Fath El Bab, 1977a). Herbert & Hayashida (1974) identified GH cells in the rhesus monkey, predominantly in posterior, lateral and postero-lateral regions. More recently Antunes et al. (1980) described the GH cells as being in cords and acini. Herbert & Silverman (1983) showed that GH cells in the baboon predominate at the superior and inferior poles and described them as round or oval in nests or clusters.

The remaining acidophils – the prolactin cells or lactotrophs – are found throughout the pars distalis of the rat, often in association with gonadotrophs. These cup-shaped cells (Fig. 2.5) are concentrated in the 'sex zone' and classically contain the largest secretory granules of the adenohypophysis at 600–900 nm diameter. The granules are ovoid or polymorphic and cluster near the nucleus. However, it is now generally accepted that prolactin is produced by two morphologically different cell-types (Horvath & Kovacs, 1988). The largest, as described above, are most common in females whilst smaller cells with less abundant organelles and small (200–300 nm) spherical granules are more frequently seen in males.

Baker & Gross (1978) described the PRL cells in the mouse as polyhedral with a general distribution except in the 'sex zone' where, in contrast to the rat, few are seen. Sasaki & Iwama (1988) confirmed that they are larger and in greater number in females, and by electron microscopy described a Type I with irregular granules and a Type II with small round granules of 100–200 nm.

In the dog, El Etreby & Fath El Bab (1977a) noted small groups of

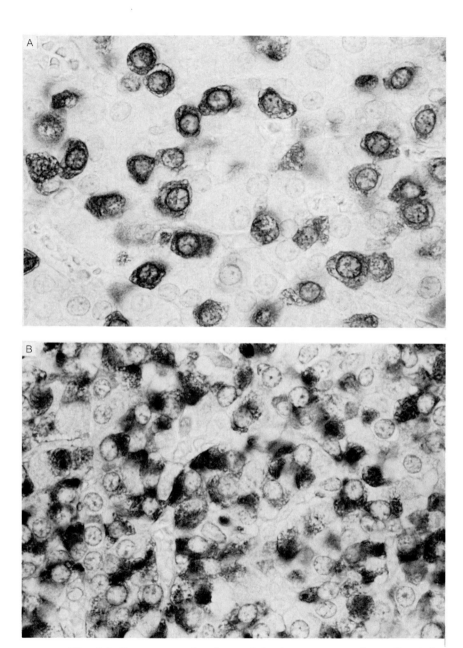

Fig. 2.5. Immunocytochemistry of the hormone-secreting cells of the pars distalis of the rat. (Peroxidase-Anti-Peroxidase Technique.) A. GH cells; B. PRL cells; C. FSH cells; D. LH cells; E. TSH cells; F. ACTH cells.

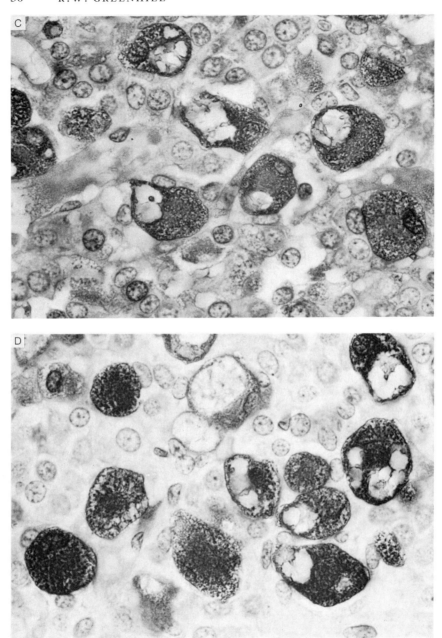

Fig. 2.5 (*cont.*)

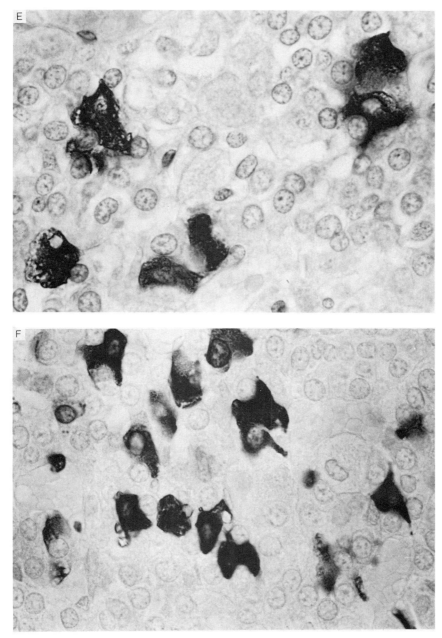

Fig. 2.5 (*cont.*)

large polygonal lactotrophs mainly in ventrocentral and cranial portions of the pituitary; dorsally they were seen both less frequently and singly. El Etreby, Richter & Gunzel (1973) have described lactotrophs in the rhesus monkey where they were scattered irregularly, singly or in clusters. Herbert & Hayashida (1974) mapped their distribution in this species as principally anterior, medial or inferior. Prolactin cells in the baboon show a similar morphology and distribution to that described for GH cells by Herbert & Silverman in 1983.

The dynamics of the plurihormonal gonadotrophs have always been a source of great interest. Horvath & Kovacs (1988) cite the extensive work of Childs in concluding that the true gonadotroph distribution in the rat probably lies between the monohormonal and bihormonal concepts. That is, in the female about 50% are bihormonal and 20–25% contain only FSH or LH, a situation which changes rapidly through the oestrus cycle. In males, about 70% are bihormonal and the rest are divided between monohormonal cell types. By light microscopy the gonadotrophs are large- to middle-sized and ovoid or polyhedral in shape (Fig. 2.5). Ultrastructurally, secretory granules have generally been described as between 200 and 300 nm but morphological variants have been recognized and, while this type is more common in females, a second type containing small (200–300 nm) and large (450–700 nm) granules is more prevalent in males.

According to Baker & Gross (1978) bihormonal gonadotrophs are most common in the mouse showing a general distribution but forming aggregations in the 'sex zone'. Watanabe (1985) noted that most LH-cells are closely surrounded by somatotrophs and are only occasionally seen in juxtaposition to lactotrophs. Similarly in the dog, most gonadotrophs are described as bihormonal (El Etreby & Fath El Bab, 1977b); they are oval to polyhedral cells with round, generally eccentric, nuclei. They are seen singly and are found particularly in the dorsocranial region ('sex zone') and its caudal extensions alongside the pars intermedia. Herbert (1976) demonstrated the bihormonal concept for the gonadotrophs in the rhesus monkey in which they are distributed singly throughout the pars distalis and described later (Herbert, 1978) as ovoid or spherical with a slightly eccentric nucleus. The gonadotrophs have a similar appearance in the baboon (Herbert & Silverman, 1983).

The TSH-cells, or thyrotrophs, of the rat share many features of the gonadotrophs in rounded nuclei, slightly dilated rough endoplasmic reticulum and prominent large spherical Golgi. The glycoprotein hormones produced by the thyrotrophs and gonadotrophs are composed of two subunits, $\alpha$ and $\beta$; they share common $\alpha$ subunits but each possess specific $\beta$ subunits that control their specific structure and function. Specificity of antisera for identification of the three cell types can only be ensured by using β subunit antigens for antibody preparation. In the rat, TSH cells are the least common and least well characterized cell-type of the pars distalis. They are seen in clusters in the centre of the gland and may be angular, elongated or stellate, or even small and ovoid (Fig. 2.5). They contain the smallest secretory granules (140 nm) scattered throughout the cytoplasm or at the periphery. In the mouse, these large polyhedral cells are restricted almost solely to the ventral region (Baker & Gross, 1978). Thyrotrophs of similar morphology are seen ventrocentrally in the dog (El Etreby & Fath El Bab, 1978) with large round or oval vesicular nuclei, which are generally eccentric. However, they are scarce close to the pars intermedia and cranially. A restricted central distribution of groups of TSH-cells is also seen in the rhesus monkey (Herbert, 1978) and baboon (Herbert & Silverman, 1983) and are described as ovoid and pleomorphic, respectively.

Cells producing ACTH in the rat – the corticotrophs – are widely distributed in the pars distalis where they appear elongated, stellate, or angular in shape; the nucleus is similarly flattened or crescent-shaped (Fig. 2.5). Cytoplasmic projections are often in contact with capillaries and the cells are often in close association with somatotrophs. A single row of dense-cored secretory granules of about 200 nm diameter is seen along the plasma membrane. Corticotrophs in the mouse resemble those of the rat (Baker & Gross, 1978; Yoshimura *et al.*, 1982). They are seen most commonly near the ventral surface and form bilateral centromedial groups in the lateral wings. Morphologically-similar ACTH cells are seen in the rhesus monkey (Yoshimura *et al.*, 1982), singly or in small groups, particularly superficially, and in a wedge-shaped area on the mid-line (Antunes *et al.*, 1980). In the dog, corticotrophs are described as poly-hedral to round, sparsely granulated and with a round, hyperchromatic usually eccentric nucleus (El Etreby & Dubois, 1980), and are most numerous in the ventrocentral and cranial portions of the distalis, where they occur in large groups.

Discussion thus far has concentrated on the morphological aspects of the cells of the pars distalis; some quantitative work has been done and will become increasingly important as computerized morphometric analyses are more widely used. Poole & Kornegay (1982) and Dada, Campbell & Blake (1984) have carried out quantitative studies in the young female rat during dioestrus (relatively inactive). With respect to relative numbers of each cell type, although there is variation between absolute numbers and regional variations, the authors are in general agreement that PRL/GH>FSH/LH/chromophobes>ACTH/TSH. Dada *et al.* (1984) reports that a similar distribution is seen in the male and similar ratios are seen with respect to total volume of each cell type although, in the female only, PRL>GH. However, Poole notes that the ratio of individual cell volume is FSH/LH/ACTH>PRL/GH>TSH/ chromophobes. Earlier work by Dada, Campbell & Blake (1983) had shown that during the oestrus cycle absolute numbers and size of FSH/LH cells do not change. In the mouse, Sasaki & Iwama (1988) have shown that in the female PRL cells are 45% of the total and GH 36%, in the male the figures are 23% and 52%, respectively.

## Pars tuberalis

The pars tuberalis is a dorsal extension of the pars distalis along the infundibular stalk, often enclosing it. However, despite its widespread occurrence in mammals and the fact that its volume, relative to the entire adenohypophysis, is as great or greater than that of the pars intermedia, the functional significance of the pars tuberalis remains obscure.

Microscopically the pars tuberalis consists of a network of non-granular chromophobe cells which are roughly cuboidal, slightly basophilic and have small pyknotic nuclei. A number of cell types, morphologically similar to those of the pars distalis, have been demonstrated over the years and a comprehensive immunocytochemical study of the laboratory species has recently been reported by Gross (1984). This shows that gonadotrophs and thyrotrophs are a consistent feature as is the absence of GH, PRL and ACTH cells.

In the rodent species, the pars tuberalis appears as a layer of 2–4 cells thick along the ventral and lateral sides of the infundibular stalk and extending rostrally on the ventral surface of the median eminence and basal hypothalamus. In the rat, Gross (1984) identified all cells present; the majority (95%) were small ovoid thyrotrophs, a few small gonadotrophs staining for LH and FSH were the only other population. In contrast, the majority (55%) of the cells in the mouse pars tuberalis did not react with any of the comprehensive range of antisera used. Gonadotrophs showed a similar distribution to the rat but were in greater numbers, and about 20% of the cells were small, ovoid lightly stained thyrotrophs.

In the rhesus monkey, Gross (1984) confirmed the findings of Baker et al. (1977) that the pars tuberalis comprises clusters of 10 to 20 cells arranged in cords along the pituitary stalk and includes large ovoid gonadotrophs, staining for both LH and FSH, and small polygonal thyrotrophs but, as in the mouse, the majority of cells (50%) are non-immunoreactive. Like the rat, and indeed human, all cells are identified in the pars tuberalis of the baboon. Layers of 2 to 5 cells thick surround the pituitary stalk, the majority (about 75%) are large ovoid cells staining for both LH and FSH. The remainder are thyrotrophs scattered singly around the stalk and median eminence.

The pars tuberalis of the dog has been less extensively studied; however, El Etreby & Fath El Bab (1977b) and El Etreby & Dubois (1980) noted the presence of clusters of cells staining for both LH and FSH, and for ACTH and MSH. The latter were described as similar to those found in the pars distalis and would seem to be rarely seen in the pars tuberalis of other mammals.

By way of warning, because of its small size and location in the rat, it is possible for the pars tuberalis to survive intact following hypophysectomy and indeed to then contain not only cells producing LH/FSH and TSH but also GH, PRL and ACTH (Petrusz & Ordronneau, 1983). This response occurs within two days and may maintain minimal amounts of adeno-hypophyseal hormones in a model considered to be free of pituitary hormones.

## Pars intermedia

The pars intermedia forms the junction between the pars distalis and the pars nervosa. As discussed earlier, grossly it shows a variety of form and size in the laboratory species. By comparison, in man it is found in the foetus but regresses in adult life to a series of follicles and cysts, and the hormone secreting cells generally associated with this zone are to be found in the pars distalis, possibly following migration from the inter-media (Ham, 1974). In humans and the baboon, where there is little glandular development, the pars intermedia is correspondingly poorly vascularized. However, in the rat, a well developed capillary plexus serves the more abundant, lobulated parenchyma. Innervation of this zone also varies greatly between species (Weatherhead, 1983). In his comprehensive review of the pars intermedia Weatherhead notes that the secretory products found there are derived from the precursor molecule pro-opiomelanocortin (POMC), as described earlier. Consequently if region specific antibodies directed to any of the characteristic amino-acid sequences of α-MSH, CLIP, ACTH, β-LPH or β-endorphin are used, these peptides can be detected in all cells of the pars intermedia (Petrusz & Ordronneau, 1983). Using antisera to ACTH, immunopositive cells are the only type in the pars intermedia of the rhesus monkey and the rat. In the former they form a continuous sheath usually 4–5 cells thick (Antunes *et al.*, 1980), in the latter they are generally described as round to ovoid cells containing many electron dense to less dense granules averaging about 200 nm in diameter. However, in the dog the immunocytology of the pars intermedia is not so monotonous, both El Etreby & Dubois (1980) and Halmi *et al.* (1981) recognized that there were two cell types present. The typical pars intermedial cell or 'A' type, representing about 90% of the cells, stains strongly for α-MSH and only weakly for ACTH and β-LPH as in the pars intermedia of other species. The remaining 10% of cells, the 'B' type, stain strongly for ACTH and β-LPH but not for α-MSH and therefore are similar to the corticotrophs of the pars distalis. The latter cells may account for the high concentrations of ACTH in the dog pars intermedia and explain why adenomas causing Cushing's syndrome in the dog may arise from the pars intermedia as well as the pars distalis (Halmi *et al.*, 1981).

### Pars nervosa

The pars nervosa consists of the endings of nonmyelinated axons from hypothalamic secretory neurones. The axons form a bundle of fibres known as the hypothalamo-hypophyseal tract which passes down the pituitary stalk to the pars nervosa. Each axon has several thousand terminals around the numerous fenestrated capillaries of the nervosa. The terminals contain dense-cored neurosecretory granules known as Herring bodies, in the rat these are 100–300 nm in diameter. These granules contain antidiuretic hormone (ADH), oxytocin and their associated neurophysins, which are synthesized in the hypothalamic neurones and are transported down the tract prior to storage and release from the axon terminals. Between the terminals are large branching spindle cells, called pituicytes, which are specialized glial cells supporting the capillaries.

## Pathology of the pituitary gland

Despite its central role in controlling the endocrine system which predisposes the pituitary to atrophy, hypertrophy, hyperplasia and tumours, pathologic conditions are relatively uncommon in most laboratory animals. As an introduction to experimental pathology, the spontaneous pathology of the pituitary will be discussed.

### Congenital abnormalities

Congenital abnormalities in the pituitary commonly manifest themselves as cystic structures. Glaister (1986) has recorded incidences of cysts in young rats, dogs, and baboons of about 3, 25 and 14% respectively. Remnants of the craniopharyngeal duct may become cystic; they are lined by a ciliated cuboidal to columnar epithelium and contain mucin. These anomalies are quite commonly seen in the dog, particularly at the periphery of the pars distalis and tuberalis (Anderson & Capen, 1978). They have also been reported in the baboon (Anderson & Capen, 1978; Skelton-Stroud & Ishmael, 1986), often as microcysts at the periphery of the distalis, and in *Macaca sinica* (Anderson & Capen, 1978). In the rodents they are not common, although an incidence of 10% has been reported, and are usually microscopic (Carlton & Gries, 1983). Cystic dilatation of the residual hypophyseal lumen of Rathké's cleft has been reported in dogs and mice (Anderson & Capen, 1978), and rats (Carlton & Gries, 1983) and shows a pseudostratified ciliated columnar epithelium that may contain goblet cells. In rats, these are more common than craniopharyngeal cysts and in dogs may occupy the entire distalis resulting in panhypopituitarism (Capen, 1988).

## Degenerative lesions

Inflammatory lesions of the pituitary are uncommon in laboratory species; however, degenerative lesions are occasionally described. In the mouse, cystoid degeneration characterized by focal cell loss in the pars distalis has been seen adjacent to neoplasms and following treatment with diethylstilboestrol, but rarely in control mice (Cameron & Sheldon, 1983). Experimentally, infarction has been seen in rats following hexadimethrine and focal degeneration has been induced with a novel anti-cancer drug (Gopinath, Prentice & Lewis, 1987).

In the pars nervosa, depletion of hormone containing vesicles, increased connective tissue around terminals, axons, and capillaries, and lipid accumulation in pituicytes can be observed in the aging rat (Greaves & Faccini, 1984).

## Disorders of growth

Disorders of growth, both non-neoplastic and neoplastic, is an important category of spontaneous adenohypophyseal lesions in laboratory animals, and will be dealt with by species.

### Rodent
Hypertrophy in the para distalis is characterized in the rodents by degranulation, enlargement and formation of cytoplasmic vacuoles (Anderson & Capen, 1978). Experimentally, hypertrophy and hyperplasia have been seen in rats (Furth, Nakane & Pasteels, 1976) and mice (Leibelt, 1979) in response to various treatments, and have progressed to tumour formation. These include deficiency of thyroid hormones (via

thyroidectomy, $I^{131}$ or goitrogenic drugs), ionizing radiation, exogenous oestrogens, and neonatal gonadectomy.

Spontaneous tumours in the mouse pituitary are relatively uncommon (Anderson & Capen, 1978), 43 were reported in the literature between 1960 and 1974 in six different strains; all but four were in females. From a similar survey Liebelt (1979) noted that mice with spontaneous tumours were invariably very old (i.e. >2 years). More recently Frith & Ward (1988) cited a relatively high incidence of tumours of the pars distalis in some strains of mice (i.e. C57BL/6), most of these, and probably those in other strains, are composed of prolactin cells. Tumours of the pars intermedia are rare.

In contrast to the low incidence of tumours seen in other laboratory animals, in the rat, spontaneous tumours of the pars distalis are a common cause of morbidity and mortality. In the second year of carcinogenicity studies in the Sprague–Dawley rat, a constant pattern of unscheduled deaths can be seen in which approximately 40% of female and 30% of male deaths will be caused by pituitary tumours (Glaister, 1986). These, generally benign, tumours may be single or multiple and range from microscopic to greater than 10 mm diameter causing compression atrophy of the brain and hydrocephalus. They are often functional resulting in other endocrine pathology, in both sexes. In fact, the clinical picture of weight loss ('pituitary cachexia'), muscle atrophy (due to protein anabolic effects of GH), neurological signs and red tear stains around the eyes is almost pathognomonic of large pituitary tumours. Furth *et al.* (1976) stated that there were no rat strains known with a proven low pituitary tumour incidence. From a survey of the recent literature, the spontaneous incidence of tumours can be as high as 83% and shows variation between the sexes and between strains (Table 2.3).

Mascoscopically, tumours are generally well defined, spherical and may be solid or have cavernous haemorrhagic spaces (Carlton & Gries, 1983). Microscopically, tumour cells vary in size and shape from small, round, oval or polyhedral to large bizarre forms. Nuclei are generally larger than those of normal cells and are pale, round to oval and usually centrally placed. For investigative purposes the tumours have been classified into three main morphological types (Berkvens, van Nesselrooy & Kroes, 1980); most are of the 'haemorrhagic type' with the cells in cords abutting large blood filled spaces. The 'spongiocytic tumours' are more solid in appearance, also consisting of cords of cells but with pale vacuolated cytoplasm and endothelium lined sinuses between the cords. The third category, the 'solid tumours', lack blood-filled spaces but have sheets of cells without any obvious structure. The classification of tumours in this way has been used in conjunction with immuno-

Table 2.3. *Spontaneous incidence of pituitary adenoma in scheduled and unscheduled deaths from two-year carcinogenicity studies in rats*

| Strain | Male | Female | Author |
|---|---|---|---|
| Long Evans | 21/50 (42%) | 25/50 (50%) | Sells & Gibson, 1987 |
| Wistar | 138/1020 (13%) | 363/1145 (32%) | Barsoum *et al.*, 1985 |
| Fischer 344 | 26/100 (26%) | 36/100 (36%) | |
| Sprague-Dawley | 10/100 (10%) | 61/100 (61%) | Sandusky *et al.*, 1988 |
| | 74/120 (62%) | 100/120 (83%) | Dodd *et al.*, 1987 |
| | 133/207 (64%) | 145/207 (70%) | Greenhill (unpub. data) |

cytochemistry in the author's laboratory to examine correlations of function and morphology from 41 male and 45 female Sprague–Dawley rats surviving to 2 years of age. The results of these studies are shown in Table 2.4.

In recent years the use of specific antisera to pituitary hormones has given us a greater understanding of the functional activity of tumour cells. The work reported here is in agreement with a number of comprehensive studies of large tumour sets using a full range of antisera (Berkvens *et al.*, 1980; McComb *et al.*, 1984; Sandusky *et al.*, 1988), and more limited studies (Trouillas *et al.*, 1982; Barsoum *et al.*, 1985) suggesting that over half of tumours of the pars distalis are positive for PRL; the majority of the remainder are either immunonegative or stain for GH/PRL (or in one study, LH) and only occasional tumours are positive for GH, TSH, ACTH or show mixed reactions. The current work also shows that the majority of tumours in the Sprague–Dawley rat are haemorrhagic and stain for prolactin, as was shown by Berkvens *et al.* (1980) in the Wistar rat. That the tumour structure is indicative of the functional type was suggested by van Putten & van Zwieten (1988) who showed positive staining for PRL in haemorrhagic tumours from animals which showed high serum PRL levels whilst solid tumours from animals with less marked increases in serum PRL, were immunonegative. This hypothesis is supported by the work of Trouillas *et al.* (1982), but was not considered substantiated by McComb *et al.* (1984). In the current study an interesting

Table 2.4. *Morphological and functional correlations in pituitary tumours from two-year old Sprague-Dawley rats*

| Immunocytochemistry | Morphology | | | Total |
| --- | --- | --- | --- | --- |
| | Haemorrhagic | Solid | Spongiocytic | |
| ♂ PRL | 19 | 5 | 0 | 24 |
| PRL/GH | 2 | 1 | 0 | 3 |
| ACTH | 0 | 0 | 0 | 0 |
| −VE | 0 | 8 | 2 | 10 |
| Total | 21 | 14 | 2 | 37 |
| ♀ PRL | 19 | 1 | 0 | 20 |
| PRL/GH | 0 | 0 | 0 | 0 |
| ACTH | 0 | 0 | 0 | 0 |
| −VE | 2 | 10 | 3 | 15 |
| Total | 21 | 11 | 3 | 35 |

PRL = prolactin; GH = growth hormone; ACTH = adrenocorticotrophic hormone

sex difference is noted in that in the female almost all solid tumours were immunonegative whilst in the male just under half were positive for PRL.

The pathogenesis of adenomas of the pars distalis is not clear; it could be a result of age-related changes in the regulatory centres of the hypothalamus or due to target organ failure causing a loss of negative feedback control or due to changes within the pituitary cells themselves. Tumours are produced experimentally in response to various treatments as described earlier. In addition, chronic treatment of male rats with a neuroleptic drug resulted in an increased incidence of pituitary tumours (Roe & Bar, 1985); this may be related to the known dopaminergic properties of some members of this class of compound, dopamine being an important inhibitor of PRL release. In association with effects on the pituitary, increased and reduced incidences of tumours in other endocrine tissues of the rat may be seen with these drugs.

Malignant tumours of the pars distalis, showing infiltration into adjacent tissues, are rare; Magnusson, Majeed & Gopinath (1979) recorded only 11 in 2609 male and female Sprague–Dawley rats (0.42%). Tumours of the pars intermedia are also rare. Berkvens *et al.* (1980) saw four in 69 tumours from 114 Wistar rats, they were chromophobic and immunonegative, and cells adjacent to sinusoids showed a characteristic empty area at the periphery of the slightly acidophilic cytoplasm. Craniopharyngiomas, cystic lesions with formations of epithelial cells are occasionally seen in the rat (Carlton & Gries, 1983). These tumours are thought to originate from squamous cell remnants of Rathké's pouch and are usually seen in young animals.

Finally, the only reported tumour of the pars nervosa is the pituicytoma, a circumscribed, non-encapsulated tumour of closely packed spindle cells arranged in indistinct cords and interlacing bundles which may cause compression of the pars distalis, and is only rarely seen in the rat (Carlton & Gries, 1983).

### Dog

In aged dogs of various breeds, El Etreby *et al.* (1980) described diffuse hyperplasia and hypertrophy of GH and PRL cells in the pars distalis and focal hyperplasia of ACTH/MSH cells in both the pars distalis and pars intermedia. Experimentally, El Etreby *et al.* (1977) and El Etreby (1981) noted diffuse hypertrophy and hyperplasia of either GH or PRL producing cells and regression of LH/FSH cells following treatment of bitches with oestrogens. Treatment with high doses of cyproterone acetate (a synthetic progesterone) or progesterone, induced atrophy of TSH and ACTH/MSH cells.

Hyperplasia of the ACTH/MSH cells often accompanies chromophobe adenomas, the most common tumour of the pituitary in the dog but rarely seen in other species (Anderson & Capen, 1978). In the dog, these may arise in the pars distalis or pars intermedia and may or may not secrete ACTH. Non-functional tumours of the pars intermedia are often associated with hypopituitarism and diabetes insipidus resulting from compression atrophy of adjacent tissues; functional tumours lead to bilateral adrenocortical hyperplasia and cortisol excess (Capen, 1988). Peterson *et al.* (1982) studied 25 dogs of various breeds with hyperadrenocorticism; 21 had pituitary adenomas, 15 in the pars distalis and six in the intermedia. By immunocytochemistry, ACTH, β-LPH and β-endorphin were seen in the majority. In addition, α-MSH was seen in many cells of the intermedial tumours but in only occasional cells in tumours of the pars distalis. Investigation of this condition in 11 dogs by McNicol, Thompson & Stewart (1983) suggests that in some cases the cause is a primary abnormality of the pituitary but in others it may result from a dysfunction of the hypothalamus or CNS.

Other tumour types are rare in the dog; pituitary carcinomas have been seen in aged animals (Carlton & Gries, 1983) and are usually endocrinologically inactive but result in functional disturbances due to destruction of adjacent tissues (Capen, 1988).

Craniopharyngiomas have been reported (Anderson & Capen, 1978), comprising cystic lesions with formations of epithelial cells, including squamous epithelium, which may extend into areas of the pars distalis.

### Primate

A recent review of the literature (Beniashvili, 1989) contains only two reports of pituitary tumours in the non-human primates. In addition, from autopsies of 450 rhesus monkeys, Kent & Pickering (1958) described one basophilic granular adenoma in the pars distalis of an animal which also showed thyroid hypoplasia. Hypertrophic and hyperplastic responses have been reported in primates in response to various experimental treatments.

## Conclusions and future prospects

The overall morphology of the pituitary gland in rodents, dog and primates is similar, but variations are seen in relative proportions and position of component tissues. The pars distalis is always the largest endocrine component producing the same hormone types in the various species. The extensive literature on the morphology, distribution, and ratios of the various cell types of the pars distalis has been reviewed and highlights a paucity of data for the mouse, beagle dog, and primate. Workers in this area have emphasized the essential role of immuno-cytochemistry for the identification of cell types at both the light micro-scopic and ultrastructural level but uncertainties still remain as to the hormone content of some cells and as to the exact genesis of the cells of the pars distalis.

Species variations are seen in the extent of the pars intermedia, from being well-developed in the rodents to rudimentary in some primates (and absent in humans) with corresponding variations in innervation and vasculature. Variations are also seen in the cell types present in the pars tuberalis, an area of unknown endocrine significance. In the rat, a preponderance of thyrotrophs is seen in contrast to gonadotrophs in most other species, including man. Some species have a high proportion of as yet unidentified cells. These variations in the pars intermedia and pars tuberalis in the rat are of particular interest in this widely used laboratory species which also shows a uniquely high incidence of pituitary tumours. The pathogenesis of these tumours is unclear but over-nutrition is recognized as a major contributory factor which could be eliminated (Roe, 1989). However, it seems that the *ad libitum* fed rat will continue to add to the growing interest in endocrine toxicology in the foreseeable future with consequent study of the pituitary playing an essential role. Immunocytochemical techniques will be of increasing interest but could be more widely used if there were readily available sources of reliable antisera for this type of work. To illustrate the usefulness of immuno-cytochemistry of the pituitary in investigations of endocrine toxicity, van Leeuwen, Franken & Loeber (1987) used studies of bromide and bis (tri-n-butyltin) oxide (TBTO) in the rat. Following treatment with bromide, increased staining intensity of TSH and ACTH cells corresponded with reduced thyroxine and corticosterone levels suggesting that the mechanisms were via direct effects on the thyroid and adrenals respectively, with consequent increases in stimulation of the pituitary by negative feedback. Conversely, reduced TSH staining in the pituitary after TBTO treatment correlated with reduced morphological evidence of thyroid activity, reduced thyroid weight and reduced serum thyroxine and TSH, suggesting that TBTO directly impaired pituitary TSH production and secretion.

Endocrinologists will also continue to utilize immunocytochemical techniques to further elucidate control mechanisms and to investigate as yet poorly defined functions of the pituitary. One such function could be its interaction with the immune system. It is now known that neurotransmitters and hormones can control cells of the immune system while lymphokines and monokines, the regulatory secretions of the immune system, can modulate the function of the neuroendocrine system (Bateman *et al.*, 1989); in fact the cells of the two systems possess some receptors that are identical. Because of these inter-relationships it has been postulated that compounds that affect the neuroendocrine system will also affect the immune system; TBTO, as cited above, may be an example of this. Snyder (1989) has gone a stage further to suggest that tests of immune function could be useful tools in the study of compounds that affect neuroendocrine components while extending our knowledge of the interactions of these two important systems.

## Acknowledgements

I wish to thank Dr C.J. Powell, D.H. Department of Toxicology, St Bartholomew's Hospital Medical College, for the supply of specimens stained for TSH and gonadotrophins. (Anti-sera supplied by the National Institute of Diabetes, Digestive and Kidney Diseases.) I am indebted to my colleagues at SmithKline Beecham Pharmaceuticals for their helpful comments and discussion, and to Miss W.J. Almond for her patience in typing this manuscript.

## References

Anderson, M.P. & Capen, C.C. (1978). The endocrine system. In *Pathology of Laboratory Animals*, vol. I, ed. K. Benirscke, F.M. Garner & T.C. Jones, pp. 424–508. New York: Springer.

Antunes, J.L., Louis, K., Cogen, P., Zimmerman, E.A. & Ferin, M. (1980). Section of the pituitary stalk in the rhesus monkey. II Morphological studies. *Neuroendocrinology*, **30**, 76–82.

Baker, B.L., Midgley, A.R., Gersten, B.E. & Yu, Y.Y. (1969). Differentiation of growth hormone and prolactin-containing acidophils with peroxidase-labelled antibody. *Anatomical Record*, **164**, 163–72.

Baker, B.L., Karsch, E.J., Hoffman, D.L. & Beckman, W.C. (1977). The presence of gonadotrophic and thyrotrophic cells in the pituitary pars tuberalis of the monkey (*Macaca mulatta*). *Biology of Reproduction*, **17**, 232–40.

Baker, B.L. & Gross, D.S. (1978). Cytology and distribution of secretory cell types in the mouse hypophysis as demonstrated with immunocytochemistry. *American Journal of Anatomy*, **153**, 193–216.

Barsoum, N.J., Moore, J.D., Gough, A.W., Sturgess, J.M. & De La Iglesia, F.A. (1985). Morphofunctional investigations on spontaneous pituitary tumours in Wistar Rats. *Toxicologic Pathology*, **13**(3), 200–8.

Bateman, A., Singh, A., Kral, T. & Solomon, S. (1989). The immune-hypothalamic-pituitary-adrenal axis. *Endocrine Reviews*, **10**(1), 92–112.

Beniashvili, D.Sh. (1989). An overview of the world literature on spontaneous tumours in nonhuman primates. *Journal of Medical Primatology*, **18**, 423–37.

Berkvens, J.M., van Nesselrooy, J.H.J. & Kroes, R. (1980). Spontaneous tumours in the pituitary gland of old Wistar rats. A morphological and immunocytochemical study. *Journal of Pathology*, **130**, 179–91.

Cameron, A.M. & Sheldon, W.G. (1983). Cystoid degeneration, anterior pituitary, mouse. In *Endocrine System*, ed. T.C. Jones, U. Mohr & R.D. Hunt, pp. 165–8. Monographs on Pathology of Laboratory Animals, (International Life Science Institute). Berlin: Springer-Verlag.

Capen, C.C. (1983). Functional and pathologic interrelationships of the pituitary gland and the hypothalamus. In *Endocrine System*, ed. T.C. Jones, U. Mohr & R.D. Hunt, pp. 103–20. Monographs on Pathology of Laboratory Animals (International Life Science Institute). Berlin: Springer-Verlag.

Capen, C.C. (1988). Endocrine system. In *Special Veterinary Pathology*, ed. R.G. Thompson, pp. 369–435. Toronto: B.C. Decker Inc.

Carlton, W.W. & Gries, C.L. (1983). Adenoma and carcinoma, pars distalis, rat, pp. 134–45. Adenoma, pars intermedia, anterior pituitary, rat, pp. 145–9. Craniopharyngioma, pituitary gland, rat, pp. 149–53. Pituicytoma, neurohypophysis, rat, pp. 156–60. Cysts, pituitary, rat, mouse and hamster, pp. 161–3. In *Endocrine System*, ed. T.C. Jones, U. Mohr & R.D. Hunt. Monographs on Pathology of

Laboratory Animals (International Life Science Institute). Berlin: Springer-Verlag.

Childs, G.V., Unabia, G. & Ellison, D. (1986). Immunocytochemical studies of pituitary hormones with PAP, ABC and immunogold techniques: evolution of technology to best fit the antigen. *The American Journal of Anatomy*, **175**, 307–30.

Dada, M.O., Campbell, G.T. & Blake, C.A. (1983). A quantitative immunocytochemical study of luteinizing hormone and follicle-stimulating hormone cells in the adenohypophysis of adult male rats and adult female rats throughout the oestrous cycle. *Endocrinology*, **113**(3), 970–83.

Dada, M.O., Campbell, G.T. & Blake, C.A. (1984). Pars distalis cell quantification in normal adult male and female rats. *Journal of Endocrinology*, **101**, 87–94.

Dodd, D.C., Port, C.D., Deslex, P., Regnier, B., Sanders, P. & Indacochea-Redmond, N. (1987). Two-year evaluation of misoprostol for carcinogenicity in CD Sprague–Dawley rats. *Toxicologic Pathology*, **15**(2), 125–33.

El Etreby, M.F. (1981). Practical applications of immunocytochemistry to the pharmacology and toxicology of the endocrine system. *Histochemical Journal*, **13**, 821–37.

El Etreby, M.F. & Dubois, M.P. (1980). The utility of antisera to different synthetic adrenocorticotrophins (ACTH) and melanotrophins (MSH) for immunocytochemical staining of the dog pituitary gland. *Histochemistry*, **66**, 245–60.

El Etreby, M.F. & Fath El Bab, M.R. (1977a). The utility of antisera to canine growth hormone and canine prolactin for immunocytochemical staining of the dog pituitary gland. *Histochemistry*, **53**, 1–15.

El Etreby, M.F. & Fath El Bab, M.R. (1977b). Localization of gonadotrophic hormones in the dog pituitary gland. *Cell and Tissue Research*, **183**, 167–75.

El Etreby, M.F. & Fath El Bab, M.R. (1978). Localisation of thyrotropin (TSH) in the dog pituitary gland. *Cell and Tissue Research*, **186**, 399–412.

El Etreby, M.F., Muller-Peddinghaus, R., Bhargava, A.S. & Trautwein, G. (1980). Functional morphology of spontaneous hyperplastic and neoplastic lesions in the canine pituitary gland. *Veterinary Pathology*, **17**, 109–22.

El Etreby, M.F., Richter, K.D. & Gunzel, P. (1973). Sexual hormones and prolactin cells in rat, dog, monkey and man. *Excerpta Medica International Congress Series*, **308**, 65–9.

El Etreby, M.F., Schilk, B., Soulioti, G., Tushaus, U., Wiemann, H. & Gunzel, P. (1977). Effect of 17β-estradiol on cells of the pars distalis of the adenohypophysis in the beagle bitch: an immunocytochemical and morphometric study. *Endocrinologie*, **69**(2), 202–16.

Frith, C.H. & Ward, J.M. (1988). Endocrine system. In *Colour Atlas of*

*Neoplastic and Non-neoplastic Lesions in Aging Mice*, pp. 33–48. Amsterdam: Elsevier.

Furth, J., Nakane, P. & Pasteels, J.L. (1976). Tumours of the pituitary gland. In *Pathology of Tumours in Laboratory Animals*, vol. 1. *Tumours of the Rat*, part 2, ed. V. S. Turusov, pp. 201–37. Lyon: IARC Scientific Publication.

Glaister, J.R. (1986). Laboratory animal pathology. In *Principles of Toxicological Pathology*, pp. 131–203. London: Taylor and Francis.

Gopinath, C., Prentice, D.E. & Lewis, D.J. (1987). The endocrine glands. In *Atlas of Experimental Toxicological Pathology. Current Histopathology*, vol. 13, ed. G.A. Gresham, pp. 104–21. Lancaster: MTP Press Ltd.

Greaves, P. & Faccini, J.M. (1984). Endocrine glands. In *Rat Histopathology*, pp. 187–97. Amsterdam: Elsevier.

Gross, D.S. (1984). The mammalian hypophyseal pars tuberalis: a comparative immunocytochemical study. *General and Comparative Endocrinology*, **56**, 283–98.

Halmi, N.S., Peterson, M.E., Colurso, G.J., Liotta, A.S. & Krieger, D.T. (1981). Pituitary intermediate lobe in dog: two cell types and high bioactive adrenocorticotropin content. *Science*, **211**, 72–4.

Ham, A.W. (1974). The endocrine system. In *Histology*, 7th edn, pp. 782–846. Philadelphia: Lippincott.

Hanstrom, B. (1966). Gross anatomy of the hypophysis in mammals. In *The Pituitary Gland*, vol. 1, *Anterior Pituitary*, ed. G.W. Harris & B.T. Donovan, pp. 1–57. London: Butterworth.

Herbert, D.C. (1976). Immunocytochemical evidence that luteinizing hormone (LH) and follicle stimulating hormone (FSH) are present in the same cell type in the rhesus monkey pituitary gland. *Endocrinology*, **98**, 1554–7.

Herbert, D.C. (1978). Identification of the LH and TSH-secreting cells in the pituitary gland of the rhesus monkey. *Cell and Tissue Research*, **190**, 151–61.

Herbert, D.C. & Hayashida, T. (1974). Histologic identification and immunochemical studies of prolactin and growth hormone in the primate pituitary gland. *General and Comparative Endocrinology*, **24**, 381–97.

Herbert, D.C. & Silverman, A.Y. (1983). Topographical distribution of the gonadotrophs, mammotrophs, somatotrophs and thyrotrophs in the pituitary gland of the baboon (*Papio cynocephalus*). *Cell and Tissue Research*, **230**, 233–8.

Holmes, R.L. & Ball, J.N. (1974). A general consideration of the pituitary gland, pp. 5–15. Comparative morphology of the mammalian pituitary, pp. 16–25. In *Biological Structure and Function*, vol. 4, *The Pituitary Gland – A Comparative Account*. Cambridge: Cambridge University Press.

Horvath, E. & Kovacs, K. (1988). Fine structural cytology of the adeno-hypophysis in rat and man. *Journal of Electron Microscopy Technique*, **8**, 401–32.

Kaufman, J. (1987). The pituitary and hypothalamus. In *Small Animal Endocrinology*, ed. F.H. Drazner, pp. 47–81. Edinburgh: Churchill Livingstone.

Kent, S.P. & Pickering, J.E. (1958). Neoplasms in monkeys (*Macaca mulatta*): spontaneous and irradiation induced. *Cancer*, **11**(1), 138–47.

Kurosumi, K. (1986). Cell classification of the rat anterior pituitary by means of immunoelectron microscopy. *Journal of Clinical Electron Microscopy*, **19**(4), 299–319.

Lechan, R.M. (1987). Neuroendocrinology of pituitary hormone regulation. *Endocrinology and Metabolism Clinics*, **16**(3), 475–501.

van Leeuwen, F.X.R., Franken, M.A.M. & Loeber, J.G. (1987). The endocrine system in experimental toxicology. In *Advances in Veterinary Science and Comparative Medicine*, vol. 31, *Experimental and Comparative Toxicology*, ed. A. Rico, pp. 121–49. San Diego: Academic Press.

Liebelt, A.G. (1979). Tumours of the pituitary gland. In *Pathology of Tumours in Laboratory Animals*, vol. II, *Tumours of the Mouse*, ed. V.S. Turusov, pp. 411–50. Lyon: IARC Scientific Publication.

Losinski, N.E., Horvath, E. & Kovacs, K. (1989). Double-labelling immunogold electron microscopic study of hormonal colocalization in nontumorous and adenomatous rat pituitaries. *The American Journal of Anatomy*, **185**, 236–43.

McComb, D.J., Kovacs, K., Beri, J. & Zak, F. (1984). Pituitary adenomas in old Sprague–Dawley rats: a histologic, ultrastructural, and immunocytochemical study. *Journal of the National Cancer Institute*, **73**(5), 1143–66.

McNicol, A.M., Thompson, H. & Stewart, C.J.R. (1983). The corticotrophic cells of the canine pituitary gland in pituitary-dependent hyperadrenocorticism. *Journal of Endocrinology*, **96**, 303–9.

Magnusson, G., Majeed, S.K. & Gopinath, C. (1979). Infiltrating pituitary neoplasms in the rat. *Laboratory Animals*, **13**, 111–13.

Middleton, D.J., Rijnberk, A., Bevers, M.M., Goos, H.J.T.L., Beeftink, E.A., Thijssen, J.H.H. & Croughs, R.J.M. (1987). Some functional aspects of canine corticotrophs. *Hormone Metabolism Research*, **19**, 632–5.

Murakami, T., Kikuta, A., Taguchi, T., Ohtsuka, A. & Ohtani, O. (1987). Blood vascular architecture of the rat cerebral hypophysis and hypothalamus. A dissection/scanning electron microscopy of vascular casts. *Archives of Histology, Japan*, **50**(2), 133–76.

Nakane, P.K. (1970). Classification of anterior pituitary cell types with immunoenzyme histochemistry. *The Journal of Histochemistry and Cytochemistry*, **18**(1), 9–20.

Nakane, P.K. (1975). Identification of anterior pituitary cells by immunoelectron microscopy. In *The Anterior Pituitary*, ed. A. Tixer-Vidal, pp. 45–61. San Diego: Academic Press.

Page, R.B. (1988). The anatomy of the hypothalamo-hypophyseal complex. In *The Physiology of Reproduction*, ed. E. Knobil, J.D. Neil, L.L. Ewing, G.S. Greenwald, C.L. Market & D.W. Pfaff, pp. 1161–233. New York: Raven Press.

Pelletier, G. (1984). The secretory process in the anterior hypophysis. In *Cell Biology of the Secretory Process*, ed. M. Cantin, pp. 196–213. Basel: Karger.

Peterson, M.E., Krieger, D.T., Drucker, W.D. & Halmi, N.S. (1982). Immunocytochemical study of the hypophysis in 25 dogs with pituitary-dependent hyperadrenocorticism. *Acta Endocrinologica*, **101**, 15–24.

Petrusz, P. & Ordronneau, P. (1983). Immunocytochemistry of pituitary hormones. In *Immunocytochemistry. Practical Applications in Pathology and Biology*, ed. J.M. Polak & S. van Noorden, pp. 212–32. Bristol: John Wright and Sons Ltd.

Poole, M.C. & Kornegay, W.D. (1982). Cellular distribution within the rat adenohypophysis: a morphometric study. *The Anatomical Record*, **204**, 45–53.

van Putten, L.J.A. & van Zwieten, M.J. (1988). Studies on prolactin-secreting cells in aging rats of different strains. II Selected morphological and immunocytochemical features of pituitary tumours correlated with serum prolactin levels. *Mechanisms of Aging and Development*, **42**, 115–27.

Reichlin, S. (1989). Neuroendocrinology of the pituitary gland. *Toxicologic Pathology*, **17**(2), 250–5.

Roe, F.J.C. & Bar, A. (1985). Enzootic and epizootic adrenal medullary proliferative disease of rats: influence of dietary factors which affect calcium absorption. *Human Toxicology*, **4**, 27–52.

Roe, F.J.C. (1989). Non-genotoxic carcinogenesis: implications for testing and extrapolation to man. *Mutagenesis*, **4**(6), 407–11.

Sandusky, G.E., Van Pelt, C.S., Todd, G.C. & Wightman, K. (1988). An immunocytochemical study of pituitary adenomas and focal hyperplasias in old Sprague-Dawley and Fischer 344 rats. *Toxicologic Pathology*, **16**(3), 376–80.

Sasaki, F. & Iwama, Y. (1988). Sex difference in prolactin and growth hormone cells in mouse adenohypophysis: stereological, morphometric and immunohistochemical studies by light and electron microscopy. *Endocrinology*, **123**(2), 905–12.

Sells, D.M. & Gibson, J.P. (1987). Carcinogenicity studies with medroxalol hydrochloride in rats and mice. *Toxicologic Pathology*, **15**(4), 457–67.

Skelton-Stroud, P.M. & Ishmael, J. (1986). Naturally occurring lesions in some endocrine glands of laboratory maintained baboons (*Papio* sp). *Veterinary Pathology*, **23**, 380–5.

Snyder, C.A. (1989). The neuroendocrine system, an opportunity for immunotoxicologists. *Environmental Health Perspectives*, **81**, 165–6.

Soji, T. & Herbert, D.C. (1989). Intercellular communication between rat anterior pituitary cells. *The Anatomical Record*, **224**, 523–33.

Trouillas, J., Girod, C., Claustrat, B., Cure, M. & Dubois, M.P. (1982). Spontaneous pituitary tumours in the Wistar/Furth/Ico rat strain. *American Journal of Pathology*, **109**(1), 57–70.

Watanabe, Y.G. (1985). An immunohistochemical study on the mouse adenohypophysis with reference to the spatial relationship between GH cells and other types of hormone-producing cells. *Anatomy and Embryology*, **172**, 277–80.

Weatherhead, B. (1983). The pars intermedia of the pituitary gland. In *Progress in Anatomy*, vol. 3, ed. R.J. Harrison & E. Navaratram, pp. 1–32. Cambridge: Cambridge University Press.

Yoshimura, F. (1986). A new concept of anterior pituitary cell classification in the rat based on both cell differentiation and the secretory cycle. In *Pars Distalis of the Pituitary Gland – Structure, Function and Regulation*, ed. F. Yoshimura & A. Gorbman, pp. 59–69. Amsterdam: Elsevier.

Yoshimura, F., Nogami, H., Yashiro, T. & Aoyama, T. (1982). Comparative immunohistochemical study of the mammalian pituitary corticotrophs. *Okajimas Folia Anatomy, Japan*, **56**(4–6), 709–28.

RICHARD F. WALKER AND RALPH L.
COOPER

# 3 Toxic effects of xenobiotics on the pituitary gland

## Introduction

The pituitary gland occupies a central position in the endocrine system,
regulating the activity of several peripheral glands and influencing metabolism throughout the body. Hypothetically, perturbations of pituitary
function could adversely affect organismal homeostasis, causing diffuse
systemic toxicity. Despite this potential, there are relatively few
published studies that specifically investigate toxic effects of xenobiotics
on the pituitary gland. Factors contributing to the paucity of specific
studies include:

1 the relatively low exposure of pituitary cells to xenobiotics as
the vascular supply and concentrating ability of the gland are
considerably less than major organs of excretion and
metabolism,
2 the low frequency of published reports describing
histopathologic lesions in the pituitary compared to other
endocrine glands, especially the gonads, and perhaps most
importantly,
3 the fact that manifestations of pituitary toxicity often expressed in terms of functional and structural changes in peripheral
endocrine glands under its control, thus shifting attention
from the pituitary to its target tissues such as the gonads,
adrenals, thyroid and mammary glands.

Specific pituitary cell populations have been quantified in rats by
immunocytochemical techniques (Dada, Campbell & Blake, 1984) and
include lactotrophs (prolactin [PRL] containing cells), somatotrophs
(growth hormone [GH] cells), gonadotrophs (luteinizing hormone [LH]
and follicle stimulating hormone [FSH] cells), and thyrotrophs (thyroid
stimulating hormone [TSH] cells). These specific cell types constituted
approximately 51, 21, 9 and 2% of cells in the anterior pituitary, respec-

tively. The remaining cells did not show specific immunocytochemical reactivity, and sex differences in the ratios of cell types were not apparent. The incidence of published studies reporting pituitary toxicity reflects the frequency distribution of the different anterior pituitary cell types quantified by Dada *et al.* (1984). Thus, there is a preponderance of reports on hyperprolactinaemia and lactotroph adenomas. However, it is unclear whether the large number of reports involving PRL cell toxicity reflects a greater sensitivity of lactotrophs to toxicants, or if their greater occurrence in the pituitary makes the consequences of hypertrophy, hyperplasia and adenoma formation more apparent.

All adenohypophyseal cell types can give rise to pituitary neoplasms that generally produce endocrine dysfunction. However, some pituitary tumours, do not cause local or endocrine symptoms (McComb *et al.*, 1983). Because they are more easily recognized, adenohypophyseal cells associated with abnormal hormone secretion receive more attention in defining the pituitary as a locus of toxicity.

Lactotroph adenomas are the most common pituitary tumour, responsible in approximately one third of all cases of hyperprolactinemia (Martin & Reichlin, 1987). The other pituitary tumours that occur in high frequency are GH- and adrenocorticotrophin (ACTH)-secreting. The reasons for the predominance of PRL, GH and ACTH secreting tumours are unknown; however, all three hormones are similar in that they are released in response to physical and emotional stress, meals, arginine infusion, hypoglycaemia, sleep and oestrogen administration. Also, these hormones are often co-localized in pituitary cells demonstrating that certain adenohypophyseal cell types produce more than one of each of the three hormones, and suggesting that the phenotype (in terms of hormone production) of these cells may change in response to certain conditions, including xenobiotic exposure.

Pituitary lesions involving thyrotrophs pass through several stages, the first of which involves the appearance of large swollen 'thyroidectomy' cells. These hypertrophic cells contain dilated and ballooned rough endoplasmic reticulum which becomes distended with flocculate material. The rapid discharge of TSH associated with the initial stimulation of the thyrotrophs leads to depletion of cytoplasmic secretory granules. Subsequently, secretory material increases in the rough endoplasmic reticulum causing distension. Hyperplasia of the thyrotroph population then results from continued stimulation. Upon severe and continued stimulation, there is a progression to 'exhaustion' cells which are grossly vacuolated with small shrunken dense nuclei (Gopinath, Prentice & Lewis, 1987). Thyrotroph adenomas are rare, but when they occur, contain high concentrations of TSH.

Gonadotroph adenomas are uncommon, appear chromophobic by conventional staining and contain FSH and/or LH as determined by immunoperoxidase methodology.

Histopathologic evidence of pituitary toxicity can be divided into two broad categories depending upon which cells in the gland are affected by xenobiotic exposure. The lesions may be non-specific, occurring throughout the gland without predilection for specific cell populations. The non-specific lesions include infarction, necrosis, vacuolation or apoptosis, and have a relatively low incidence. In contrast, specific lesions localized to discrete regions of the pituitary, and involving cells responsible for the production and release of specific trophic hormone are commonly reported. The specific lesions are characterized by proliferative changes that generally pass through distinct stages (Capen, 1983) including:

- degranulation, resulting from the rapid release of secretory granules,
- hypertrophy of the degranulated cells following several days of persistent stimulation,
- hyperplasia, when hypertrophy persists for days and weeks,
- and finally, cellular vacuolation and nuclear displacement if treatment with the toxic agent continues for weeks or months.
- Adenomas involving specific cell types have been associated with hyperplastic changes; however, it is unclear whether hyperplasia proceeds to neoplasia or if the two conditions are independent of each other.

Compared to hyperplasia and hypertrophy, pituitary tumours are relatively uncommon. In humans, the incidence of all pituitary tumours diagnosed during life represent approximately 10 per cent of intracranial tumours (Martin & Reichlin, 1987). However, despite the relatively infrequent clinical presentation of patients with symptoms of pituitary tumours, as many as 8 to 27% of routine autopsies in which serial sections of the adenohypophysis were performed, revealed pituitary adenomas (Costello, 1936; McCormick & Halmi, 1971; Burrow *et al.*, 1981). These observations suggest that the incidence of pituitary pathology is higher than evident from clinical observations. While some of the lesions may be spontaneous, others may result from xenobiotic exposure. In animals, especially rats, pituitary adenomas occur commonly during aging, and affect females to a greater extent than males (Meites & Nicoll, 1966; Kovacs *et al.*, 1977; Kroes *et al.*, 1981; Walker, Weideman & Wheeldon, 1988). Thus, the background of spontaneously occurring pituitary tumours, especially in chronic studies with rodents, and the ambiguity or absence of clinical signs associated with pituitary toxicity in humans, contributes to possible underestimates of their occurrence as the result of xenobiotic exposure.

Three major symptoms associated with pituitary pathology, especially tumours, are endocrine dysfunctions, loss of vision and headaches (Krieger, 1980a). Although endocrine dysfunctions predominate as a symptom of pituitary tumours, visual symptoms precede the other complaints in about 30–35% of cases. The visual symptoms are experienced as haziness or dimness of either eye, and although compression of the optic chiasma could occur during growth of the tumour, double vision is relatively rare.

Multiple endocrine dysfunction is a fairly good indicator of pituitary toxicity *per se*, especially if the dysfunctions appear in a specific sequence (Krieger, 1980a). Endocrine dysfunction tends to follow certain patterns that are set, in part, by the location and nature of the pituitary tumour. Slow growing tumours in the sella tend to first produce clinical abnormalities related to gonadotropins, followed by thyroid and adrenal dysfunctions. This order may be reversed in rapidly progressive pituitary failure as may occur during acute haemorrhage into the pituitary gland. In addition, signs of increased or decreased growth, and increased PRL secretion (galactorrhae) may accompany changes in reproductive, thyroid and adrenal functions.

The etiologies of pituitary toxicity resulting from exposure to xenobiotics are summarized in Table 3.1. As seen in Fig. 3.1, synthesis and release of pituitary hormones are influenced by stimulatory and inhibitory signals from the brain (primarily peptides and dopamine, respectively), the activity of which is in turn modified by a complex network of feedback relationships involving hormones of peripheral origin as well as from the pituitary itself (Tepperman & Tepperman, 1987). The feedback matrix regulating the endocrine system can thus be disrupted at many levels, including the brain, pituitary and/or peripheral endocrine glands. For example, xenobiotic-induced gonadal dysfunction might occur directly by inhibiting steroidogenesis, or indirectly by reducing the output of gonadotrophins or gonadotrophin-releasing hormones (GnRH) from the pituitary or brain, respectively. While the effects on the gonads might be the same, the perturbations within the matrix would be different depending upon the locus of toxicity. Thus, hypophyseal toxicities must be identified by analysis of intrinsic pituitary function as well as by evaluating changes in the activities of tissues that it controls.

Table 3.1. *Etiology of common pituitary lesions*

Toxic substances can affect pituitary structure and/or function by:
- disrupting pituitary function through a direct action upon cells within the gland,

- changing the availability or influence of peripheral hormones that provide negative feedback control upon the pituitary, or

- altering the neurogenic signals (neurotransmitters/neuropeptides) that regulate the activity of adenohypophyseal cells, thus, leading to hypersecretion and hyperplasia or hyposecretion and atrophy,

- compromising blood flow to the pituitary and thereby causing necrosis,

- a combination of effects that may include more than one of the above.

## Etiology of common pituitary lesions

The occurrence of functional and/or structural abnormalities in the pituitary can be designated as primary, secondary or tertiary toxicities. Primary toxicity occurs when a xenobiotic injures hypophyseal cells directly; that is, independent of regulatory feedback responses within the neuroendocrine system. Secondary and tertiary toxicites result from adverse effects on long-loop feedback hormones produced by peripheral endocrine glands, or on regulatory neurotransmitters or peptides from the brain, respectively.

## Direct pituitary effects

Pituitary toxicity may result from a direct insult to cellular components of the gland by xenobiotics. Some compounds are non-specific in terms of the pituitary cell types to which they are toxic. For example, pituitary infarction and necrosis occur in rats administered hexadimethrine (Kovacs, Caroll & Tapp, 1966). In another case, an unidentified 'novel anticancer drug' produced vacuolation of monkey anterior pituitary cells without predilection for any single cell type. The vacuolation was associated with apoptosis – focal single cell degeneration (Gopinath *et al.*, 1987).

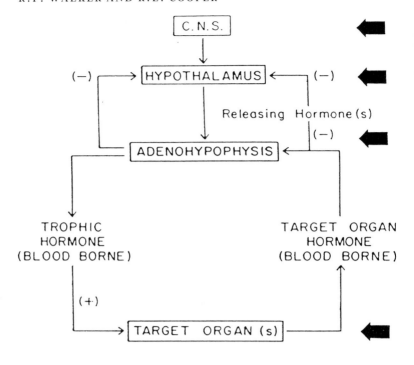

Fig. 3.1. Diagrammatic representation of a neuroendocrine axis showing the central position of the pituitary, hormonal feedback relationships, and sites of at which xenobiotics could cause pituitary toxicity. (From Thomas *et al.*, 1989.)

Circulatory disorders

Sometimes, xenobiotics may precipitate clinical symptoms of pituitary toxicity secondary to a pre-existing adenoma. For example, pituitary apoplexy (haemorrhage into the pituitary gland) almost always occurs in glands in which adenomas are present (Locke & Tyler, 1961; Taylor, 1968; Dawson & Kothandaram, 1972), and most commonly with somatotroph, lactotroph or corticotroph adenomas. It is precipitated by various events, including administration of anticoagulants or oestrogens (Veldhuis & Hammond, 1980).

Hypopituitarism may also result from ischemic necrosis of the pituitary. This disorder results most frequently from severe haemorrhage of the pituitary capillary network during parturition, but may also result from exposure to anesthesia or poisoning (Doniach & Walker, 1946; Smith & Howard, 1959; Murdoch, 1962; Harlin & Givins, 1968).

### Metals

There are few examples of compounds that have been shown to be directly toxic to cells of the pituitary gland. Accumulations of metal selenide were demonstrated by light and electron microscopy in the rat anterior pituitary after administration of sodium selenite via drinking water or i.p. injections (Schamberger, 1983; Thorlacius-Ussing & Danscher, 1985). The toxic effects of selenium recognized in animals and humans include reduced growth and ovarian dysfunction, both of which can be attributed to a selenium-induced pituitary lesion. Although the mechanism of selenium pituitary toxicity is unknown, a substitution with sulphur or zinc was proposed as a means by which the metal could alter secretion of PRL, GH and perhaps other hormones (Thorlacius-Ussing & Danscher, 1985).

The possibility of nickel involvement in pituitary dysfunction has been suggested because of its preferential uptake by pituitary tissue, second in magnitude only to renal tissue (Smith & Hackley, 1968; Parker & Sunderman, 1974; Clary, 1979). An expression of potential nickel toxicity in the pituitary was reported as an inhibitory effect upon PRL release when added to incubation medium containing bovine pituitary slices (LaBella *et al.*, 1973). Under these conditions, the inhibitory effect did not alter release of other hormones. Somewhat conflicting results were reported in another study in which pituitaries taken from rats administered nickel 48 hours prior to necropsy, released more PRL *in vitro*, than those from untreated rats (Clemons & Garcia, 1981). The cause of the differential effect of nickel upon bovine pituitary cells *in vitro* and rat pituitaries *ex vivo* is not known, but for the latter case, a central locus of toxicity (e.g. altered dopamine release from the hypothalamus) may be involved as proposed below. In a more recent study, baseline and stimulated PRL, LH and TSH release from perifused rat pituitaries was not affected by addition of nickel (50 μM) to the perifusion medium (Fig. 3.2; Cooper *et al.*, 1987). However, similar treatment with zinc (50 μM) or cadmium (50 μM) altered release of all three pituitary hormones evaluated. The addition of zinc to the perifusion medium suppressed baseline PRL release, as well as stimulated (KCl challenge) PRL release. Under these

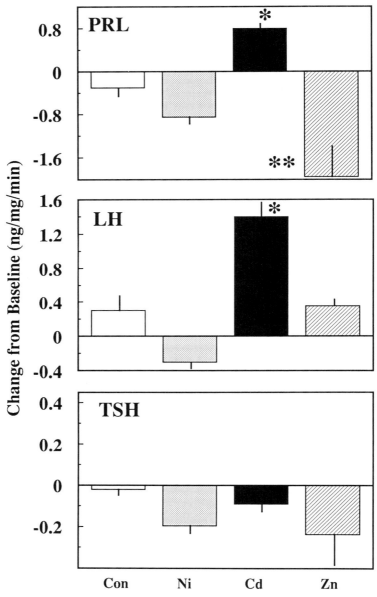

Fig. 3.2. Spontaneous release of PRL (prolactin), LH (luteinizing hormone) and TSH (thyroid stimulating hormone) from rat pituitaries *in vitro*, following addition of nickel (Ni), cadmium (Cd) or zinc (Zn) to the perifusion media. Con=saline control. Bars represent the difference

conditions, LH and TSH were not altered. However, after the removal of zinc from the perifusion medium, the stimulated release of all three hormones was significantly enhanced (Fig. 3.3). This 'rebound' effect of zinc on PRL release was also reported by Judd, MacLeod & Login (1984). The addition of cadmium to the incubation medium resulted in an increased baseline release of LH. PRL secretion was not altered. However, Lorenson, Robson & Jacobs (1983a; 1983b) found that pituitary exposure to a number of cations altered PRL secretion.

Recently, Camoratto *et al.* (1990) reported that pituitaries from rats treated chronically with lead for seven weeks postnatally released 64% less GH in response to growth hormone releasing hormone (GHRH) stimulation *in vitro*, and bound less radiolabelled GHRH than controls. The content of pituitary GH was not altered by lead, indicating that the metal had a direct effect on somatotroph release mechanisms.

### Natural and synthetic oestrogens

In contrast to metals which may affect more than one pituitary cell type, xenobiotics appear to be more specific in their toxicity to hypophyseal cell populations. Perhaps the most common example is the result of lactotroph stimulation leading to hypertrophy, hyperplasia and possibly to neoplasia.

Hypertrophy and hyperplasia of lactotrophs have been observed in rats, mice, beagle dogs and non-human primates administered natural or synthetic oestrogens (El Etreby *et al.*, 1979; El Etreby, 1981; Lloyd, 1983). This effect may be analogous to pituitary enlargement that occurs during pregnancy when endogenous oestrogens are produced in large quantities. The locus of toxicity of oestrogenic substances has been suggested to be the pituitary (Lloyd, 1983), since local oestrogen receptors have been demonstrated by several laboratories.

In rats, pituitary cells stimulated by oestrogen pass through a stage of hyperplasia to adenoma formation, and eventually may become malignant and metastasize. Although the cells were initially oestrogen dependent, they may become autonomous and capable of proliferation when transplanted to other animals. In humans, oestrogen treatment also stimulates lactotroph hypertrophy and hyperplasia and may enlarge pre-existing prolactinomas; however, the steroid does not induce tumour formation *de novo* in man (Reichlin, 1980).

Caption for Fig. 3.2. (*cont.*)
in cumulative release (mean±SEM, N=6), of pituitary hormones compared to a 30 minute period of prior exposure (*p≤0.05; **p≤0.01). (From Cooper *et al.*, 1987.)

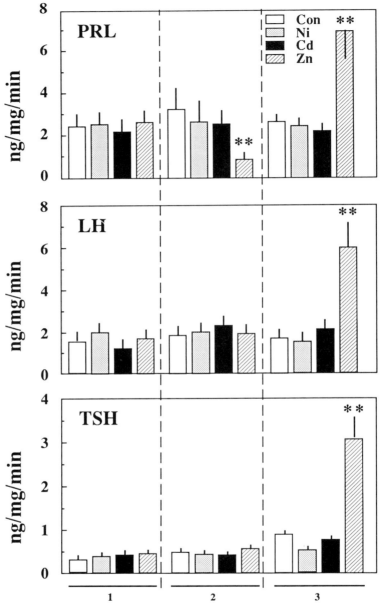

Fig. 3.3. Stimulated release of PRL (prolactin), LH (luteinising hormone) and TSH (thyroid stimulating hormone) in response to 60 nM KCl (1) prior to, (2) during, and (3) after exposure to perifusion buffers

Another change in lactotrophs that may be mediated by a direct action upon the pituitary is a form of autophagy termed 'acrinophagy' that occurs in oestradiol-primed rats within minutes of somatostatin administration. Apparently somatostatin causes sequestration of PRL into intracellular bodies associated with concentric cisternae resulting from rearrangement of the rough endoplasmic reticulum (Saunders, Reifel & Shin, 1983). Somatostatin may have a similar effect in man because the peptide has been reported to inhibit PRL release clinically in patients primed with oestrogen and cyproterone acetate (Gooren, Harmsen-Louman & van Keswel, 1984).

Pesticides

Chlordecone (kepone), a chlorinated polycyclic ketone insecticide that is known to adversely affect reproduction in laboratory animals and humans may produce its toxicity, at least in part, through direct inhibition of gonadotrophin release from the pituitary (Huang & Nelson, 1986). Rat pituitary cell cultures were treated with chlordecone before a six-hour challenge with GnRH, and secretion of LH and FSH were measured. Although no effect on basal gonadotrophin release was observed, chlordecone significantly suppressed FSH and LH release in response to GnRH and also antagonized the potentiated response to GnRH produced by oestrogen. In contrast, Mirex, a compound with similar chemical structure to chlordecone, did not block GnRH-stimulated gonadotrophin release. This study demonstrated that although chlordecone has oestrogenic activity in the ovary and uterus, it is anti-oestrogenic in the pituitary. The action undoubtedly contributes to the reproductive toxicity of chlordecone.

Another weakly oestrogenic pesticide, methoxychlor, has also been shown to alter pituitary weight and PRL secretion. Pituitaries from male rats treated with methoxychlor had elevated PRL concentrations and released more PRL *in vitro* than controls (Fig. 3.4; Goldman *et al.*, 1986). This effect of methoxychlor on PRL was observed at doses that did not alter the serum or pituitary concentrations of other hormones assayed (e.g. LH, FSH and testosterone). This alteration in pituitary release of PRL agrees with the hyperprolactinemic effects reported for oestradiol and diethylstibestrol (DES) (Fig. 3.5; Cooper *et al.*, 1985). Since there is strong evidence for a relationship between elevated oestrogen levels and tumour activity (Cooper, 1983), this effect may be involved in the

Caption for Fig. 3.3 (*cont.*)
containing nickel (Ni), cadmium (Cd) or zinc (Zn). Con=saline control.
Values represent means±SEM, N=6. (From Cooper *et al.*, 1987.)

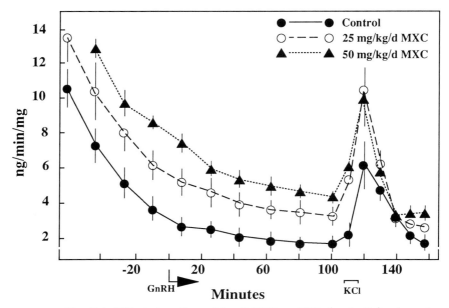

Fig. 3.4. Effect of methoxychlor (MXC) on PRL (prolactin) release by rat hemi-pituitaries *in vivo* in response to gonadotrophin releasing hormone (GnRH). The arrow depicts point (0 time) at which continuous GnRH challenge was begun. The 9 minute KCl stimulus is represented by the short bar under the right portion of the horizontal axis. Release is in ng/mg anterior pituitary±SEM. (From Goldman *et al.*, 1986.)

previously reported tumourigenic response to methoxychlor. However, in contrast to the effect of oestrogen or DES treatment which increased pituitary weight (Cooper *et al.*, 1985), methoxychlor treatment resulted in a significant decrease in pituitary weight (Gray *et al.*, 1986).

Unlike the anti-oestrogenic effect of chlordecone on gonadotrophins described above, an oestrogen-like activity of this insecticide has been reported on the pituitary enkephalin system (Hudson *et al.*, 1984). Injections of chlordecone for up to 10 days caused a time and dose-related decrease in pituitary [Met[5]]-enkephalin-like immunoreactivity (ME-LI) in adult rats similar to that produced by oestrogen. However, the authors pointed out that unlike oestrogens, chlordecone did not increase protein content or peroxidase activity in the pituitary. Thus, it was possible that chlordecone only mimicked the oestrogenic effect on ME-LI in the pituitary. In any event, it was concluded that while the effect was real, a pituitary locus of toxicity could not be unequivocally defined.

The gamma isomer of 1,2,3,4,5,6-hexachlorocyclohexane (γHCH),

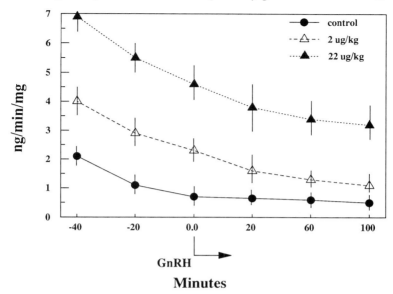

Fig. 3.5. Pituitary PRL (prolactin) release during perifusion from pituitary glands obtained from male rats that received 0, 1, or 22 µg/kg DES (diethylstilbestrol), s.c. for a 7 day period. Pituitaries were challenged with GnRH (gonadotrophin releasing hormone) at time 0 to evaluate LH (luteinizing hormone) release. Data not shown. N=10/group. (From Cooper *et al.*, 1985.)

lindane, which causes reproductive dysfunction, may also reduce gonadotrophin release at least in part, as an expression of its pituitary toxicity (Cooper *et al.*, 1989). Oral administration of lindane to female rat pups for approximately 100 consecutive days (from 21 to 125 days of age) significantly reduced serum and pituitary LH and PRL concentrations (Fig. 3.6), as well as relative pituitary weights. Furthermore, lindane attenuated oestradiol-stimulated LH release, an effect previously reported for chlordecone in rat pituitary cells *in vitro* (Huang & Nelson, 1986).

Other xenobiotics

A possible effect of bis(tri-n-butyltin) oxide (TBTO) on the endocrine system was reported by Funahashi *et al.* (1980), who observed histopathological abnormalities in the pituitary glands of treated male rats. Consistent with a pituitary effect were alterations in serum TSH and thyroxine. In a subsequent study, TBTO was administered as a dietary supplement to rats for four weeks (Krajnc *et al.*, 1984). Pituitary release

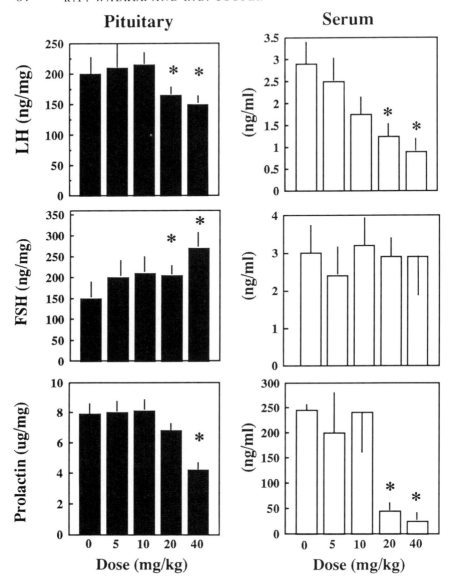

Fig. 3.6. Effects of lindane on pituitary concentrations of LH (luteinizing hormone), FSH (follicle stimulating hormone) and prolactin. All rats were killed at 1300 h on the day of vaginal proestrus (*p<0.05). (From Cooper *et al.*, 1989.)

of LH was increased in TBTO-treated rats, as were the number of cells identified immunohistochemically as containing LH. In contrast, a dose-related reduction in the number and staining intensity of TSH-producing cells was observed. These studies did not evaluate possible changes in hypophysiotrophic peptides following TBTO exposure, but since end-organ as well as pituitary activity were altered in the same directions, the data suggest that the pituitary was the target for TBTO toxicity. If this hypothesis is true, the effect is unusual in that hypersecretion of gonadotrophins is not a common effect of compounds with pituitary toxicity. More often, xenobiotics reduce pituitary gonadotrophin activity. For example, the cytotoxic chemotherapeutic agent cisplatin is embryotoxic in rats by altering PRL and LH release (Bajt & Aggarwal, 1985).

In another study, malignant neoplasms of the pituitary were observed in male and female rats administered vinyl acetate in drinking water for two years at concentrations of 2500 or 1000 mg/l (Lijinsky & Reuber, 1983). The neoplasms were poorly differentiated or undifferentiated carcinomas, and there is not sufficient data to determine whether the effect resulted from a direct or indirect action of vinyl acetate upon the pituitary.

## Pituitary toxicity following changes in negative feedback relationships

Pituitary hormone-secreting tumours can develop, in some cases, following exposure to toxicants that disrupt the negative feedback relationships normally suppressing hypophyseal hypersecretion. Generally, these changes result from toxicant-mediated deficiences in endocrine gland hormones, which allow stimulated or autonomous hyperactivity of certain pituitary cell populations. For example, TSH-secreting tumours which gain variable degrees of autonomy and increased resistance to feedback inhibition by thyroxine, may develop in thyroidectomized rats (Furth & Clifton, 1966; Reichlin, 1980). Anti-thyroid compounds such as amitrole, ethylenethiourea, thiouracil, methylithiouracil, 2,4-diaminoanisol or propylthiouracil (Evarts & Brown, 1981; Farquahar, 1969; Osamura & Takayhama, 1983; Tsuda, 1983) will cause hypertrophy and hyperplasia of thyrotrophs by inhibiting the production and release of thyroid hormones which maintain an inhibitory tone upon the pituitary.

The reverse effect of compounds that produce 'stimulatory' lesions in populations of thyrotrophs can be produced by thyroxine or triiodothyronine, which increase negative feedback upon the thyroid neuroendocrine axis (Gopinath *et al.*, 1987; Jones *et al.*, 1988). In thyroxine-treated rats, secretory materials and granules accumulate in the cytoplasm of thyrotrophs due to reduced release of TSH. Eventually the rough endoplasmic reticulum regresses in rats treated with thyroxine and the cells may involute. Similar atrophy and regression of thyrotrophs have been reported in dogs administered cyproterone and progesterone (El Etreby, 1981) which also appear to reduce thyrotrophic stimulation of the pituitary.

Oral administration of the leukotriene antagonist, L-649,923, (Sanders *et al.*, 1988) or phenobarbital, PCB and TCDD (2,3,7,8-tetrachloro-dibenzo-p-dioxin) (Japundzic, 1969; Bastomsky, 1977; Collins *et al.*, 1977; Potter *et al.*, 1986) was associated with hypersecretion of TSH. The factor common to each of these compounds was that they increased the rate of hepatic metabolism and clearance of thyroid hormones, thus reducing their negative feedback influence on the pituitary and increasing its secretion of TSH. Akoso *et al.* (1982) examined the pituitary-thyroid axis in rats administered polybrominated biphenyl (PBB) congeners and described the pituitary changes as those resulting from severe hyper-stimulation, that is, the chromophobes were swollen and vacuolated, with a marked foamy appearance of the cytoplalsm. Increased concentrations of pituitary TSH and lowered concentrations of serum thyroid hormones in PBB-treated rats supported the view that histopathologic changes in exposed rats were the result of hyperstimulation of the pituitary, due to a loss of negative feedback influence from thyroxine and triiodothyronine (Allen-Rowlands *et al.*, 1981).

Since there is no specific target organ for GH, secretion of this pituitary hormone is less readily manipulated experimentally than other pituitary hormones whose production and secretion is regulated within well-defined negative feedback loops. However, somatotroph lysosomes with recognizable secretory granules are sometimes increased in animals a few days after thyroidectomy or adrenalectomy (Gopinath *et al.*, 1987). Fur-thermore, diffuse hypertrophy of GH producing hypophyseal cells have been described in dogs treated with oestrogen, progesterone or combina-tions of these sex steroids (El Etreby *et al.*, 1979; El Etreby, 1981). However, since GH is often co-localized with PRL in 'somato-lac-totrophs', it is difficult to unequivocally discern the effects of the steroids on the PRL phenotype as distinct from GH phenotype.

Castration or exposure to compounds that cause gonadal atrophy and concomittant defects in gonadal hormone production will cause histopathological changes in adenohypophyseal gonadotrophs. Due to release of negative feedback influence, hypothalamic hypophysiotrophic factors hyperstimulate the pituitary, causing 'castration cells' which are vacuolated and assume a typical 'signet-ring' appearance (Gopinath *et al.*, 1987).

Corticotrophs are under negative feedback control from hormones produced and secreted by the adrenal cortex. However, changes in pituitary corticotrophs attributable to xenobiotics are rarely encountered in routine toxicity studies.

Loss of negative feedback following 'endocrinectomy' is often a cause of abnormal pituitary changes in rodents. However, loss of target organ feedback does not seem to be very important in the great majority of human adenomas. Although pituitary enlargement is commonly observed clinically in patients with chronic hypothyroidism, tumours rarely develop (Samaan *et al.*, 1977). Similarly, the occurrence of gonadotrophin-secreting tumours in gonadally deficient humans is a relatively rare occurrence. Adrenocorticotroph adenomas may grow aggressively after adrenalectomy and subsequent loss of feedback inhibition on ACTH secretion in patients with Cushing's disease. However, in such patients, the tumour is present before perturbation of feedback relationships. Thus, in humans, defects responsible for development and/ or maintenance of most pituitary hormone-secreting tumours appear to act directly upon the pituitary or by altering hypothalamic influence on the gland.

## Pituitary toxicity following altered hypothalamic function

Since virtually all adenohypophyseal cell types are influenced by regulatory factors from the hypothalamus, toxicant-mediated hypothalamic dysfunction has the potential to promote pituitary tumour growth and/or altered pituitary activity (Krieger, 1978; Krieger, 1980b). In most cases the toxic agent would be expected to enhance secretion of trophic factors, causing hypertrophy, hyperplasia and perhaps adenoma formation. However, for lactotrophs, toxic perturbations of the brain that reduce or eliminate the inhibitory influence of dopamine upon the pituitary provide an environment favouring the development of PRL secreting tumours.

### Pathological conditions
Certain disease states provide examples that resemble the toxic effects of certain compounds upon the pituitary via a hypothalamic locus of toxicity. For example, in acromegaly, hypothalamic control mechanisms for GH release are qualitatively and quantitatively abnormal (Reichlin & Moltich, 1984) resulting in 'paradoxical' increases in GH release follow-

ing glucose loading, loss of sleep-related GH release, decreased rather than increased release of GH in response to dopamine agonists, and GH release in response to thyroid hormone releasing hormone (TRH; Lawrence, Goldfine & Kirsteins, 1970; Maeda, 1976; Hanew *et al.*, 1977; Besser, Wass & Thorner, 1978; Tolis, Koutsilieris & Bertrand, 1984). These abnormal changes in pituitary function do not appear to be intrinsic defects, since surgical correction of the excessive GHRH secretion also reversed the paradoxical responses (Tolis *et al.*, 1984). Relevant is the finding that in some of these patients, pituitary cell hyperplasia and adenomas were present, suggesting that prolonged stimulation of the somatotrophs by GHRH induced tumours of GH secreting cells. Thus, these examples from disease states suggest that drugs or chemicals with side effects including enhanced GHRH secretion from hypothalamic or ectopic loci (peripheral tumours) may indirectly cause pituitary toxicity.

Similarly ACTH hypersecretion, characteristic of Cushing's disease can be caused by excessive secretion of hypothalamic corticotropin releasing hormone (CRH) from hypothalamic or ectopic loci (Belsky *et al.*, 1985; Martin & Reichlin, 1987). Between 40–64% of Cushingoid patients with inappropriate elevation of ACTH secretion have pituitary adenomas as determined by radiologic or histologic examination (Plotz, Knowlton & Ragan, 1952; Burke & Beardwell, 1973).

Prolactin-secreting tumours may arise through a toxic insult causing defects in hypothalamic catecholamine secretion (Van Loon, 1978), or through possible alterations in regional vascular perfusion of the pituitary resulting in reduced local concentrations of dopamine (Elias & Weiner, 1984).

### Individual drugs and chemicals

TCDD produces a wasting syndrome that is characteristic of its toxicity in all species studies (Harris *et al.*, 1973; Kociba *et al.*, 1976; Gasiewicz & Neal, 1979; Seefeld, Albrecht & Peterson, 1979). Because PRL has been shown to be an important developmental and immunomodulatory hormone, circadian alterations in serum PRL, as well as the activity of ornithine decarboxylase, a physiological marker for changes in PRL receptor-mediated coupling, were studied in TCDD-treated rats (Jones *et al.*, 1987). Disturbances in PRL circadian rhythmicity associated with altered activity of the thyroid and adrenal glands were observed in TCDD-treated rats. Changes in thyroid and adrenal gland function were attributed to altered PRL which is reported to modulate function of the peripheral endocrine glands. In support of this hypothesis, PRL-stimulated ornithine decarboxylase activity was significantly reduced in adrenal tissue from TCDD-treated rats. Thus, TCDD-mediated changes in PRL release may subserve certain aspects of pituitary toxicity underlying growth retardation attributed to the insecticide. The data from this study were not sufficient to determine a locus of toxicity, but in a subsequent study a hypothalamic site of action for TCDD was identified (Russell *et al.*, 1988). When TCDD was administered to rats, serum PRL concentrations were significantly reduced. This effect was reversed by pimozide, a dopamine antagonist, suggesting that TCDD decreased PRL release by a dopaminergic action upon the pituitary, or by reducing the amount of dopamine released from the hypothalamus. When TCDD was incubated with rat pituitaries *in vitro*, PRL release was not reduced, supporting a hypothalamic locus of toxicity for TCDD.

Degranulation of thyrotrophs and reduced pituitary TSH content indicative of hypostimulation was observed in pyridoxine-deficient rats (Dakshinamurti, Paulose & Vriend, 1986). In that study, reduced hypothalamic serotonin levels were associated with pyridoxine deficiency, suggesting a diencephalic locus of toxicity for the pituitary lesion.

Similarly, the anti-hypertensive agent losulazine, produced reproductive dysfunction in female rats by increasing serum PRL (Mesfin *et al.*, 1987). The hyperprolactinemia and reproductive dysfunction caused by losulazine were reversed by bromocriptine, a dopamine agonist. Since hypothalamic catecholamines were depleted by losulazine, the data suggest that the drug had a hypothalamic locus of toxicity which altered the release of pituitary prolactin and subsequently caused reproductive dysfunction. This view is consistent with the occurrence of proliferative adenohypophyseal lesions involving lactotrophs in animals treated with neuroleptics of the phenothiazine or butyrophenone type, which are dopamine antagonists (Horowski & Graf, 1979).

### Oestrogen effects

Pituitary toxicity is sometimes expressed clinically at a peripheral site as in renal carcinoma, induced by prolonged administration of oestrogen to male hamsters (Kirkman, 1959). Hamilton *et al.* (1977) suggested that this effect is mediated by the pituitary gland through secretion of melanocyte stimulating hormone (MSH), because the pars intermedia in hamsters with renal carcinoma had hyperplastic and neoplastic changes. In a subsequent study, Saluja *et al.* (1979) demonstrated that the onset of pituitary enlargement and serum MSH elevation in hamsters administered DES coincided with the appearance of renal tumours, suggesting the possibility that hypersecretion of MSH was involved in renal carcinogenesis.

Another case in which pituitary toxicity was expressed clinically at a different site involved mammary cancer resulting from exposure to 7,12-

dimethylbenz(a)anthracene (DMBA). Growth of mammary tumours induced by exposure of rats to DMBA was retarded and in some cases, the tumours disappeared following treatments that reduced PRL hypersecretion by the pituitary. To the contrary, tumour growth was accelerated by drugs that enhanced PRL secretion. Thus, administration of dopaminergic compounds such as ergot drugs, iproniazid, l-dopa or pargyline decreased DMBA-induced mammary tumours, while bilateral lesions of the median eminence, or administration of haloperidol, reserpine, methyldopa or oestrogens increased them (Klaiber *et al.*, 1969; Quadri, Clark & Meites, 1973; Quadri, Kledzik & Meites, 1973, 1974).

Oestrogenic compounds support the induction and growth of DMBA-mammary tumours in large part by stimulating PRL secretion from the pituitary. This view is supported by the absence of oestrogenic effects on mammary tumours in hypophysectomized animals (Meites, 1972). Thus, oestrogenic compounds have the potential for pituitary toxicity and may promote tumour formation and/or pituitary dysfunction. For example, DES and other potent oestrogens induced PRL-secreting pituitary tumours in ovariectomized Fischer 344/N rats (Wiklund *et al.*, 1981). Similarly, cyclic siloxanes such as $2,6$-cis-$[(PhMeSiO)_2(Me_2SiO)_2]$ exhibited oestrogen-like activity and were reported to cause pituitary enlargement with increased concentrations of pituitary PRL, LH and FSH (Le Vier & Jankowiak, 1972; Bulger & Kupfer, 1985). However, the tumourigenic effect is not expressed for all compounds with oestrogenic actions, since in contrast to DES, chlordecone, did not trigger development or adenohypophyseal prolactinomas when administered to rats for eight weeks (Mastri & Lucier, 1985). On the other hand, chlordecone, like DES, effectively inhibited pituitary secretion of FSH and LH.

### Monoamines

In some cases, pituitary toxicity of xenobiotics is enhanced by other substances through additive or synergistic actions. These effects may occur at the pituitary level. For example, the serotonin content of pituitaries from aged, female rats in constant oestrus (an oestrogenic condition) was significantly higher than aged females that were ovariectomized or from young females (Table 3.2, Walker & Cooper, 1985). The relevance of this finding is the fact that ovariectomy reduces the incidence of spontaneous pituitary tumours in ageing rats, and that serum oestrogen concentrations increase with age in rats with constant oestrus. Since oestrogen exposure increases the development of pituitary tumours in certain rat strains, it was of interest to determine if serotonin contributes to this phenomenon. To test this hypothesis, zimelidine or quipazine, serotonin receptor agonists were administered alone or in combination

Table 3.2. *Anterior pituitary 5-HT content in rats of different age and reproductive status*

| Group | N | Anterior pituitary weight (mg ± SEM) | Anterior pituitary 5-HT (pg + SEM) | |
|---|---|---|---|---|
| | | | Content | Concentration |
| Young | | | | |
| Estrus | 9 | 14.3 ± 0.77 | 1973 ± 410 | 136.7 ± 28 |
| Diestrus | 6 | 13.5 ± 0.89 | 1710 ± 349 | 126.5 ± 25 |
| Middle-aged | | | | |
| Diestrus | 6 | 14.1 ± 0.95 | 2323 ± 386 | 164.8 ± 27 |
| Constant Estrus | 7 | 17.8 ± 1.14* | 3394 ± 840† | 190.6 ± 47 |

*Pituitaries significantly ($p<0.05$) heavier than all other groups.
†Pituitary serotonin content significantly ($p<0.05$) greater than two young groups.
(From Walker & Cooper, 1985.)

with oestrogen to determine the tumourogenic potential of serotonin in the pituitary. Prolonged stimulation of serotonin receptors by quipazine or zimelidine accelerated the hypertrophic effect of oestrogen on the pituitary. Larger pituitaries and more macroadenomas occurred in rats administered oestrogen in combination with the serotonin receptor agonists than in rats treated with oestrogen alone (Table 3.3, Walker & Cooper, 1985). Treatment with zimelidine or quipazine alone did not cause pituitary hypertrophy, suggesting that the tumourogenic effect of the serotonin receptor agonists were complementary to, not independent of stimulation by oestrogen. It is possible that the effect of serotonin may also be mediated by other compounds, since corticoids, administered in addition to oestrogen have a synergistic effect on pituitary hyperstimulation (El Etreby *et al.*, 1979), and serotonin stimulates the release of glucocoticoids in rats. Synergisms between xenobiotics that cause pituitary toxicity may be clinically relevant, since the hyperstimulatory effect of oestrogens on PRL release in women taking oral contraceptives was exacerbated by phenothiazines, compounds that alter the release of neurotransmitters including serotonin (Buckman & Peake, 1973). In contrast to the effects of serotonin, maintenance of catecholamine tone throughout life is antagonistic to the spontaneous development of pituitary tumours. For example, age-associated decay of central nervous system dopamine function which contributes to hyperprolactinemia, and perhaps lactotroph tumourigenesis, is delayed by dietary restriction

Table 3.3. *Effects of 5-HT receptor agonists and oestrogen on pituitary hypertrophy and tumourigenesis in 4-month-old, ovariectomized rats*

| Treatment | N | Pituitary weight (mg ± SEM) | Number of rats with macroadenomas |
|---|---|---|---|
| OVX* | 4 | 12.0 ± 0.82† | 0 |
| Oestrogen | 5 | 36.6 ± 3.95 | 0 |
| Oestrogen + PCPA | 6 | 32.2 ± 2.87 | 0 |
| Oestrogen + 5-HTP | 7 | 38.4 ± 3.54 | 0 |
| Oestrogen + Zimelidine | 7 | 78.6 ± 18.00‡ | 3 |
| Oestrogen + Quipazine | 5 | 53.2 ± 13.60 | 1 |
| Zimelidine* | 4 | 14.2 ± 0.71† | 0 |
| Quipazine* | 4 | 12.6 ± 0.69† | 0 |

*Animals had empty Silastic capsules implanted subcutaneously.
†The pituitary weight of these three groups was significantly smaller ($p < 0.05$) than those groups receiving oestrogen implants.
‡Significantly larger ($p < 0.05$) than all other groups except oestrogen + Quipazine.
(From Walker & Cooper, 1985.)

(Atterwill *et al.*, 1989). In a more direct test, the catecholaminergic drug ibopamine (N-methyl dopamine, 0,0'-diisobutyroyl ester HCl) was administered orally to rats for two years (Walker *et al.*, 1987). The incidence of benign, malignant and multiple neoplasmas was reduced in ibopamine-treated rats (Table 3.4). Six neoplastic lesions including pituitary adenomas, and five non-neoplastic lesions were significantly reduced in a dose-related fashion. Since ibopamine is dopaminergic, its anti-tumourigenic effect was undoubtedly mediated in part, by a direct effect upon lactotrophs to inhibit hypersecretion of PRL. However, the additional palliative effects on lesions not associated with hypersecretion of prolactin, for example, adrenal cortical adenoma, suggest that ibopamine also had a hypothalamic influence to reduce hyperstimulation of the pituitary by other trophic factors such as ACTH-releasing hormone.

## Genetic factors

Although relatively rare, certain family pedigrees predispose their members to the development of pituitary neoplasms. For example, genetic or familial hyperparathyroidism, pancreatic islet-cell tumours, tumours of the adrenal cortex and thyroid, carcinoids, renal cortical tumours and

Table 3.4. *Effect of ibopamine on the incidence of neoplasms in rats*

| | Incidence (% of animals) | | | |
| | Male | | Female | |
| | Control | Ibopamine* | Control | Ibopamine* |
|---|---|---|---|---|
| Number of Animals | 200 | 100 | 200 | 100 |
| Neoplasms | 88 | 76‡ | 97 | 86‡ |
| Benign Neoplasms | 80 | 63‡ | 96 | 83‡ |
| Malignant Neoplasms | 53 | 33‡ | 39 | 25‡ |
| Multiple Neoplasms | 62 | 34‡ | 75 | 48‡ |

*Ibopamine was administered in doses of 180 mg/kg/day.
†Comparison with control group is statistically significant ($p<0.01$).
‡Comparison with control group is statistically significant ($p<0.001$).
(From Walker *et al.*, 1987.)

lipomas, inherited as an autosomal dominant, is associated in some pedigrees, up to 65% with concomittant pituitary tumours (Baylin, 1978; Vandewegh *et al.*, 1978; Delellis & Wolfe, 1979). Evidence for genetic predisposition of pituitary tumours in animal models derives from the fact that the incidence of these pathological changes are higher in certain strains of mice than others. Genetic disposition for the spontaneous development of pituitary tumours has been deduced from their considerable variation in frequency rate in the various strains that have been studied (El Etreby *et al.*, 1979). Prolonged administration of high doses of oestrogen will induce pituitary tumours in mice but only in genetically susceptible strains (Gardner & Strong, 1940; Furth & Clifton, 1966). In rats, DES induced PRL-secreting pituitary tumours in ovariectomized Fischer 344/N rats but not in Holtzman rats (Wiklund, Wertz & Gorski, 1981). The implications for hormonal expression of a genetic predisposition to pituitary tumours, led to the evaluation of different contraceptives for carcinogenic activity by dietary administration to mice and rats for 80 and 104 weeks, respectively, in doses ranging from 2 to 400 times the human contraceptive dose. The results of that study suggested that high doses of certain steroids and their combinations may stimulate the development of pituitary tumours, especially in mice (El Etreby *et al.*, 1979). Although studies ranking the exact sensitivity of different strains of laboratory animals to xenobiotic induction of pituitary tumours is lacking, the genetic predisposition for certain types has been demonstrated and should be recognized as a risk factor for xenobiotic-induced pituitary toxicity.

## Conclusion

The purpose of this overview is to provide a summary of adverse effects of xenobiotics upon the pituitary, an endocrine gland that has not heretofore been examined in review format, as a specific target tissue of toxicity. Drugs and chemicals infrequently accumulate in the pituitary, hence, necrotic, degenerative and regenerative changes (seen typically in the liver or kidney) are rarely encountered. The most common histopathological pituitary lesion is hyperplasia, sometimes associated with adenoma, that generally results from perturbation of homeostatic balance within neuroendocrine axes where the pituitary occupies a central position. While these changes can result from a direct pituitary action, they often occur indirectly following loss of negative feedback control and/or increased presentation of hypophysiotrophic factors that stimulate specific cell types within the pituitary. Thus, while morphological changes within the pituitary could produce clinically relevant signs of toxicity resulting from compression of the hypothalmus or optic chiasm, pituitary toxicity is more often clinically indicated by physiological disturbances that vary from changes in body temperature regulation to mammary tumours. It was in recognition of that diversity, that we have attempted to provide a thread of continuity to those interested in endocrine toxicology, and specifically to put into perspective the pituitary as a target tissue.

## References

Afrasiabi, A., Valenta, L. & Gwinup, G. (1979). A TSH-secreting pituitary tumour causing hyperthyroidism: Presentation of a case and review of the literature. *Acta Endocrinol.* **72**, 448–60.

Akoso, B.T., Sleight, S.D., Nachreiner, R.F. & Aust, S.D. (1982). Effects of purified polybrominated biphenyl congeners on the thyroid and pituitary glands in rats. *J. Amer. Coll. Toxicol.*, **1**, 23–6.

Allen-Rowlands, C.F., Castracane, V.D., Hamilton, M.G. & Seifter, J. (1981). Effect of polybrominated biphenyls (PBB) on the pituitary-thyroid axis of the rat. *Proc. Soc. Exp. Biol. Med.*, **166**, 500–14.

Atterwill, C.K., Brown, C.G., Conybeare, G., Holland, C.W. & Jones, C.A. (1989). Relation between dopaminergic control of pituitary lactotroph function and deceleration of age-related changes in serum prolactin of diet-restricted rats. *Fd. Chem. Toxic.*, **27**, 97–103.

Bajt, M.L. & Aggarwal, S.K. (1985). An analysis of factors responsible for resorption of embryos in cisplatin-treated rats. *Toxicol. Appl. Pharmacol.*, **80**, 97–107.

Bastomsky, C.H. (1977). Enhanced thyroxine metabolism and high uptake goiters in rats after a single dose of 2,3,7,8-tetrachlorodibenzo-p-dioxin. *Endocrinology* **1001**, 292–6.

Baylin, S.B. (1978). The multiple endocrine neoplasia syndromes: implications for the study of inherited tumors. *Semin. Oncol.*, **5**, 35–45.

Belsky, J.L., Cuello, B., Swanson, L.W., Simmons, D.M., Jarrett, R.M. & Braza, F. (1985). Cushing's syndrome due to ectopic production of corticotropin-releasing factor. *J. Clin. Endocrinol. Metab.*, **60**, 496–500.

Besser, G.M., Wass, J.A.H. & Thorner, M.O. (1978). Acromegaly – results of long term treatment with bromocriptine. *Acta Endocrinol.*, **88**, (Suppl) 1897–198.

Buckmann, M.T. & Peake, G.T. (1973). Estrogen potentiation of phenothiazine-induced prolactin secretion in man. *J. Clin. Endocrinol. Metab.*, **37**, 977–821.

Bulger, W.H. & Kupfer, D. (1985). Estrogenic activity of pesticides and other xenobiotics on the uterus and male reproductive tract. In *Endocrine Toxicology*, ed. J.A. Thomas, K.S. Korach & J.A. MclLachlan, pp. 1–33. New York: Raven Press.

Burke, C.W. & Beardwell, C.G. (1973). Cushing's syndrome. An evaluation of the clinical usefulness of urinary free cortisol and other urinary steroid measurements in diagnosis. *Q. J. Med.*, **42**, 175–204.

Burrow, G.N., Wortzman, G., Rewcastle, N.B., Holgate, P.C. & Kovacs, K. (1981). Microadenomas of the pituitary and abnormal sellar tomograms in an unselected autopsy series. *N. Engl. J. Med.*, **304**, 156–8.

Camoratto, A.M., White, L.M., Lau, Y.S. & Moriarty, C.M. (1990). Inhibition of rat pituitary growth hormone release by subclinical levels of lead. *Toxicologist*, **10**, 641.

Capen, C.C. (1983). Functional pathological interrelationships of the pituitary gland and the hypothalamus. In *The Endocrine System. Monographs on Pathology of Laboratory Animals*, ed. T.C. Jones, U. Mohr & R.D. Hunt, pp. 101–20. Heidelberg: Springer-Verlag.

Clary, J.J. (1979). Nickel chloride-induced metabolic changes in the rat and guinea pig. *Toxicol. Appl. Pharmacol.*, **31**, 55–65.

Clemons, G. & Garcia, J.F. (1981). Neuroendocrine effects of acute nickel chloride administration in rats. *Toxicol. Appl. Pharmacol.*, **61**, 3343–8.

Collins, W.T., Capen, C.C., Kasza, L., Carter, C. & Daily, R.E. (1977). Effect of polychlorinated biphenyl (PCB) on the thyroid gland: ultrastructural and biochemical investigations. *Amer. J. Pathol.*, **89**, 119–36.

Cooper, R.L. (1983). Pharmacological and dietary manipulations of reproductive aging in the rat: Significance to central nervous system aging. In *Clinical and Experimental Interventions In Aging*, ed. R.F. Walker & R.L. Cooper, pp. 27–44. New York: Marcel Dekker.

Cooper, R.L., Chadwick, R.W., Rehnberg, G.L., Goldman, M., Booth, K.C., Hein, J.F. & McElroy, W.K. (1989). Effect of lindane on hormonal control of reproductive function in the female rat. *Toxicol. Appl. Pharmacol.*, **99**, 384–94.

Cooper, R.L., Goldman, J.M., Gray, L.E., Lyles, K.W. & Ellison, D.L. (1985). Assessment of pituitary function. *Toxicologist*, **5**, 182.

Cooper, R.L., Goldman, J.M., Rehnberg, G.L., McElroy, W.K. & Hein, J.F. (1987). Effects of metal cations on pituitary hormone secretion in vitro. *J. Biochem. Toxicol.*, **2**, 241–9.

Costello, R.T. (1936). Subclinical adenomas of the pituitary gland. *Am. J. Pathol.*, **12**, 205–16.

Dada, M.O., Campbell, G.T. & Blake, C.A. (1984). Pars distalis cell quantification in normal adult male and female rats. *J. Endocrinol.*, **101**, 87–94.

Dakshinamurti, K., Paulose, C.S. & Vriend, J. (1986). Hypothyroidism of hypothalamic origin in pyridoxine-deficient rats. *J. Endocrinol.*, **109**, 345–9.

Dawson, B.H. & P. Kothandaram. (1972). Actue massive infarction of pituitary adenomas. *J. Neurosurg.*, **37**, 275.

Delellis, R.A. & Wolfe, H.J. (1979). Multiple endocrine adenomatosis syndromes: Origins and inter-relationships. In *Cancer Medicine*, 2nd edn, pp. 00–00, ed. J. Holland & E. Frei. Philadelphia: Lea and Febiger.

Doniach, I. & Walker, A.H.C. (1946). Combined anterior pituitary necrosis and bilateral corticol necrosis of kidneys following concealed accidental hemorrhage. *J. Obstet. Gynecol. Br. Emp.*, **53**, 140.

El Etreby, M.F. (1981). Practical applications of immunocytochemistry of the pharmacology and toxicology of the endocrine system. *Histochem. J.*, **13**, 821–37.

El Etreby, M.F., Graf, K.J., Gunzel, P. & Neumann, F. (1979). Evaluation of effects of sexual steroids on the hypothalamic-pituitary system of animals and man. In *Mechanisms of Toxic Actions on Some Target Organs*, ed. P.L. Chambers & P. Gunzel, pp. 11–39. Arch. Toxicol. (Suppl. 2). New York: Springer-Verlag.

Elias, K.A. & Weiner, R.I. (1984). Direct arterial vascularization of estrogen-induced prolactin-secreting anterior pituitary tumors. *Proc. Natl. Acad. Sci. (USA)*, **81**, 4549–53.

Evarts, R.P. & Brown, C.A. (1981). 2,4-diaminoanisole-induced thyroid pigmentation in rats inhibited by m-phenylene-diamine. *Toxicol. Lett.*, **8**, 257–64.

Farquahar, M.G. (1969). Lysosome function in regulating secretion: disposal of secretory granules in cells of the anterior pituitary gland. In *Lysosomes in Biology and Pathology*, ed. J.T. Dingle & H.B. Fell, pp. 462–82. North Holland, Amsterdam.

Furth, J. & Clifton, K.H. (1966). Experimental pituitary tumors. In *The Pituitary Gland*, ed. G.W. Harris & B.T. Donovan, pp. 460–97. London: Buttersworth.

Gardner, W.U. & Strong, L.C. (1940). Strain-limited development of tumors of the pituitary gland in mice receiving estrogens. *Yale J. Biol. Med.*, **12**, 543–8.

Gasiewicz, T.A. & Neal, R.A. (1979). TCDD: tissue distribution, excretion and effects on clinical chemical parameters in guinea pigs. *Toxicol. Appl. Pharmacol.*, **51**, 329–39.

Gray, L.E., Jr., Ferrell, J., Ostby, J., Gray, K., Rehnberg, G., Linder, R., Cooper, R., Goldman, J., Slott, V. & Laskey, J. (1989). A dose response analysis of methoxychlor-induced alteration of reproductive development and function in the rat. *Fund. Appl. Toxicol.*, **12**, 92–108.

Gooren, L.J.G., Harmsen-Louman, W. & van Keswsel, H. (1984). Somatostatin inhibits prolactin release from the lactotrophs primed with oestrogen and cyproterone acetate in man. *J. Endocrinol.*, **103**, 333–5.

Gopinath, C., Prentice, D.E. & Lewis, D.J. (1987). *Atlas of Experimental Toxicological Pathology*, vol. 13, pp. 104–21. Boston: MTP Press.

Hamilton, J.M., Sluja, P.G., Thody, A.J. & Flaks, A. (1977). The pars intermedia and renal carcinogenesis in hamsters. *Euro. J. Cancer*, **13**, 29–32.

Hanew, K., Aida, M., Tano, T. & Yoshinaga, K. (1977). Abnormal growth hormone responses to L-Dopa and thyrotropin releasing hormone in patients with acromegaly. *Tohoku J. Exp. Med.* **121**, 197–206.

Harlin, R.S. & Givens, J.R. (1968). Sheehan's syndrome associated with eclampsia and small sella turcica. *South Med. J.*, **61**, 900.

Harris, M.W., Moore, J.G., Vos, J.G. & Gupta, B.N. (1973). General biological effects of TCDD in laboratory animals. *Environ. Health. Perspect.*, **5**, 101–9.

Horowski, R. & Graf, K.J. (1979). Neuroendocrine effects of neuropsychotrophic drugs and their possible influence on toxic reactions in animals and man – the role of dopamine-prolactin system. *Arch. Toxicol.*, Suppl. 2, 93–104.

Huang, E.S.-R. & Nelson, F.R. (1986). Anti-estrogenic action of chlordecone in rat pituitary gonadotrophs *in vitro*. *Toxicol. Appl. Pharmacol.*, **82**, 62–9.

Hudson, P.M., Yoshikawa, K., Fatehyab Ali, S., Lamb, J.C., Reel, J.R. & Hong, J.-S. (1984). Estrogen-like activity of chlordecone (kepone) on the hypothalamo-pituitary axis: effects on the pituitary enkephalin system. *Toxicol. Appl. Pharmacol.*, **74**, 383–9.

Japundzic, M.M. (1969). The goitrogenic effect of phenobarbital-Na on the rat thyroid. *Acta Anat.* **74**, 88–96.

Jones, C.A., Brown, C.G., Dickens, T.A. & Atterwill, C.K. (1988). Differential effects of D- and L-isomers of triiodothyronine on pituitary TSH: secretion and peripheral deiodinase activity in the rat. *Toxicology*, **48**, 273–84.

Jones, M.K., Weisenburger, W.P., Sipes, I.G. & Russell, D.H. (1987).

Circadian alterations in prolactin, corticosterone, and thyroid hormone levels and down-regulation of prolactin receptor activity by 2,3,7,8-tetrachlorodibenzo-p-dioxin. *Toxicol. Appl. Pharmacol.*, **87**, 337–50.

Judd, A.M., MacLeod, R.M. & Login, I.S. (1984). Zinc acutely, selectively and reversibly inhibits pituitary prolactin secretion. *Brain Res.*, **294**, 190–2.

Kociba, R.J., Keeler, P.A., Park, C.N. & Gehring, P.J. (1976). 2,3,7,8-tetrachlorodibenzo-p-dioxin (TCDD): Results of a 13 week oral toxicity study in rats. *Toxicol. Appl. Pharmacol.*, **35**, 553–74.

Kovacs, K., Carroll, R. & Tapp, E. (1966). The pathogenesis of hexadimethrine necrosis of the pituitary and adrenal. *Arzneim.-Forsch.*, **16**, 516–19.

Kovacs, K., Horwath, E., Ilse, G., Ezrin, C. & Ilze, D. (1977). Spontaneous pituitary adenomas in aging rats. *Bietrage zur Pathologie*, **161**, 1–16.

Kirkman, H. (1959). Estrogen-induced tumours of the kidney in the Syrian hamster. *Natl. Cancer Inst. Monogr.*, **1**, 1–139.

Klaiber, M.S., Gruenstin, M., Meranze, D.R. & Shimkin, M.B. (1969). Influence of hypothalamic lesions on the induction and growth of mammary cancers in Sprague-Dawley rats receiving 7,12-dimethylbenz(a)anthracene. *Canc. Res.*, **29**, 999–1001.

Krajnc, E.I., Wester, P.W., Loeber, J.G., van Leeuwen, F.X.R., Vos, J.G., Vaessen, H.A.M.G. & van der Jeijden, C.A. (1984). Toxicity of bis(tri-n-butyltin)oxide in the rat. *Toxicol. Appl. Pharmacol.*, **75**, 363–86.

Krieger, D.T. (1978). The central nervous system and Cushing's disease. *Med. Clin. North Am.*, **62**, 268–85.

Krieger, D.T. (1980a). The hypothalamus and neuroendocrine pathology. In *Neuroendocrinology*, ed. D.T. Krieger & J.C. Hughes, pp. 13–22. Sunderland, MA: Sinauer Associates, Inc.

Krieger, H.P. (1980b). Sellar and juxtasellar disease: A neurologic viewpoint. In *Neuroendocrinology*, ed. D.T. Krieger & J.C. Hughes, pp. 275–83. Sunderland, MA: Sinauer Associates, Inc.

Kroes, R., Gabris-Berkvens, J.M., de Vries, T. & van Nesselrooy, J.H.J. (1981). Histopathological profiles of Wistar rat stock including a survey of the literature. *J. Gerontol.*, **36**, 259–79.

LaBella, F.S., Dular, R., Lemons, P., Vivian, S. & Wueen, M. (1973). Prolactin secretion is specifically inhibited by nickel. *Nature*, **245**, 330–2.

Lawrence, A.M., Goldfine, I.D. & Kirsteins, L. (1970). Growth hormone dynamics in acromegaly. *J. Clin. Endocrinol. Metab.*, **31**, 239–47.

LeVier, R.R. and Jankowiak, M.E. (1972). Effects of oral 2,6-cis-diphenylhexamethylcyclotetrasiloxane on the reproductive system of the male rat. *Toxicol. Appl. Pharmacol.*, **21**, 80–8.

Lijinsy W. & Reuber, M.D. (1983). Chronic toxicity studies of vinyl acetate in Fischer rats. *Toxicol. Appl. Pharmacol.*, **68**, 43–53.

Lloyd, R.V. (1983). Estrogen-induced hyperplasia and neoplasia in the rat anterior pituitary gland. *Am. J. Pathol.*, **113**, 198–206.

Locke, S. & H.R. Tyler. (1961). Pituitary apoplexy. *Am. J. Med.*, **30**, 643.

Lorenson, M.Y., Robson, D.L. & Jacobs, L.S. (1983a). Detectability of pituitary PRL and GH by immunoassay is increased by thiols and suppressed by divalent cations. *Endocrinology*, **112**, 1880–2.

Lorenson, M.Y., Robson, D.L. & Jacobs, L.S. (1983b). Divalent cation inhibition of hormone release from isolated adenohypophyseal secretory granules. *J. Biol. Chem.*, **258**, 8618–2.

Maeda, K. (1976). Critical review: effects of thyrotropin releasing hormone on growth hormone release in normal subjects and in patients with depression, anorexia nervosa and acromegaly. *Kobe J. Med. Sci.*, **22**, 263–70.

Martin, J.B. & Reichlin, S. (1987). *Clinical Neuroendocrinology*, pp. 423–44. Philadelphia: F.A. Davis, Co.

Mastri, C. & Lucier, G. (1985). Actions of hormonally active chemicals in the liver. In *Endocrine Toxicology*, ed. J.A. Thomas, K.S. Korach & J.A. McLachlan, pp. 335–92. New York: Raven Press.

McComb, D.J., Ryan, N., Horvath, E. & K. Kovacs. (1983). Subclinical adenomas of the human pituitary: new light on old problems. *Arch. Pathol. Lab. Med.*, **107**, 488–91.

McCormick, W.F. & Halmi, N.S. (1971). Absence of chromophobe adenomas from a large series of pituitary tumors. *Arch. Pathol.*, **92**, 231–8.

Meites, J. (1972). Relation of prolactin and estrogen to mammary tumorigenesis in the rat. *J. Natl. Cancer Inst.*, **48**, 1217–24.

Meites, J. & Nicoll, C.S. (1966). Adenohypophysis prolactin. *Annual Rev. Physiol.*, **28**, 57–88.

Murdoch, R. (1962). Sheehan's syndrome. Survey of 57 cases since 1950. *Lancet*, **1**, 1327.

Mesfin, G.M., Johnson, G.A., Higgins, M.J. & Morris, D.F. (1987). Mechanism of anestrus in rats treated with an antihypertensive agent, losulazine hydrochloride. *Toxicol. Appl. Pharmacol.*, **87**, 91–101.

Osamura, R.Y. & Takayama, S. (1983). Histochemical identification of hormones in pituitary tumors, rat. In *Endocrine System. Monographs on Pathology of Laboratory Animals*, ed. T.C. Jones, U. Mohr & R.D. Hunt, pp. 130–4. Berlin: Springer-Verlag.

Parker, K. & Sunderman, F.W. (1974). Distribution of $^{63}$Ni in rabbit tissues following intravenous injections of $^{63}$NiCl$_2$. *Res. Commun. Chem. Pathol. Pharmacol.*, **7**, 755–62.

Pieters, G.F.F.M., Hermus, A.R.M.M., Smals, A.G.H. & Kloppenborg, P.W.C. (1984). Paradoxical responsiveness of growth hormone to corticotrophin-releasing factor in acromegaly. *J. Clin. Endocr. Metab.*, **58**, 560–2.

Plotz, C.M., Knowlton, A.I. & Ragan, C. (1952). Natural history of Cushing's syndrome. *Am. J. Med.*, **13**, 596–614.

Potter, C.L., Moore, R.W., Inhorn, S.L., Hagen, T.C. & Peterson, R.E. (1986). Thyroid status and thermogenesis in rats treated with 2,3,7,8-tetrachlorodibenzo-p-dioxin. *Toxicol. Appl. Pharm.*, **84**, 45–55.

Quadri, S.K., Clark, J.L. & Meites, J. (1973). Effects of LSD, pargyline and haloperidol on mammary tumor growth in rats. *Proc. Soc. exp. Biol Med.*, **142**, 22–6.

Quadri, S.K., Kledzik, G.S. & Meites, J. (1973). Effects of l-dopa and methyldopa on growth of mammary cancers in rats. *Proc. Soc. exp. Biol. Med.*, **142**, 759–61.

Quadri, S.K., Kledzik, G.S. & Meites, J. (1974). Enhanced regression of DMBA-induced mammary cancers in rats by combination of ergocornine with ovariectomy or high doses of estrogen. *Canc. Res.*, **34**, 499–501.

Reichlin, S. (1980). Etiology of pituitary adenomas. In *The Pituitary Adenoma*, ed. K.D. Post, I.M.D., Jackson & S. Reichlin, pp. 29–45. New York: Plenum Press.

Reichlin, S. & Moltich, M.E. (1984). Neuroendocrine aspects of pituitary adenoma. In *Pituitary Hyperfunction*, ed. F. Camanni & E.E. Muller, pp. 47–70. New York: Raven Press.

Russell, D.H., Buckley, A.R., Shah, G.N., Sipes, I.G., Blask, D.E. & Benson, B. (1988). Hypothalamic site of action of 2,3,7,8-tetrachlorodibenzo-p-dioxin (TCDD). *Toxicol. Appl. Pharmacol.*, **94**, 496–502.

Saluja, P.G., Hamilton, J.M., Thody, A.J., Ismail, A.A. & Knowles, J. (1979). Ultrastructure of intermediate lobe of the pituitary and melanocyte-stimulating hormone secretion in oestrogen-induced kidney tumours in male hamsters. In: *Mechanism of Toxic Action on Some Target Organs*, ed. P.L. Chambers & P. Gunzel, pp. 41–5, *Arch. Toxicol.* (Suppl. 2). New York: Springer-Verlag.

Samaan, N.A., Osborne, B.M., MacKay, B., Leavens, M.E., Duello, T.M. & Halmi, N.S. (1977). Endocrine and morphologic studies of pituitary adenomas secondary to primary hypothyroidism. *J. Clin. Endocrinol. Metab.*, **45**, 903–11.

Sanders, J.D., Eigenberg, D.A., Bracht, L.J., Wang, W.R. & vanZwieten, J.J. (1988). Thyroid and liver trophic changes in rats secondary to liver microsomal enzyme induction caused by an experimental leukotriene antagonist (L-649,923). *Toxicol. Appl. Pharmacol.*, **95**, 378–87.

Saunders, S.L., Reifel, C.W. & Shin, S.H. (1983). Ultrastructural changes rapidly induced by somatostatin may inhibit prolactin release in estrogen-primed rat adenohypophysis. *Cell Tiss. Res.*, **232**, 21–34.

Schamberger, T.J. (1983). Metabolism of selenium. In *Biochemistry of Selenium*, ed. E. Frieden, pp. 59–75. New York: Plenum Press.

Seefeld, M.D., Albrecht, R.M. & Peterson, R.E. (1979). Effects of TCDD on indocyanine green, blood clearance in rhesus monkeys. *Toxicology*, **14**, 263–72.

Smith, C.W., Jr. & Howard, R.P. (1959). Variations in endocrine gland function in postpartum pituitary necrosis. *J. Clin. Endocrinol.*, **19**, 1420.

Smith, J.C. & Hackley, B. (1968). Distribution and excretion of nickel 63 administered intravenously to rats. *J. Nutr.*, **95**, 541–6.

Taylor, A.L. (1968). Pituitary apoplexy in acromegaly. *J. Clin. Endocr.*, **28**, 1784.

Tepperman, J. & Tepperman, H.M. (1987). In *Metabolic and Endocrine Physiology*, 5th edn, pp. 57–94. Chicago: Year Book Medical Publishers, Inc.

Thomas, J.A., Thomas, M.J. & Thomas, D.J. (1989). Hormone assay and endocrine function. In *Principals and Methods of Toxicology*, 2nd edn, ed. A.W. Hays, pp. 677–98. New York: Raven Press.

Thorlacius-Ussing, O. & Danscher, G. (1985). Selenium in the anterior pituitary of rats exposed to sodium selenite: light and electron microscopic localization. *Toxicol. Appl. Pharmacol.*, **81**, 67–74.

Tolis, G., Bird, C. & Bertrand, G. (1978). Pituitary hyperthyroidism: case report and review of the literature. *Am. J. Med.*, **64**, 177–83.

Tolis, G., Koutsilieris, M. & Bertrand, G. (1984). Endocrine diagnosis of growth hormone secreting pituitary tumors. In *Secretory Tumors of the Pituitary Gland*, ed. P.M. Black, N.T. Zervas, E.C. Ridgway & J.B. Martin, pp. 145–54. New York: Raven Press.

Tsuda, H. (1983). Goiter, adenoma and carcinoma of the thyroid induced by amitrole and ethylenthiourea, rat. In *Endocrine System. Monographs on Pathology of Laboratory Animals*, ed. T.C. Jones, U. Mohr & R.D. Hunt, pp. 204–11. Berlin: Springer-Verlag.

Vandewegh, M., Braxel, K., Schutyser, J. & Vermuelen, A. (1978). A case of multiple endocrine adenomatosis with primary amenorrhea. *Postgrad. Med. J.*, **54**, 618–22.

Van Loon, G.R. (1978). A defect in catecholamine neurons in patients with prolactin-secreting pituitary adenoma. *Lancet*, **2**, 868–71.

Veldhuis, J.D. and Hammond, J.M. (1980). Endocrine function after spontaneous infarction of the human pituitary: Report, review and reappraisal. *Endo. Rev.*, **1**, 100.

Walker, R.F. & Cooper, R.L. (1985). Synergistic effects of estrogen and serotonin-receptor agonists on the development of pituitary tumors in aging rats. *Neurobiol. Aging*, **6**, 107–11.

Walker, R.F., Weideman, C.A. & Wheeldon, E.B. (1987). Reduced disease in aged rats treated chronically with Ibopamine, a catecholaminergic drug. *Neurobiol. Aging*, **9**, 291–301.

Wiklund, J., Wertz, N. & Gorski, J. (1981). A comparison of estrogen effects on uterine and pituitary growth and prolactin synthesis in F344 and Holtzman rats. *Endocrinology*, **109**, 1700–7.

JULIA C. BUCKINGHAM AND GLENDA E.
GILLIES

# 4  Hypothalamus and pituitary gland – xenobiotic induced toxicity and models for its investigation

The essential role of the hypothalamo-pituitary axis in the maintenance of homeostasis is well established. Unless carefully controlled, pituitary insufficiency invariably results in a spectrum of disorders of growth, development, metabolism and reproductive function as too does excessive or 'inappropriate' pituitary hormone release. Such conditions are normally the consequence of pathological lesions but they may also be induced iatrogenically. The present chapter aims to illustrate points within the complex mechanisms controlling hypothalamo-pituitary activity where drugs may produce their potentially hazardous actions and to outline methods whereby their effects may be identified and characterized.

## The hypothalamo-pituitary axis

### Anatomy and function of the pituitary gland

The pituitary gland is a small bilobed structure lying immediately below the median eminence area of the hypothalamus to which it is connected by the pituitary stalk. The two lobes are distinct anatomically and physiologically, having different embryological origins and separate control mechanisms (Everitt & Hokfelt, 1986). The anterior lobe or adenohypophysis is derived from ectodermal tissue of the oral epithelium and is differentiated into three distinct zones, the pars distalis, the pars intermedia and the pars tuberalis. Although the pars intermedia is sparsely innervated by fibres of hypothalamic origin, the adenohypophysis is largely devoid of nerve fibres. It is, however, linked to the hypothalamus by a highly specialized portal vascular system from which it receives the bulk of its blood supply. The posterior lobe (pars nervosa or neurohypophysis) by contrast is derived from neural tissues of the diencephalon and is essentially a down growth of the hypothalamus. It comprises the axons and terminals of neurosecretory cells, whose perikarya are located in the supraoptic and paraventricular nuclei of the hypothalamus, and modified glial cells – the pituicytes. Unlike the adenohypophysis, its blood supply is not derived primarily from the hypothalamus but from the posterior hypophysial arteries which form a capillary plexus in the gland into which the neurosecretory cells release their products.

The endocrine function of the adenohypophysis is contained primarily within the pars distalis which is responsible for the secretion of at least seven hormones of which the physiological functions are generally well understood. These include growth hormone (GH, normal growth and development), thyrotrophin (TSH, control of thyroid function), corticotrophin (ACTH, regulation of adrenocortical activity), β-lipotrophin (β-LPH)/β-endorphin (functions largely unknown but may include regulation of duodenal bicarbonate), prolactin (lactation), and the gonadotrophins, luteinizing hormone (LH) and follicle stimulating hormone (FSH; gonadal function). The pars intermedia (which is well developed in lower vertebrates and some mammals, but which in man regresses post-natally and is absent in adult) produces α-melanocyte stimulating hormone (α-MSH, camouflage/pigmentation and, possibly, regulation of the foetal adrenal) while the pars tuberalis appears to be devoid of endocrine activity. The majority of the adenohypophysial hormones are single-chain polypeptides but thyrotrophin and the two gonadotrophins each comprise two glycoprotein chains. Histological studies have revealed that GH, prolactin and thyrotrophin are each synthesized by separate, specific cell types. Corticotrophin and β-LPH/β-endorphin are derived from the same precursor molecule (pro-opiomelanocortin, POMC) and are thus co-released from the same cells (corticotrophs) while LH and FSH are both produced by gonadotrophs (Table 4.1)

The posterior pituitary gland is primarily responsible for the secretion of two neurohormones each of which is a nonapeptide: vasopressin, the antidiuretic hormone, is concerned with osmotic balance and the maintenance of blood pressure in, for example, haemorrhage, while oxytocin regulates uterine contractility and milk ejection (Table 4.1). The two peptides are produced by separate populations of hypothalamic neurosecretory cells and subject to independent control mechanisms.

## Biosynthesis and release of pituitary hormones

The pituitary hormones are formed from large precursor molecules termed pre-prohormones which undergo proteolytic cleavage and, sometimes, further modification (e.g. acetylation, glycosylation) to yield the active hormone (Mains et al., 1990). For example, ACTH and related peptides (β-LPH/β-endorphin) are formed in the corticotrophs from a

Table 4.1. *Pituitary hormones: cellular origin, chemistry and functions*

**Pars distalis**

| Cell type | Products | Chemical nature | Major physiological functions | Hyposecretion | Inappropriate hypersecretion |
|---|---|---|---|---|---|
| Thyrotrophs | thyrotrophin (TSH) | glycoprotein (two chains, α + β) mol. wt ≃ 22500 | ↑ synthesis and release of thyroxine ($T_4$) and triiodothyronine ($T_3$) | Foetus and neonate; impaired mental and physical development (cretinism). Adult: hypothyroidism, characterized by ↓ BMR, lethargy, etc. | Thyrotoxicosis |
| Gonadotrophs | follicle stimulating hormone (FSH) | glycoprotein (two chains, α + β) mol. wt ≃ 34000 | ♂ ↑ inhibin secretion ?facilitation of early stages of spermatogenesis<br><br>♀ follicular development aromatization androgen → oestrogen ↑ inhibin secretion facilitation of ovulation (with LH) | Pubertal period: delayed puberty Adult: hypogonadism, infertility and regression of secondary sex characteristics | Pre-puberty: precocious puberty Adult: disturbances of reproductive function |
| Gonadotrophs | luteinizing hormone (LH) | glycoprotein (two chains, α + β) mol. wt. ≃ 28000 | ♂ ↑ testicular steroidogenesis (testosterone)<br><br>♀ initiation of ovulation development of corpus luteum ↑ progesterone secretion ↑ androgen synthesis (oestradiol precursor) | | |

Table 4.1. (*Cont.*)

| | Cell type | Products | Chemical nature | Major physiological functions | Hyposecretion | Inappropriate hypersecretion |
|---|---|---|---|---|---|---|
| **Pars distalis** cont. | Somatotrophs | growth hormone (GH) | polypeptide (mol. wt $\simeq$ 27000) | growth of soft tissues, cartilage and bone ↑ protein synthesis, lipolysis, blood sugar ↑ somatomedin production | Pre-puberty: dwarfism | Pre-puberty: gigantism Adult: acromegaly |
| | Lactotrophs | prolactin (PRL) | polypeptide (mol. wt ≈ 25000) | ♀ initiation and maintenance of lactation ♂ no established role | Failure of lactation | Galactorrhoea Infertility |
| | Corticotrophs | ACTH | polypeptides (mol. wt $\simeq$ 4500) | ↑ synthesis and release of adrenal glucocorticoids ↑ adrenal blood flow hypertrophy of adrenocortical cells | Adrenal insufficiency | Cushing's disease Immunosuppression |
| | | β-lipotrophin (β-LPH)/β-endorphin | polypeptides (mol. wt $\simeq$ 12000/3500) | functions unknown – | | |
| | | N-POMC peptides | polypeptides (mol. wt $\simeq$ 16000 and less) | ? ↑ duodenal bicarbonate adrenocortical mitogenesis hydrolysis of cholesterol ester in adrenocortical cells | | |

| | | | | | | |
|---|---|---|---|---|---|---|
| **Pars intermedia** | | | | | | |
| | Corticotrophs | α-MSH | polypeptide (mol. wt ≃ 1500) | pigmentation ?regulation of foetal adrenal cortex | Failure of camouflage (lower vertebrates) | Pigmentation |
| | | CLIP | polypeptide (mol. wt ≃ 2500) | functions unknown | | |
| | | β-endorphin | polypeptide (mol. wt ≃ 3500) | functions unknown | | |
| | | N-POMC peptides | polypeptides (mol. wt ≃ 16000 and less) | functions unknown | | |
| **Pars nervosa** | | | | | | |
| | Vasopressinergic neurones | arginine vasopressin (AVP) | nonapeptide | ↑ permeability of renal collecting ducts → ↑ water reabsorption vasoconstriction | Diabetes insipidus Failure to maintain blood pressure in e.g. haemorrhage | $H_2O$ and $Na^+$ retention Hypertension |
| | Oxytocinergic neurones | oxytocin (OT) | nonapeptide | milk ejection uterine contraction | Milk ejection reflex impaired ?prolonged labour | ? |

ACTH = adrenocorticotrophic hormone; N–POMC = N-terminal pro-opiomelanocortin; α–MSH = melanocyte stimulating hormone; CLIP = corticotrophin-like intermediate lobe peptide; BMR = basal metabolic rate.

well characterized prohormone (POMC). The human and bovine genes encoding for POMC have a characteristic split eukaryotic structure (Fig. 4.1) comprising three mRNA-coding regions (exons 1, 2, and 3) separated by two introns (A and B). Following transcription of the gene and post-transcriptional processing, the resultant mRNA is translated on the ribosomes to yield pre-POMC. The newly formed polypeptide is translocated via the endoplasmic reticulum (where the signal peptide is removed) to the Golgi apparatus, packaged into secretory vesicles and subjected to further processing. Post-translational proleolytic cleavage occurs between paired basic amino acid residues (normally lysine and arginine) and, in the pars distalis, results primarily in the generation of four polypeptides, N-POMC$_{1-76}$, ACTH, $\beta$-LPH and a 31-residue peptide located between N-POMC$_{1-76}$ and ACTH (J peptide). Approximately 30% of the $\beta$-LPH is cleaved further to $\beta$- and $\gamma$-endorphin while, in certain pathophysiological conditions (e.g. following adrenal enucleation in the rat) more extensive processing may occur at the N-terminal resulting in the formation of N-POMC$_{1-48}$ and N-POMC$_{51-76}$ ($\gamma_3$-MSH). Interestingly, these two peptides have profound effects on the adrenal cortex: $\gamma$-MSH facilitates the hydrolysis of cholesterol esters and hence, by increasing substrate availability, potentiates the steroidogenic actions of ACTH while N-POMC$_{1-48}$ promotes adrenocortical mitogenesis. It is important to note that the POMC gene is expressed in tissues other than the pars distalis (e.g. pars intermedia, hypothalamus, gonads, placenta) where tissue specific, generally more extensive post-translational processing results in the formation of a different spectrum of peptides. For example, in the pars intermedia, hydrolysis of the lysine-arginine sequences in ACTH and $\beta$-LPH is complete giving rise to $\alpha$-MSH (which is subsequently acetylated at the carboxy terminus) and the corticotrophin-like intermediate lobe peptide (ACTH 18–39, CLIP) and to $\gamma$-LPH and $\beta$-endorphin, respectively (Fig. 4.1). Further processing may also occur in some species (Lowry, 1984).

Similar processes are involved in the biosynthesis of the other monomeric peptides produced by the pituitary gland, that is GH, prolactin, oxytocin and vasopressin (Mains et al., 1990). The synthesis of each of the double-chained glycoproteins (TSH, LH and FSH) is more complex and invokes the activation of two genes. The $\alpha$-chain or sub unit, which is common to all three hormones, is encoded by a single gene expressed by both thyrotrophs and gonadotrophs. Hormone specificity is conferred by the respective $\beta$-sub units each of which is encoded by a separate gene and expressed only by the appropriate cell type. Following post-translational proteolytic cleavage, the two sub-units are united and stored in a glycosylated form (Wilson, Leigh & Chapman, 1990). Further

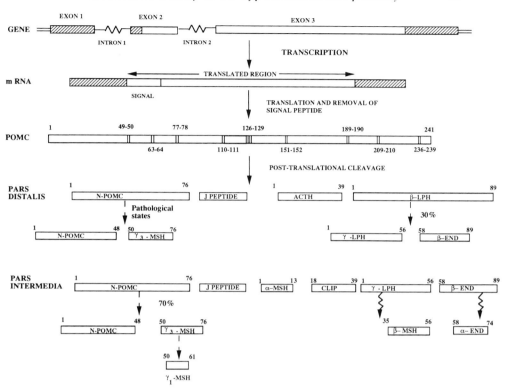

Fig. 4.1. Synthesis and post-translational processing of pro-opiomelano-cortin (POMC) in the corticotrophs of the pars distalis and pars intermedia.

▨ =untranslated nucleic acid sequences;
‖ =sites of paired basic amino acids (i.e. potential cleavage sites) in the pro-hormone;
– ► =incomplete processing;
⋀► =species specific incomplete processing.

modification of the sugar residues may occur immediately before release and the small changes occurring, for example at the mid-cycle, influence markedly the biological potency of the molecule.

## Control of adenohypophysial function

In view of the essential role of adenohypophysial hormones in the maintenance of homeostasis, it is not surprising that their release is subject to fine control. *In vivo*, the pituitary cells exhibit bursts of secretory activity resulting in characteristic 'episodic' patterns of secretion. The frequency and amplitude of pulses in, for example, corticotrophs and somatotrophs, vary according to a circadian pattern while in gonadotrophs and, in some species, lactotrophs, they are related to the ovarian cycle. Superimposed on these cyclic patterns of activity are cell specific responses to a wide spectrum and stimuli including, for example, environmental changes, emotional trauma, auditory and visual stimuli, pain, alterations in body temperature, metabolic (e.g. alterations in blood glucose or arginine) and osmotic changes.

It is now firmly established that the secretion of the hormones of the pars distalis is controlled by chemical transmitter substances liberated by hypothalamic neurones into the primary capillary plexus of the median eminence and transported to the target cells via the hypothalamo-hypophysial portal vessels (Harris, 1955). Hypothalamic hormones also control the secretory activity of the pars intermedia; some may be conveyed via the portal vessels but others may be released from neurones terminating in the vicinity of the secretory cells. Initially, it was assumed that (a) the hypothalamic regulatory hormones would be similar or identical to the classical transmitter substances of the autonomic nervous system and (b) that each pituitary hormone would be controlled by one hypothalamic factor (i.e. there would be five releasing factors initiating the secretion of GH, ACTH, LH, FSH and TSH respectively, and a release inhibiting factor effecting the tonic inhibition of prolactin secretion). Both assumptions proved incorrect. While classical transmitters (e.g. catecholamines) undoubtedly contribute to the control of anterior pituitary function, the majority of 'releasing factors' or 'releasing inhibiting factors' identified to date are neuropeptides. Moreover, it is now evident that one pituitary hormone may be influenced by two or more hypothalamic hormones whose actions may be complementary (e.g. corticotrophin releasing factor, CRF-41, and arginine vasopressin, AVP, on corticotrophs) or antagonistic (e.g. somatostatin and growth hormone releasing, GHRH, on the somatotrophs). Similarly, one hypothalamic hormone may regulate the secretion of two (and possibly more) pituitary hormones (e.g. gonadotrophin releasing hormone, GnRH, initiates the release of LH and FSH). Table 4.2 summarizes the major regulatory factors identified to date. Each of these substances has been shown, *in vivo* and *in vitro*, to exert specific effects on the secretory activity of the adenohypophysis. Further evidence in support of their physiological importance has been derived from demonstrations of their presence both in nerve terminals impinging on the capillary beds of the median eminence and in high concentrations in hypophysial portal blood, and from functional studies in which marked alterations of

Table 4.2. Regulation of adenohypophyseal cell function by hypothalamic hormones

| Hypothalamic hormone | Chemical nature | Locus of cell body | Pituitary second messenger | Effects on pituitary cell secretion |
|---|---|---|---|---|
| **Thyrotrophs** | | | | |
| TRH | Peptide (3AA) | Paraventricular and Arcuate nuclei | PI ($\uparrow$) | Increase |
| Somatostatin | Peptide (14AA) | Paraventricular nucleus | cAMP ($\downarrow$) | Decrease |
| **Gonadotrophs** | | | | |
| GnRH | Peptide (10AA) | Preoptic area | PI ($\uparrow$) | Increase |
| Acetylcholine | Choline ester | ? | PI ($\uparrow$) (muscarinic receptor) | |
| **Somatotrophs** | | | | |
| GHRH | Peptide (44AA) | Arcuate nucleus | cAMP ($\uparrow$) | Increase |
| Acetylcholine | Choline ester | ? | PI ($\uparrow$) (muscarinic receptor) | |
| Somatostatin | Peptide (14AA) | Periventricular nucleus | cAMP ($\downarrow$) | Decrease |
| Dopamine | Catecholamine | Arcuate nucleus | cAMP ($\downarrow$) $K^+$ efflux ($\uparrow$) (DA$_2$receptor) | |
| **Lactotrophs** | | | | |
| Dopamine | Catecholamine | Arcuate nucleus | $K^+$ efflux ($\uparrow$) + cAMP ($\downarrow$) (DA$_{2A}$ receptor) | Decrease |
| GABA | Amino acid | | Cl-influx ($\uparrow$) GABA$_A$) receptor | |
| TRH | Peptide (3AA) | Paraventricular nucleus | PI ($\uparrow$) | Increase |
| VIP | Peptide (28AA) | | cAMP ($\uparrow$) | |
| **Corticotrophs (pars distalis)** | | | | |
| CRF-41 | Peptide (41AA) | Paraventricular nucleus | cAMP ($\uparrow$) | Increase |
| Vasopressin | Peptide (9AA) | | PI ($\uparrow$) | |
| Oxytocin | Peptide (9AA) | ? | PI ($\uparrow$) | |
| Adrenaline | Catecholamine | | PI ($\uparrow$) ($\alpha_1$-adrenoceptor) | |
| Atriopeptin III | Peptide (24AA) | Para- and periventricular nuclei | cGMP ($\uparrow$) | Decrease |
| Substance P | Peptide (11AA) | ? | ?cAMP ($\downarrow$) | |
| **Corticotrophs (pars intermedia)** | | | | |
| Dopamine | Catecholamine | Arcuate nucleus | cAMP ($\downarrow$) (DA$_{2B}$ receptor) | Decrease |
| Adrenaline | Catecholamine | ? | cAMP ($\uparrow$) ($\beta$-Adrenoceptor) | Increase |

TRH = thyrotrophin releasing hormone; GnRH = gonadotrophin releasing hormone; GHRH = growth hormone releasing hormone; GABA = gamma-amino butyric acid; VIP = vasoactive intestinal peptide, CRF-41 = corticotrophin releasing factor pituitary activity have been observed following neutralization of their activity by administration of specific antisera or antagonists. Immuno-cytochemical studies have mapped the cell bodies and axonal pathways of many of the relevant hypothalamic neurones and demonstrated that while most of the hypophysiotrophic hormones are synthesized by separate neuronal populations some (e.g. CRF-41 and AVP) may be produced by the same cells. The neuropeptides, like the adeno-hypophysial hormones, are formed from large precursor molecules; gene transcription and the production and packaging of the pro-hor-mone occurs in the cell body while post-translational processing pro-ceeds as the storage vesicle passes down the nerve axon. By contrast, non-peptide hypothalamic regulatory hormones (e.g. dopamine) are synthesized and packaged primarily in the nerve terminal utilizing enzymes synthesized in the cell body and transported to the terminal by axoplasmic flow. In both cases, release of the transmitter is evoked neurochemically and involves a process of $Ca^{++}$ dependent exocytosis.

The actions of the hypothalamic hormones on their respective pituitary cells are complex and may involve not only alterations in the rate of hormone release (a process effected by $Ca^{++}$ dependent exocytosis) but also regulation of hormone synthesis (transcription and translation), post-translational processing (proteolysis, glycosylation, etc.) and margination of secretory granules. Effects on release occur rapidly and are normally maximal within one minute of cell stimulation. The other effects occur more slowly and are usually apparent only after repeated stimulation of the cells. The responses to each of the hypothalamic hormones are medi-ated by specific membrane bound receptors on the target cells (Table 4.2). Some of the receptors (e.g. gamma-amino butyric acid, $GABA_A$ receptor on lactotrophs) are linked to ion channels and thus when stimulated alter the excitability of the membrane. The majority, however, invoke intracellular second messenger systems. Of particular importance in this respect are inositol trisphosphate ($IP_3$) and diacylgly-cerol (DAG) liberated from membrane phospholipids by the action of phospholipase C (Berridge, 1984) and cyclic adenosine monophosphate (cAMP) formed from AMP by adenylcyclase (Aguilera et al., 1983). Other second messenger systems are also involved including arachidonic acid and its metabolites (prostanoids, leukotrienes, epoxides), which may be derived intracellularly from membrane phospholipids by the action of phospholipase $A_2$ or by degradation of DAG by lipases (Cowell & Buck-ingham, 1989), cyclic GMP and the polyamines (e.g. spermidine) (Jones & Gillham, 1988).

Stimulation of the membrane bound receptor may culminate in phos-phorylation and internalization of the receptor-ligand complex. The receptor may be degraded, a process important in the regulation of receptor number/turnover, or recycled. Until comparatively recently it was assumed that the internalized ligand was metabolized rapidly. Recent studies, however, demonstrating the presence of immunoreactive TRH in the nuclei of thyrotrophs suggest that this is not necessarily the case but that the process of internalization may provide an effective means of translocating the ligand to a site within the cell where it may exert further biological actions, for example modulation of genomic activity.

Several factors may modulate the magnitude of the pituitary responses to the various hypothalamic hormones. The pattern of stimulation appears to be of particular importance. Adenohypophysial hormones are normally released in short pulses, the frequency and amplitude of which vary according to the physiological/pathological state. The episodic mode of pituitary secretion is dependent on complementary pulsatile secretion of the appropriate hypothalamic hormones. The frequency of pulses is critical because continuous or too frequent exposure to the hypothalamic hormone may render the cells tolerant while a marked reduction in pulse frequency may be insufficient to maintain the cells' secretory activity. Thus, for example, prolonged infusions of GnRH or administration of long acting GnRH analogues render the gonadotrophs refractory to further stimulation with the releasing hormone. By contrast, when given in a pulsatile manner (1 pulse/90 min, s.c.), so as to mimic the physiological pattern of secretion, GnRH effectively maintains gonadal function both in experimental animals in which the GnRH neurones are ablated surgically and in human subjects with infertility/hypogonadism of hypothalamic origin (Marshall, Monroe & Jaffe, 1988). Several workers have claimed that the desensitization evoked by GnRH is due to a reduction in the number of pituitary receptors. Others, however, have found that alterations in cell sensitivity are not always positively correlated with receptor number and have provided evidence that other factors (resulting in uncoupling of stimulus secretion coupling) may be more important in this respect (Clayton, 1989).

The secretion of pituitary hormones may also be subject to 'feedback effects', positive and negative, exerted by target organ hormones (Fink, 1988). Importantly, the thyroid hormones, thyroxine ($T_4$) and triiodothyronine ($T_3$), exert powerful inhibitory actions on the thyrotrophs and impair markedly their secretory responses to TRH, a phenomenon exploited clinically to differentiate between primary and secondary thyroid disease. Similarly, the adrenocortical steroids (cortisol, corticosterone) and the gonadal hormones (androgens, oestrogens, progestogens, inhibin) may respectively attenuate the neurochemically evoked secretory activity of the corticotrophs and gonadotrophs although their actions at the pituitary level, unlike those of $T_3$ and $T_4$ on the thyrotrophs, are relatively weak. Indeed, in some cases, oestradiol may effect a positive feedback action on the gonadotrophs facilitating at, for example, the mid-cycle 'GnRH self-priming', a protein synthesis dependent process, whereby the magnitude of the secretory response to GnRH is increased progressively. Oestradiol may also facilitate prolactin release.

In the case of pituitary cells under the control of mutually antagonistic hypothalamic hormones (e.g. somatotrophs) the magnitude of the response to one factor will depend on the prevailing tone exerted by the other. For example, a single injection of GHRH may precipitate a marked rise in serum GH. A second injection, administered two hours later may be relatively ineffective not because the cells are refractory to the releasing factor but because the degree of somatostatin tone is increased (Tannenbaum, 1988). Interactions between releasing factors whose actions are complementary may also occur. For example, the effects of CRF-41 and AVP on ACTH secretion are not additive but powerfully synergistic (Gillies et al., 1982). Thus the secretory responses to CRF-41 depend largely on the degree of vasopressinergic tone to the corticotrophs and vice versa.

## Regulation of releasing factor neurones

The secretion of each of the hypophysiotrophic hormones is controlled primarily by a complex of intra- and extra-hypothalamic neural pathways which relay essential information concerning the circadian periodicity, metabolic and osmotic status, enviromental changes, emotional trauma, etc. In addition, secretory activity may be influenced by feedback effects exerted by gonadal, adrenocortical and thyroid hormones, by the pituitary hormones and, possibly, by the hypothalamic hormones themselves (Fig. 4.2).

Attempts to characterize the neural pathways have involved a variety of experimental approaches including anatomical investigations at light and electron microscope levels, biochemical correlates of transmitter turnover with hypothalamo-pituitary activity, functional studies following electrical stimulation or lesioning of 'specific' pathways or pharmacological manipulation of neurochemical transmission and in vitro studies utilizing acutely removed or cultured hypothalamic tissue (Jones et al., 1987; Taleisnik & Sawyer, 1986). The data so accrued indicate that many of the numerous ascending and descending pathways converging on the hypothalamus are involved. Of particular importance, appear to be the noradrenergic fibres originating in the $A_1$ and $A_6$ (locus coeruleus) loci, 5-hydroxytryptaminergic pathways arising in the raphe nucleus, cholinergic

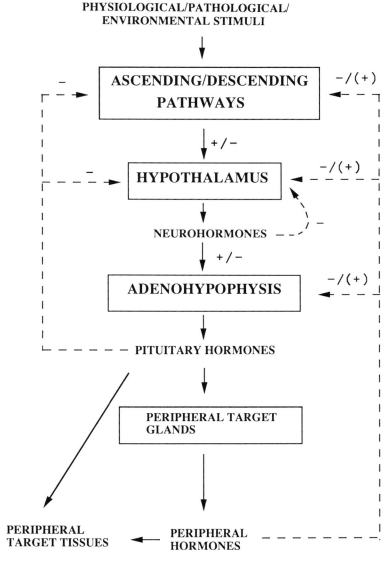

Fig. 4.2. Mechanisms controlling the secretion of hypothalamic regulatory hormones.

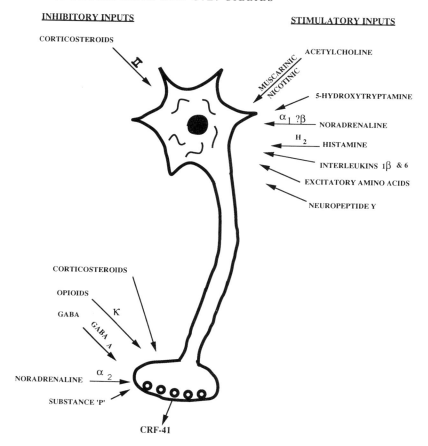

Fig. 4.3. Postulated mechanisms controlling the secretion of CRF-41 (corticotrophin releasing factor) by parvocellular neurones in the paraventricular median eminence tract.

fibres from the lateral pre-optic area, the parabrachial nuleus, the stria terminalis and the nucleus of the diagonal band plus other, less well characterized pathways originating in the cortex and limbic system. In addition, innumerable neurotransmitter/neuromodulator substances produced by interneurones within the hypothalamus (e.g. GABA, dopamine, opioid peptides, neuropeptide Y, excitatory amino acids) are also of considerable importance in this respect. The picture is far from complete. A detailed description of the current 'state of the art' is beyond the scope of this chapter but the schematic diagram (Fig. 4.3) depicting postulated mechanisms controlling the CRF-41 producing neurones should serve to illustrate the complexity of the system (Jones *et al.*, 1987).

With respect to the feedback control, corticosteroids exert potent inhibitory actions on the secretion of CRF-41 and AVP by parvocellular neurones in the paraventricular nucleus. Their actions involve an immediate, short lasting response associated with impaired $Ca^{++}$ transport and a delayed, more sustained effect involving inhibition of the synthesis and release of the neuropeptides, apparently by genomic mechanisms (Jones & Gillham, 1988). Gonadal steroids (androgens, oestrogens and progesterone) modulate the release of GnRH (Fink, 1988). Their potent actions are generally inhibitory although at the mid-cycle the ovarian steroids may facilitate GnRH release. TRH secretion is also subject to feedback inhibition but the effects of $T_3$ and $T_4$ on the hypothalamus are weak compared to those exerted at the pituitary level. The actions of the target organ hormones are exerted on specific receptors located not only in the relevant neurohormone secreting cells but also in intra- and extra-hypothalamic neurones controlling their activity, for example CA1 and CA2 regions of the hippocampus (corticosteroid receptors) and GABA-ergic and noradrenergic neurones (oestrogen receptors). It is widely believed that the pituitary hormones also exert regulatory effects on the secretion of their respective hypothalamic controlling factors. Since these hormones do not readily penetrate the blood-brain barrier, it is probable that their effects are exerted at the level of the median eminence. There is also some evidence that the neurohormones may influence their own secretion. Moreover, some degree of interplay between neurones may occur. Certainly interactions between somatostatin and GHRH-neurones have been described. Furthermore, the stress-induced inhibition of GnRH appears to be secondary to the intrahypothalamic release of CRF-41.

## Control of neurohypophysial hormones

The neurohypophysial hormones, oxytocin and vasopressin, are synthesized in the magnocellular neurosecretory cells of the paraventricular and supra-optic nuclei by mechanisms analogous to those described earlier for other neuropeptides (Robinson, 1986). Despite their structural similarities, the two neuropeptides are formed from different pro-hormones in separate neurones which can be distinguished readily on histo-logical and electrophysiological grounds and which are subject to independent control mechanisms. Vasopressin release is triggered by a number of physiological stimuli including (a) volume depletion detected by the baroreceptors in the left atrium and pulmonary vein as well as those in the carotid sinus and aortic arch (which are also sensitive to chemical stimulants, e.g. hypoxia) and relayed via the nucleus tractus solitarius and dorsal vagal nuclei to the hypothalamus, (b) increases in serum osmolarity detected by osmoreceptors located on the circumventricular organs (subfornical organ and organ vasculosum of the lamina terminalis) and/or cell bodies of vasopressinergic neurones and (c) stressful, emotional and nociceptive stimuli apparently relayed via limbic afferents originating primarily from the amygdala and septum. Numerous transmitter substances have been implicated in these processes including noradrenaline (from fibres originating primarily in the $A_1$ but also $A_2$ and $A_6$ loci), acetylcholine (via nicotinic and muscarinic receptors), excitatory amino acids and GABA which exerts powerful inhibitory actions in both the brain stem and the hypothalamus (Cowley, Laird & Ansiello, 1988). Oxytocin is produced primarily during labour and in lactation (Leng & Bicknell, 1986). In the latter, release is provoked by suckling which initiates the passage of impulses via the spinal afferents and brain stem to the hypothalamus. The consequent burst of oxytocin release triggers contraction of the mammary myoepithelial cells and a rise in intra-mammary pressure which, together, precipitate milk ejection (milk ejection reflex). The mechanisms facilitating oxytocin release in labour are less well understood. They may involve sensory stimuli arising from the cervix and vagina and, possibly, a reduction in circulating relaxin, a polypeptide reputed to depress oxytocin secretion in late pregnancy. Oxytocin release is also precipitated by gastric distension and, like vasopressin, is sensitive to osmotic stimuli and depressed by alcohol.

Control of both oxytocinergic and vasopressinergic fibres appears to be effected primarily at the level of the cell body. However, in both cell types, some degree of modulation may occur in the nerve terminal where the degree of $Ca^{++}$ dependent exocytosis triggered by action potentials passing down the neurone may be tempered by opioid peptides and other locally produced neuromodulators.

## Interactions between the immune system and the hypothalamo-pituitary axis

Although the potentially toxic effects of glucocorticoids on immune function have been known for many years, the high degree of communication between the immune and endocrine systems is only now becoming apparent (Cotman et al., 1987). Evidence is accumulating rapidly that various immune cell products (cytokines) exert profound effects on hypothalamo-pituitary function. For example, interleukin I (IL-I) stimulates the release of CRF-41 and other hypothalamic neuropeptides while IL-6 and tumour necrosis factor (TNF) modulate the secretory activity of the pars distalis. Thymic hormones are also important in this respect and for example, CRF release is modulated by thymosin $\alpha_1$ while thymosin $\beta_4$ and thymulin promote the release of GnRH and LH, respectively. Similarly several hormones of the hypothalamo-pituitary axis, some or all of which may also be produced by immune cells, have been shown to influence specifically the secretion of various cytokines and thymic hormones. This exciting area is clearly ripe for further investigation.

## Disorders of the hypothalamo-pituitary system

### Naturally occurring disorders

Endocrine malfunctions of the hypothalamus and pituitary gland manifest themselves largely as hyper- or hypo-function of the peripheral target organs. Clinical conditions arising as a result include infertility (disruption within the hypothalamo-pituitary-gonadal, HPG, axis), gigantism (excess GH secretion in childhood), acromegaly (excess GH secretion in the adult) and dwarfism (reduction of GH in childhood), hyper- and hypothyroidism (enhanced or reduced activity, respectively, within the hypothalamo-pituitary-thyroid, HPT, axis) and Cushing's syndrome or adrenal insufficiency (malfunction within the hypothalamo-pituitary-adrenal, HPA, axis) resulting in hyper- or hypo-cortisolism, respectively. These conditions are fully described in a number of excellent texts (e.g. Besser & Cudworth, 1987). Effective therapy of such conditions depends on the accurate diagnosis of the prime site of malfunction, viz the hypothalamus, pituitary gland or peripheral organ. For example, hypothyroidism (low circulating levels of thyroid hormones), manifesting itself in lethargy, low metabolic rate, sensitivity to cold and mental impairment, could arise from reduced synthesis of the thyroid hormones within the thyroid gland, reduced secretion of TSH from the anterior pituitary gland or reduced drive to the pituitary gland caused by hyposecretion of TRH due to hypothalamic pathology or altered influence from higher central nervous system (CNS) centres on TRH-producing neurons. Tests for the differential diagnosis of a peripheral, pituitary or hypothalamic perturbation of function are available and are fully described elsewhere (Besser & Cudworth, 1987). A number of endocrine disorders are also the result of over production of hypothalamic or pituitary hormones by tumours situated within these glands or by ectopic tumours which, for example, have been found to cause Cushing's syndrome (ACTH production by oat cell carcinomas of the lung) or acromegaly (secretion of GHRH from a pancreatic tumour).

## Drug induced disorders

Drugs may influence the neuroendocrine function of the hypothalamus by modifying levels of the neurotransmitters or neuromodulators which control the release of the hypothalamic regulatory factors, by interacting with intracellular second messenger systems (e.g. the adenylate cyclase, phosphatidyl inositol and Ca-calmodium systems) involved in the transduction of receptor activation into hormone release or by altering the all-important negative feedback of peripheral endocrine organ hormones at both the hypothalamic and the pituitary level. A number of centrally acting psychoactive drugs, for example, may influence the endocrine system via their action at the dopamine receptor. Chlorpromazine, a drug used to treat psychoses, may impair the tuberoinfundibular dopaminergic inhibitory control of prolactin release leading to an increase in circulating prolactin levels. A likely consequence, and hence a potential toxic effect, is therefore infertility. Clomiphene, a drug used in the treatment of infertility, appears to act by inhibiting oestrogen binding in the hypothalamus. As a result, the normal feedback inhibition is prevented, thus causing increased secretion of the releasing hormone and the gonadotrophins which, in turn, increase the drive to the ovaries and induce ovulation. However, it is critical that such drugs are given for a short period only during the early follicular phase of the cycle (typically within the first five days for a menstruating subject) as over-stimulation will result in down regulation at the pituitary and exacerbate the infertility. In some circumstances, however, the phenomenon of down regulation has been exploited clinically. Continuous rather than pulsatile administration of GnRH suppresses pituitary gonadotrophin secretion and this has been used to treat conditions such as precocious puberty in children, prostatic carcinoma in men and to block ovulation in normal women (Fig. 4.4). Infertility is, therefore, a potential consequence of any drug acting centrally to alter the neural control of GnRH, gonadotrophins or dopamine (and hence prolactin) secretion.

Hypersecretion of cortisol and the resultant physical characteristics so often diagnosed as Cushing's syndrome (moonface, wasting of muscles in the limbs, swollen abdomen) are often present in pseudo-Cushing's states which could be drug-induced, for example by psychoactive drugs. Hypercortisolism may also be present in patients with alcoholism and in a number of psychiatric states, including depression, anorexia nervosa, bulimia and obsessive conditions. A diagnosis which differentiates these from true Cushing's syndrome is essential (Chrousos et al., 1989; Grossman et al., 1988).

Xenobiotic induced toxicity at the hypothalamic or pituitary level are,

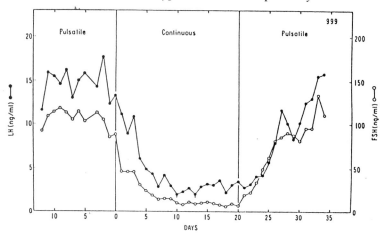

Fig. 4.4. Inhibition of gonadotropin secretion in a rhesus monkey with a hypothalamic lesion when an intermittent gonadotropin releasing hormone (GnRH) replacement regimen (1 µg/minute for 6 minutes every hour) was replaced by a continuous infusion of the decapeptide beginning on day 0. This inhibition was gradually reversed when the pulsatile mode of GnRH administration was reinstituted on day 20. The small vertical lines below some data points indicate levels below the sensitivity of the assay. LH – luteinising hormone; FSH – follicle stimulating hormone. (From Belchetz *et al.*, 1978, with permission.)

fortunately, rarely life-threatening and, in the adult, homeostasis of the natural endocrine balance is usually restored after removal of the foreign influence. For example, hyper- or hypothyroidism are consequences of drug treatments for hypo- and hyperthyroidism, respectively. The patient is monitored for development of a condition opposite to that from which (s)he is suffering and once the therapy is appropriately adjusted, the normal balance rapidly returns. In contrast, however, prolonged therapy with corticosteroids for anti-inflammatory or immunosuppressive purposes, for example, does present potential life-threatening situations if treatment is discontinued too rapidly. In such circumstances the patient is left in a condition of acute adrenal insufficiency as the exogenous steroid has totally suppressed the normal functioning of the HPA axis. Normal function could take 2–18 months to re-establish itself, during which time withdrawal should be carefully controlled.

The consequences of xenobiotically-induced endocrine perturbations of the foetus, neonate and child are more difficult to assess and more likely not to be reversible. For example, a lack of thyroid hormones in the foetus or neonate, caused by hypothalamic, pituitary or thyroid defect or maternal anti-thyroid therapy, could lead to an irreversible defect in neural development and growth resulting in cretinism. Inappropriate exposure to androgenic steroids during late foetal and early neonatal life may result in masculinization of the brain characterized by failure to produce an LH surge and male sexual behaviour in the genotypic female. Long-term treatment of children with corticosteroids may result in growth retardation. To our knowledge studies on possible toxic effects at hypothalamic or pituitary sites within the endocrine system of the immature animal are sparse and such potential effects on the developing individual remain to be fully assessed. We are also not aware of any studies indicating a specific xenobiotic induction of endocrine toxicity attributable to tumours secreting hypothalamic or pituitary hormones, but it is a possibility to be further investigated.

## Experimental models for investigating toxicological pharmacological perturbation of function of the hypothalamo-pituitary axis

### In vivo models

*In vivo* methods may be used to examine the acute and long-term effects of drugs on hypothalamo-pituitary function. They also provide a valuable means of assessing the potentially adverse effects of drug administration during pregnancy and in neonatal life on the development of the neuro-endocrine system. The studies normally involve assessment of pituitary function during and after the administration, by appropriate routes, of graded doses of drugs over a period of time and are invariably performed in two or more species. Various markers of pituitary function may be employed. Following long-term drug treatments, indirect indices of pituitary activity, involving for example assessment of body weight, urine volume and osmolarity, the weight and histological appearance of the pituitary gland, the peripheral endocrine glands (thyroid, adrenal and gonads) and appropriate target tissues (e.g. thymus, uterus), may provide a surprisingly accurate picture. Obviously more precise information may be obtained following both acute and repeated dosage by direct estimates of the pituitary hormones in the blood by specific radioimmunological, biological or immunoradiometric assay methods.

In designing studies and interpreting data several important points must be taken into consideration. Diet, housing, lighting and handling regimes may all influence pituitary function. Techniques of blood sampling are also important. In some cases animals may be bled repeatedly at appropriate time-intervals via indwelling cannulae; in others the combined stressful effects of the sampling procedure and volume depletion may necessitate collection post-mortem. Drug-induced alterations in 'basal' hormone concentrations may be due to changes in secretion and/ or metabolism and excretion. The latter possibility may be examined by comparing the plasma half-life of exogenous hormone in drug-treated and control rats in which endogenous pituitary function is impaired surgically or pharmacologically. Often the adverse effects of drugs on the neuro-endocrine system are manifested not by marked changes in 'basal' hormone concentrations but by inappropriate secretory responses to provocative (physiological) stimuli, for example hypoglycaemia, stress, etc. or by disruption of rhythmic (e.g. circadian) secretory patterns. For example, opiate drugs have minimal effects on gonadotrophin release in the dioestrous rat but, given in the critical period, they readily prevent the pre-ovulatory LH surge. Similarly, basal ACTH levels are restored rapidly following withdrawal of long-term corticosteroid treatment but a considerable time delay ensues before the life-maintaining pituitary-adrenal response to stress is reinstated fully (Buckingham & Hodges, 1976). Thus, it is not sufficient to determine 'resting' hormone levels following drug-treatment. Functional studies, in which the ability of the hypothalamo-pituitary axis to maintain its normal rhythmic patterns of secretory activity (e.g. circadian, those related to the ovarian cycle) and to respond to appropriate stimuli (e.g. ACTH response to stress, TSH response to cold) are assessed.

Marked differences often occur between the hypothalamo-pituitary responses to single and repeated doses of drugs, thus emphasizing the need for both acute and long-term studies. With some substances, for example anti-inflammatory/immunosuppressive steroids, the untoward effects are intensified with successive treatments and may persist for considerable periods after the drug is withdrawn. Others (e.g. opiates) may initiate a dramatic first dose effect but produce only weak responses thereafter either because cellular (receptor down regulation and/or disruption of post-receptor mechanisms) or metabolic (increased degradation and/or excretion) resistance develops or, more frequently, because compensatory mechanisms are invoked which enable the pituitary gland to fulfil its essential role in the maintenance of homeostasis.

*In vivo* studies may also provide limited information about the site and mode of drug action within the hypothalamo-pituitary axis. Evidence for an action at the pituitary level may be obtained from studies involving injection of the drug into the gland itself or estimation of pituitary function in median-eminence lesioned animals following drug administration by conventional routes. The latter approach will reveal direct actions of the drug on the secretory activity of the cells only, as also will similar studies in which the activity of the hypothalamic hormones is inhibited immunologically (administration of anti-sera) or pharmacologically (administration of antagonists). Additional studies, in which the pituitary responses to each of the hypothalamic hormones are monitored in drug-treated median eminence-lesioned animals are required in order to ascertain whether the drug effect involves modulation (synergistic or antagonistic) of the pituitary response to neurochemical stimulation (e.g. TSH response to TRH).

Implantation techniques may also be used to identify drug action at the hypothalamic level. However, the data should be interpreted with caution for substances given via the third ventricle may readily diffuse to other brain areas. Similarly, those injected into the hypothalamus, particularly in areas adjacent to the capillary plexus, may reach the pituitary gland. The latter problem may be overcome by making direct estimates of the hypothalamic hormones in the portal blood. However, this procedure is inappropriate for routine studies since it requires great skill. More valuable information concerning both the site and the mode of action of drugs at the molecular level may be obtained from *in vitro* studies using hypothalamic and pituitary tissue from both drug-treated and untreated rats and techniques outlined in the following section.

## *In vitro* models

As the hypothalamo-pituitary axis is part of a tightly controlled homeostatic unit, there are obvious advantages of studying directly the function of either the hypothalamus or pituitary *in vitro* in order to ascertain the locus within any endocrine axis at which foreign influences might act. In principle, the animal may be exposed to any potentially toxic condition *in vivo* and the respective glands removed and investigated directly *in vitro*, or the glands may be removed from a normal animal and exposed to the factors under investigation *in vitro*. The strategy adopted and the *in vitro* model chosen (short vs. long term) depends upon whether acute or chronic effects are to be investigated, although the most accurate results are obviously likely to be obtained from a combination of several methods. Brief descriptions of the models available are given in Tables 4.3 and 4.4 and further details may be obtained within the references cited.

The methods for assessment of hypothalamic or pituitary function *in vitro* generally depend on the measurement of hormone released into the medium under conditions known to infuence its release *in vivo*. Acute methods involving incubation of tissue fragments (see Tables 4.3 and 4.4) have the advantage that three-dimensional cellular contacts are main-

Table 4.3. *In vitro models suitable for investigating xenobiotic induced toxicity at hypothalamic level*

| Brief description | Survival of preparation | Approx. no. stimuli per preparation | Advantages | Disadvantages | Reference |
|---|---|---|---|---|---|
| **Acute preparations** | | | | | |
| Incubation of adult rat hypothalami in CSF-like solution | 3–5 hours | 2 | Cellular organization maintained. Most hormone levels easily measurable by RIA. Little inter-animal variation in responses to neurochemical stimuli | Relatively poor diffusion of nutrients, metabolites, secretagogues and released products. Significant inter-animal variation in non-stimulated release | Buckingham & Hodges, 1977a |
| Superfusion of adult rat hypothalami with balanced salt solution. | 3–5 hours | 2–3 | ,, <br> Dynamics of responses may be studied | Diffusion problems reduced. Responses decline with repeated stimulations | Gallardo & Ramirez, 1977; Gillies *et al.*, 1984 |
| **Long-term preparations** | | | | | |
| Organ/explant culture in serum-supplemented medium | Days (adult); months (neonate tissue). | | Intra-hypothalamic connections maintained. | Neurite outgrowth occurs mainly at edges of tissue mass. Potential poor diffusion and central necrosis. Serum is an undefined, variable and unphysiological additive. | Gähwiler, 1981 Gregg, 1985; Earnest & Sladek, 1987 |
| Isolated cell culture (foetal/neonatal) | | | | | |
| (a) serum-supplemented medium. | 2–6 weeks | 2–>10 | Long-term preparation – may be studied repeatedly. Minimal biological variation from pooled cell suspension. | Cellular inter-connections initially disrupted (but may re-form histotypically). Foetal/neonatal tissue contains low levels of hormones under investigation. Presence of serum, an unknown and uncontrollable variable. | Clarke, Lowry & Gillies, 1987 |
| (b) defined medium | 6 weeks | >10 | Chemical environment accurately controlled. Consequences of chronic *in vitro* treatments on subsequent responses may be studied more accurately. | Physiological relevance of behaviour of cultured cells must be borne in mind. | Clarke & Gillies, 1988 |

RIA = radioimmunoassay

Table 4.4. *In vitro models suitable for investigating xenobiotic induced toxicity at pituitary level*

| Brief description | Survival of preparation | Approx. no. stimuli per preparation | Advantages | Disadvantages | Reference |
|---|---|---|---|---|---|
| **Acute preparations** | | | | | |
| Incubation of anterior pituitary | 3 hours | 2–3 | Relatively simple to perform with minimal specialist apparatus. Highly reproducible. | Diffusion problems as time proceeds. | Buckingham & Hodges, 1977b |
| Superfusion of isolated cells with balanced salt solution. | >10 hours | >30 | Simple, rapid and highly sensitive. Diffusion problems eliminated. Dynamics of responses may be studied. | Responses may vary with repeated stimulations. Loss of cell–cell connections. | Gillies & Lowry, 1978 |
| Superfused hemipituitaries | 2 hours | 1–3 | Cell–cell contacts maintained. | Less sensitive to secretagogues than isolated cell superfusions. | Gillies *et al.*, 1984 |
| Static incubation of isolated cells | 5 hours | 2 | Diffusion problems reduced. | Loss of sensitivity. Loss of cell–cell connections. | Negro-Vilar & Lapetina, 1985 |
| **Long-term (adult tissue) preparations** | | | | | |
| Culture of isolated cells | up to 7 days | 3–6 | Chronic treatments *in vitro*. | De-differentiation and loss of responsiveness, e.g. AVP on cultured corticotrophs. Serum used in most instances. | Vale *et al.*, 1983 |

AVP = arginine vasopressin

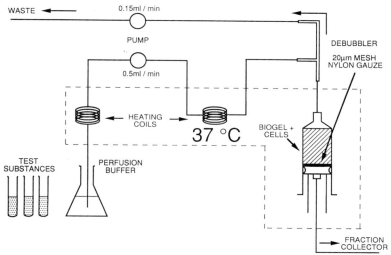

Fig. 4.5. Apparatus for the superfusion of isolated rat anterior pituitary cells. Briefly, cells are isolated by agitation and trituration in a trypsin solution, mixed with an inert matrix (0.5 G pre-swollen Bio-Gel P2) and the slurry packed into a 2 ml column constructed from a 2 ml sterile disposable syringe. The column is perfused with Earles Balanced Salt Solution containing 0.25% human serum albumin, trasylol (100 Kallikrein inactivator U/ml) 15 µg benzyl penicillin/ml and 25 µg streptomycin/ml. The substance(s) under test is diluted in this perfusion buffer and its effects on hormone release observed over times ranging from 2 mins to 10 hours. The medium is pumped at 0.5 ml/min and effluent from the cell column is collected as 2–10 minute fractions and assayed for the anterior pituitary hormone(s) of interest. (For further details see Gillies & Lowry, 1978.)

tained, but these preparations are relatively short-lived because, as time proceeds, they may suffer from diffusion artefacts. The latter are minimized when using isolated cell preparations, especially when they are superfused as described in Fig. 4.5. A typical way in which such a system may be used is illustrated for prolactin (Fig. 4.6). Longer term investigations *in vitro* require tissue culture techniques (see Tables 4.3 and 4.4). Until recently foetal calf serum and/or horse serum were added to all culture media to provide unidentified nutrients, growth factors and attachment factors. However, there is significant batch to batch variation in serum, which is an unphysiological fluid for bathing most tissues and, furthermore, its presence may interfere with the potential influences of any substances under test. Defined, serum free media are, therefore, being developed for a number of culture systems and some improvements

108

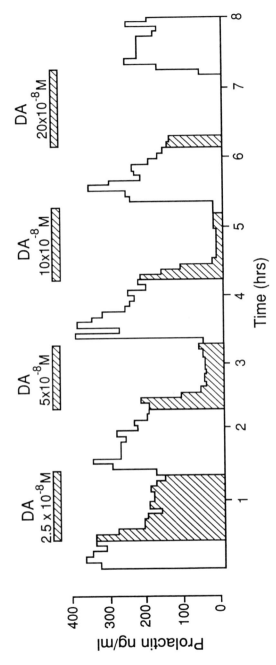

Fig. 4.6. Dose-dependent effects of dopamine (DA) on the release of prolactin from superfused rat anterior pituitary cells. Isolated rat anterior pituitary cells were packed into a column and superfused as described in Fig. 4.5. The effluent was collected as 5 minute fractions and the prolactin concentration measured by radioimmunoassay. ▨ denotes the presence of DA in the superfusion medium. (Gillies, Al-Damluji & Buckingham, unpublished observations.)

in the responses of cultured cells in such a medium is illustrated for hypothalamic neurones in Fig. 4.7. Recent studies provide evidence for a functional maturation of hypothalamic neurones in culture. From *in vivo* and *in vitro* studies, 5-HT (5-hydroxytryptamine) is regarded as a physiological neurotransmitter controlling CRF-41 release. Fig. 4.8 demonstrates that cultured CRF-41 neurones are responsive to 5-HT and that their responsiveness both to 5-HT and non-specific depolarization (Fig. 4.7) increases as time proceeds in culture. This model may therefore prove useful in long-term investigations of possible toxicological effects on developing neurones.

## Conclusions and future directions

The hypothalamus and pituitary gland form a functional endocrine unit which controls a vast array of bodily functions via a large number of hormones, the secretion of which is under tight homeostatic control. For this reason, plus the relative inaccessibility of the hypothalamus to experimental manipulation, studies on pituitary and hypothalamic function are often difficult to perform and interpret. Recently, however, various experimental models have been developed which facilitate such investigations. These have been used widely to clarify physiological parameters but their application to the study of external influences on normal functions remains to be exploited. Furthermore, while investigations in the whole animal are ultimately essential, a considerable amount of information may be accrued from *in vitro* studies, the importance of which is likely to increase in the future. With the continuing improvement of defined, serum-free media, *in vitro* preparations offer a high degree of control over the cellular environment which is obviously of prime importance when assessing the effects of foreign substances at the molecular level. *In vitro* preparations generally require fewer animals than their *in vivo* counterparts and, in the case of cultured tissues, permit repeated challenges with a test substance over a period of weeks, thus enabling the effects of prior treatments on subsequent reponses to be observed directly in a carefully controlled environment.

At the present time we do not have sufficient information to fully deduce the consequences of external influences on the development of hypothalamic and pituitary function. However, such influences appear to be likely and may have relevance to a number of pathological conditions in later life. For example, perturbations of maternal corticosteroid levels in rats can severely compromise the stress response of offspring in later life (Angelucci *et al.*, 1983; Scaccianoce, Di Sciullo & Angelucci, 1989) and malfunctions of the HPA are strongly implicated in certain

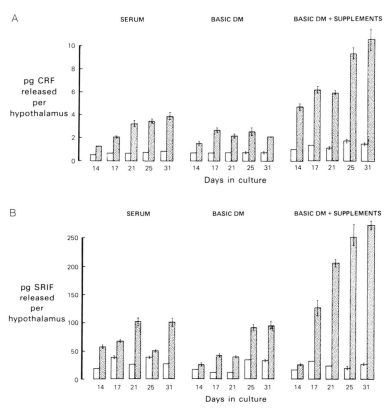

Fig. 4.7. Demonstration of the effects of medium composition on peptide release from cultured rat hypothalamic neurones. Briefly, hypothalamic neurones from foetal rats at 18 days' gestation were isolated, plated into 35 mm culture dishes and grown in a serum supplemented medium (serum), a basic defined medium which was developed for neuroblastoma cells (Bottenstein & Sato, 1979 [Basic DM]) or Basic DM plus triiodothyronine, docosahexaenoic acid and arachidonic acid (Basic DM and supplements). Over a period of several weeks the basal (☐) and 56 mM K + stimulated (▨) release of (A) CRF-41 (corticotrophin releasing factor) and (B) somatostatin (SRIF) during 1 h incubations were measured by radioimmunoassay. In supplemented DM an enhancement of neuropeptide release is observed and responses increase with time in culture, suggesting a level of maturation *in vitro*. (From Clarke & Gillies, 1988.)

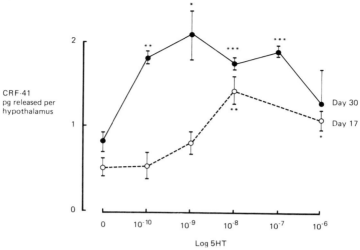

Fig. 4.8. Effect of 5-HT (5-hydroxy-tryptamine or serotonin) on the release of CRF-41 (corticotrophin releasing factor) from rat hypothalamic neurones in culture. The cells on day 30 respond with greater sensitivity and magnitude than on day 17, suggesting a maturation of neuronal function as time proceeds. (From Clarke & Gillies, 1988.)

psychiatric states (Chrousos *et al.*, 1989). A number of neuroendocrine and metabolic abnormalities are also a result of neonatal administration of monosodium glutamate (MSG) which largely destroys neurons of the arcuate nuclei and produces lesions of other central structures. Stunted growth (impaired release of hypothalamic GHRH), small pituitary glands, hypogonadism, hypothyroidism, altered prolactin levels and disruption of HPA axis regulation have all been reported as a consequence of MSG given to newborn rats (Dolnikoff *et al.*, 1988). A study of the endocrine function in the foetus, neonate and juvenile animal as well as in the adult is, therefore, required in the future. A number of the experimental models described in Tables 4.3 and 4.4 should prove suitable for the investigation of external influences on maturation of the endocrine hypothalamus and pituitary gland.

Many of the peptide hormones produced by the hypothalamus and pituitary gland (several of which can be mitogenic), are being found increasingly in the periphery, notably in cells of the gut, reproductive system, immune system and placenta. Their precise roles, presumably regulatory in nature, remain to be established, but once this is done, assessment of xenobiotic-induced toxicity within such systems will be essential.

# References

Angelucci, L., Patacchioli, F.R., Chierichetti, C. & Laureti, S. (1983). Changes in behaviour and brain glucocorticoid receptors detected in adult life of corticosterone-nursed rats. In *Application of Behavioural Pharmacology in Toxicology*, eds G. Zbiden, V. Cuomo, G. Racagini & B. Weiss, pp. 277–91. New York: Raven Press.

Aguilera, G. Harwood, J.P. Wilson, J.X., Morrell, J., Brown, J.H. & Catt, K.J. (1983). Mechanisms of action of corticotrophin releasing factor and other regulators of corticotrophin release in rat pituitary cells. *J. biol. Chem.*, **258**, 8039–45.

Belchetz, P., Plant, T., Nakai, Y., Keogh, E. & Knobil, E. (1978). Hypophyseal response to continuous and intermittent delivery of hypothalamic gonadotropin releasing hormone. *Science*, **202**, 631–3.

Berridge, M.J. (1984). Inositol triphosphate and diacylglycerol as second messengers. *Biochem. J.*, **220**, 345–60.

Besser, G.M. & Cudworth, A.G. (Eds.) (1987). *Clinical Endocrinology*. Chapman and Hall.

Bottenstein, J.E. & Sato, G.M. (1979). Growth of a rat neurobastoma cells line in a serum-free supplemented medium. *Proc. Natl. Acad. Sci. USA*, **76**, 514–17.

Buckingham, J.C. & Hodges, J.R. (1976). Hypothalamo-pituitary adrenocortical function in the rat after treatment with betamethasone. *Br. J. Pharmac.*, **56**, 235–9.

Buckingham, J.C. & Hodges, J.R. (1977a). Production of corticotrophin releasing hormone by the isolated hypothalamus of the rat. *J. Physiol.*, **272**, 469–79.

Buckingham, J.C. & Hodges, J.R. (1977b). The use of corticotrophin production by adenohypophyseal tissue *in vitro* for the detection and estimation of potential corticotrophin releasing factors. *J. Endocr.*, **72**, 187–93.

Chrousos, G.P., Udelsman, R., Gold, P.W., Margioris, A.N., Oldfield, E.H., Schürmeyer, T.H., Schülte, H.M., Doppman, J. & Loriaux, D.L. (1989). Corticotropin releasing hormone: physiological and Clinical implications. In *Neuroendocrine Perspectives*, eds. E.E. Müller & R.M. MacLeod. vol 7, pp. 49–84. Berlin: Springer-Verlag.

Clarke, M.J.O. & Gillies, G.E. (1988). Comparison of peptide release from fetal rat hypothalamic neurones cultured in defined media and serum-containing medium. *J. Endocrinology*, **116**, 349–56.

Clarke, M.J.O., Lowry, P.J. & Gillies, G.E. (1987). Assessment of corticotrophin releasing factor, vasopressin and somatostatin secretion by fetal hypothalamic neurons in culture. *Neuroendocrinology*, **46**, 147–54.

Clayton, R. (1989). Gonadotrophin releasing hormone: its actions and receptors. *J. Endocrinology*, **120**, 11–19.

Cotman, C.W., Brinton, R.E., Galaburda, A., McEwan, B. & Schneider, D.M. (Eds.) (1987). *The Neuro-Immune-Endocrine Connection.* New York: Raven Press.

Cowell, A.-M & Buckingham, J.C. (1989). Eicosanoids and the hypothalamo-pituitary axis. In *Prostaglandins, Leukotrienes and Essential Fatty Acids*, **36**, 235–50.

Cowley, A.W., Liard, J.-F. & Ansiello, D.A. (Eds) (1988). *Vasopressin Cellular and Integrative Functions.* New York: Raven Press.

Dolnikoff, M.S., Kator, C.E., Egami, M. & Andrada, I.S. (1988). Neonatal treatment with monosodium glutamate increases plasma corticosterone in the rat. *Neuroendocrinology*, **48**, 645–9.

Earnest, D.J. & Sladek, C.D. (1987). Circadian vasopressin release from perifused rat suprachiasmatic explants *in vitro*: effects of acute stimulation. *Brain Res.*, **422**, 398–402.

Everitt, B.J. & Hokfelt, T. (1986). Neuroendocrine anatomy of the hypothalamus. In *Neuroendocrinology*, eds, S.L. Lightman & B.J. Everitt. pp. 5–31. Oxford: Blackwell Scientific Publications.

Fink, G. (1988). Steroid control of brain and pituitary function. *Quart. J. exp. Physiol.*, **73**, 257–93.

Gähwiler, B.H. (1981). Organotypic monolayer cultures of nervous tissue. *J. Neurosci. Methods*, **4**, 329–42.

Gallardo, E. & Ramirez, V.D. (1977). A method for the superfusion of rat hypothalami: secretion of luteinizing hormone-releasing hormone (LH-RH). *Proc. Soc. Exp. Biol. Med.*, **155**, 79–84.

Gillies, G.E., Linton, E.A. & Lowry, P.J. (1982). Corticotrophin releasing activity of the new CRF is potentiated several times by vasopressin. *Nature*, **299**, 355–7.

Gillies, G.E. & Lowry, P.J. (1978). Perfused rat isolated anterior pituitary cell colum as a bioassay for factor(s) controlling release of adrenocorticotropin: validation of a technique. *Endocrinology*, **103**, 521–7.

Gillies, G.E., Puri, A., Hodgkinson, S. & Lowry, P.J. (1984). Involvement of rat CRF-41 and vasopressin in ACTH releasing activity from superfused rat hypothalami in vitro. *J. Endocrinol.*, **103**, 25–9.

Gregg, C.M. (1985). The compartmentalized hypothalamo-neurohypophysial system: evidence for a neurohypophysial action of acetylcholine on vasopressin release. *Neuroendocrinology*, **40**, 423–9.

Grossman, A.B., Howlett, T.A., Perry, L., Coy, D.H., Savage, M.O., Lavender, P., Rees, L.H. & Besser, G.M. (1988). CRF in the differential diagnosis of Cushing's Syndrome: a comparison with the dexamethasone suppression test. *Clinical Endocrinology*, **29**, 167–78.

Harris, G.W. (1955). *Neural Control of the Pituitary.* London: Edward Arnold.

Jones, M.T. & Gillham, B. (1988). Factors involved in the regulation of adrenocorticotropic hormone/β-lipotropic hormone. *Physiol. Rev.*, **68**, 743–818.

Jones, M.T., Gillham, B. Campbell, E.A., Al-Taher, A.R.H., Chuang, T.T. & Di Sciullo, A. (1987). Pharmacology of neural pathways affecting CRH secretion. *Ann. N.Y. Acad. Sci.*, **512**, 162–75.

Leng, G. & Bicknell, R.J. (1986). The neurohypophysis. In *Neuroendocrinology*, eds. S.L. Lightman & B.J. Everitt, pp. 177–96. Oxford: Blackwell Scientific Publications.

Lowry, P.J. (1984). Pro-opiocortin: the multiple adrenal hormone precursor. *Bioscience Reports*, **4**, 467–82.

Mains, R.E., Dickerson, I.M., May, V., Staffers, D.A., Perkins, S.N., Ouafik, L.H., Husten, E.J. & Eipper, B.A. (1990). Cellular and molecular aspects of peptide hormone synthesis. *Frontiers in Neuroendocrinology*, **11**, 52–9.

Marshall, L.A., Monroe, S.E. & Jaffe, R.B. (1988). Physiologic and therapeutic aspects of GnRH and its analogues. In *Frontiers in Neuroendocrinology* 10, eds. L. Martini, & W.F. Ganong, pp. 239–78. New York: Raven Press.

Negro-Vilar, A. & Lapetina, E.G. (1985). 1,2,-didecanoylglycerol and phorbol 12,13-dibutyrate enhance anterior pituitary hormone secretion *in vitro*. *Endocrinology*, **117**, 1559–64.

Robinson, I.C.A.F. (1986). The magnocellular and parvocellular OT and AVP systems. In *Neuroendocrinology*, eds. S.L. Lightman & B.J. Everitt, pp. 154–76. Oxford: Blackwell Scientific Publications.

Scaccianoce, S., Di Sciullo, A. & Angelucci, L. (1989). Ontogenic determinants and age-dependent changes of hypothalamo-pituitary adrenocortical axis activity in the rat: *in vitro* studies. In *The control of the Hypothalamo-Pituitary-Adrenocortical Axis*, ed. F.C. Rose, pp. 175–85. Madison: International Universities Press, Inc.

Taleisnik, S. & Sawyer, L.H. (1986). Activation of CNS adrenergic system may inhibit as well as facilitate pituitary luteinizing hormone release. *Neuroendocrinology*, **44**, 265–8.

Tannenbaum, G.S. (1988). Somatostatin as a physiological regulator of pulsatile growth hormone secretion. *Hormone Res.*, **29**, 70–4.

Vale, W., Vaughn, J., Smith, M., Yamamoto, G., Rivier, J. & Rivier, C. (1983). Effects of synthetic ovine corticotrophin-releasing factor, glucocorticodis, catecholamines, neurohypophysial peptides and other substances on cultured corticotropic cells. *Endocrinology*, **113**, 1121–30.

Wilson, C.A., Leigh, A.J. & Chapman, A.J. (1990). Gonadotrophin glycosylation and function. *J. Endocrinology*, **125**, 3–14.

# III   Thyroid and parathyroid toxicology

GERALDINE A. THOMAS AND
E. DILLWYN WILLIAMS

# 5    Thyroid gland I – physiological control and mechanisms of carcinogenesis

## Introduction

The thyroid gland is an unusual endocrine gland as not only is its function dependent on the dietary intake of a single element, but also the main epithelial component is derived embryologically from endoderm. The follicular cells still show some of the properties of intestinal mucosal cells in that they both secrete into a lumen and resorb from a lumen. The mammalian thyroid contains a minor epithelial component, the C cells, which reach the gland via the ultimobranchial body but are derived from the neural crest. The C cells secrete calcitonin and are responsive to the level of serum calcitonin. Tumours of the C cells are relatively uncommon in man but are frequently found as apparently spontaneous lesions in rodents. They are not usually of importance in carcinogenicity testing other than the need to recognize them as separate entities. This review will concentrate on the physiological control and mechanisms of carcinogenesis of the follicular cell, which is the dominant cell of the thyroid, concentrates iodide, and secretes thyroxine ($T_4$) and triiodothyronine ($T_3$).

## Structure

The follicular cells of the thyroid are arranged in closed epithelial lined spherical structures known as follicles. They possess a central lumen which contains a colloid material. The follicular cells form a single layer of normally cuboidal epithelial cells linked at their apical (inner) surfaces by tight junctions. They also show microvilli and pseudopods at their apices and are closely apposed to capillaries and to a fibroblast sheath at their basal surfaces. Thyroglobulin, which contains integral $T_3$ and $T_4$, is stored in the colloid, which serves as a reservoir of hormone which can then be used as required. The structure of the gland is of course linked to its function, and hormone synthesis and secretion can be traced from the concentration of inorganic iodide at the basal plasma membrane of the follicular cell to the storage of $T_3$ and $T_4$ as part of thyroglobulin in the colloid of the follicular lumen, and then back through the follicular cells to end with the release of $T_3$ and $T_4$ from the basal membranes of the cell.

The structure of the gland also changes with the level of thyroid stimulating hormone (TSH) stimulation. The unstimulated gland shows a flattened epithelium and dense colloid. The stimulated gland shows tall, columnar epithelium often with the follicular cells containing colloid droplets, together with a watery colloid in the follicular lumina, which, in sections of fixed tissues, shows retraction vacuoles. The colloid space is reduced and the highly stimulated gland consists largely of follicular cells forming small follicles with small colloid spaces.

Electron microscopy of follicular cells shows the presence of colloid droplets, lysosomes and phagolysosomes. The stimulated gland shows distended cisternae of the endoplasmic reticulum and prominent pseudopods at the apical surface of the cells (Halmi, 1986).

## Synthesis of thyroid hormone

Iodine is variably distributed across the earth's surface, and many complex mechanisms have evolved to cope with fluctuations in the availability of this element. Iodide is taken up into the follicular cell by an active pump mechanism which creates a gradient normally in the range of 20–40:1. This mechanism is responsive to TSH resulting in increased efficiency of uptake in times of iodide deficiency, or when there is a greater demand for thyroid hormone. This mechanism can be inhibited by anions of a similar size and charge to iodide such as $ClO_4$ and SCN. Concurrent uptake of $K^+$ occurs – drugs such as the cardiac glycosides which affect this mechanism can have an adverse effect on iodide uptake. The pump mechanism is not unique to the thyroid – it is also found in salivary glands, stomach and breast. However, the pump in these tissues is not TSH-responsive, and the concentrated iodide does not become protein bound (Bastomsky, 1984).

The next step in $T_4$ synthesis involves two thyroid-specific proteins, thyroid peroxidase (TPO) and thyroglobulin, the synthesis of which is also regulated by TSH. The inorganic iodide taken into the follicular cell by the pump mechanism is oxidized and iodinates tyrosyl residues at specialized sites on the thyroglobulin molecule. This reaction, catalysed by TPO, takes place at the apical border of the follicular cell. Iodination of tyrosyls results in the formation of mono-iodotyrosyl (MIT) and di-iodotyrosyl (DIT), and further coupling of these compounds gives rise to $T_3$ and $T_4$. All of these reactions take place on the thyroglobulin molecule and are also thought to be catalysed by TPO (see Fig. 5.1). Iodinated

THYROID HORMONE SYNTHESIS AND RELEASE

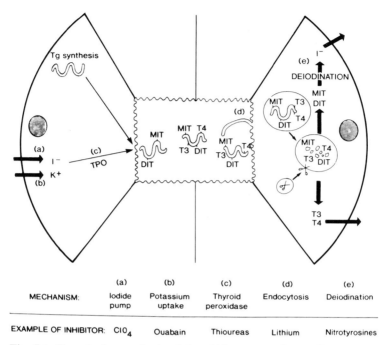

| MECHANISM: | (a)<br>Iodide<br>pump | (b)<br>Potassium<br>uptake | (c)<br>Thyroid<br>peroxidase | (d)<br>Endocytosis | (e)<br>Deiodination |
|---|---|---|---|---|---|
| EXAMPLE OF INHIBITOR: | $ClO_4$ | Ouabain | Thioureas | Lithium | Nitrotyrosines |

Fig. 5.1. Steps in the synthesis of thyroid hormones shown diagrammatically, with examples of compounds which affect these processes.

thyroglobulin is stored in the colloid which fills the follicular lumen, with the most recently synthesized thyroglobulin having the shortest half-life (van Herle, Vassart & Dumont, 1979).

### Secretion of thyroid hormone

Thyroglobulin is resorbed from the colloid into the cell through the action of pseudopods which are formed at the apical surface of the follicular cell. The rate of pseudopod formation and hence of resorption is also under TSH control and this process can be inhibited by a variety of agents including lithium (Lazarus, 1986). The endocytosis gives rise to colloid droplets within the follicular cell, these droplets then fuse with lysosomes. In the phagolysosomes so created, the thyroglobulin is broken down and $T_3$ and $T_4$ are released into the cytoplasm, as well as uncoupled MIT and DIT. The $T_3$ and $T_4$ then pass into the circulation, the iodide contained in the MIT and DIT, released by the action of deiodinase, is available for re-utilization in hormone synthesis (Stanbury & Morris, 1958). The importance of this intra-thyroid mechanism for conserving iodide is shown by the fact that absence of deiodinase activity is one of the causes of dyshormonogenesis, a rare inherited condition leading to goitrous hypothyroidism (Salvatore, Stanbury & Rall, 1980). Deiodinase deficiency is an uncommon cause; in man the most frequent cause is a defective TPO (Stanbury & Hedge, 1950); lack of the thyroid iodide pump (Stanbury & Chapman, 1960) and defective thyroglobulin (Alexander & Burrow, 1970) can also occur. The deiodinase enzyme is not confined to the thyroid.

## Circulation of thyroid hormone

The circulating thyroid hormones are very largely protein bound, the main carrier being thyroxine binding globulin (TBG), but two other proteins, thyroxine binding prealbumin and albumin itself are also involved. The function of this binding is presumably also to act as a short term buffer system which maintains the normally low levels of the free hormones that are physiologically active. The buffering system is, however, not critical. The levels of TBG, and therefore of total $T_4$, rise in pregnancy or on oestrogen treatment without any demonstrable effect on the peripheral action of thyroid hormones and conversely TBG may be congenitally absent with low total $T_4$ but again with no effect on peripheral thyroid function (Refetoff & Reed Larsen, 1989).

## Metabolism of thyroid hormones

Normally the thyroid produces much more $T_4$ than $T_3$, of the order of 10:1. $T_4$ has the longer half-life and there are much higher circulating levels of $T_4$ than $T_3$. $T_3$, however, is the more potent hormone and is formed by peripheral deiodination of $T_4$ as well as by direct production by the thyroid – this is yet another level of control (see Fig. 5.2). $T_4$ may be deiodinated either by 5′ deiodination to give the active hormone, $T_3$, or by inner ring deiodination to form reverse $T_3$ ($rT_3$) which has no known biological function (Refetoff & Reed Larsen, 1989).

Breakdown and loss of thyroid hormones, apart from the peripheral deiodination of $T_4$, occurs mainly through the liver where both $T_3$ and $T_4$ are conjugated to form either the glucuronidate or the sulphate, these are then excreted via the bile into the intestine. A proportion is hydrolyzed in the intestinal lumen, some of the $T_3$ and $T_4$ released is resorbed into the blood, but the remainder is excreted in the faeces. The rate of conjuga-

METABOLISM OF THYROID HORMONES

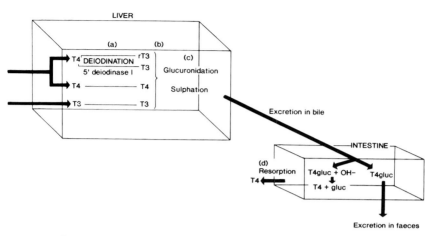

Fig. 5.2. A diagram showing the peripheral metabolism of thyroid hormones. Each of the labelled steps may be affected by xenobiotics: (a) Deiodination is inhibited by compounds such as propylthiourea. Both (b), the hepatic microsomal P450 system and (c) conjugation can be stimulated by such agents as phenobarbitone and PCBs, leading to an increased biliary clearance of thyroid hormones, resulting in a decreased plasma concentration. (d) Resorption of $T_4$ is inhibited by cholestyramine.

tion of thyroid hormone by the microsomal enzymes in the liver can be enhanced by drugs which induce enzyme synthesis (such as phenobarbital) – the importance of this regulatory level is shown by the fact that these components can increase excretion to such an extent that TSH may be elevated.

## Control of thyroid function

Key stages of thyroid hormone synthesis and secretion are under the control of TSH, and feedback control through TSH is the main mechanism in the control of thyroid function. There is a second tier of control through the action of thyrotropin releasing hormone (TRH), a tripeptide secreted by the hypothalamus which stimulates the thyrotroph in the pituitary (see Fig. 5.3A, B). This forms the route through which neural changes can modulate TSH secretion. Interestingly the main feedback control system is again complex. The nuclear binding sites within the thyrotroph that lead to the regulation of TSH secretion are $T_3$ binding

## THYROID–PITUITARY INTERACTION

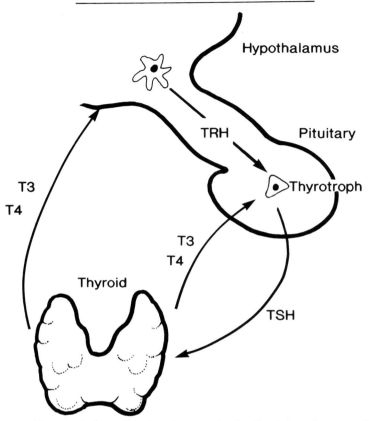

Fig. 5.3A. A diagram showing the negative feedback loop between the thyroid, the hypothalamus and the TSH-secreting cells (thyrotrophs) in the anterior pituitary.

sites, but the thyrotroph contains a deiodinase which converts $T_4$ to $T_3$ within the thyrotroph cytoplasm. As $T_4$ is present in much larger quantities than $T_3$ in the circulation, the thyrotroph is effectively responding to the level of circulating $T_4$. When $T_4$ drops, TSH secretion increases and stimulates thyroid function; when $T_4$ rises, TSH secretion is inhibited (Reed Larsen, 1982). Although the level of $T_4$ is remarkably constant under normal circumstances, there is a marked diurnal variation of TSH as with other pituitary hormones.

The three glycoprotein pituitary hormones share a common alpha chain and show considerable homology between their beta chains. It is

## THYROID–PITUITARY INTERACTION

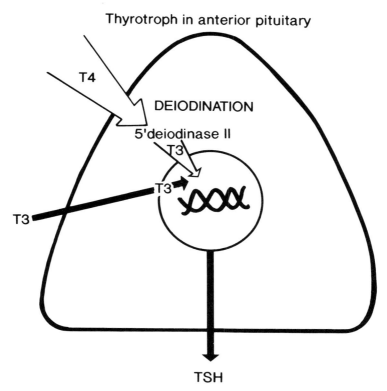

Fig. 5.3B. Diagrammatic representation of thyroid hormone metabolism by, and action on the thyrotroph.

now recognized that high levels of chorionic gonadotrophin can stimulate thyroid function, and cause the mild thyrotoxicosis that may be found with hydatiform mole or choriocarcinoma, both gonadotrophin secreting tumours of placental origin (Nisula & Talisadourus, 1980).

### Dietary iodide and control of thyroid function

The previous paragraphs have shown that the synthesis, release and metabolism of thyroid hormone is capable of modification at a number of points. Many of these controlling mechanisms seem to be related to variation in dietary iodide.

Firstly, the rate at which the thyroid concentrates iodide, the iodide pump, is TSH dependent, as is the rate of synthesis of both thyroglobulin and TPO. If iodide deficiency lowers the production of thyroid hormone, TSH rises and the thyroid becomes more efficient at collecting iodide and thus will make more thyroglobulin. This therefore, at least partly, compensates for the iodide deficiency by making more iodinated tyrosines – but the ratio of MIT to DIT increases so that there will be relatively more $T_3$ than $T_4$ produced. As $T_3$ is the more potent hormone, this too will mitigate the effect of the iodide deficiency. The unusual mechanism of the response of the pituitary thyrotroph still further adds to the compensation as it responds to $T_4$ – the more heavily iodinated but less potent hormone. A minor drop in dietary iodide will give little change in $T_3$ production but a greater drop in $T_4$. TSH therefore, responds to a very small drop in iodide intake in a way which could be regarded as precautionary. In severe iodide deficiency, when these compensatory mechanisms are not sufficient, there is of course a persistently raised TSH and thyroid growth results. The number of follicular cells, therefore, increases as well as their efficiency in thyroid hormone production. The control of growth is central to our understanding of thyroid carcinogenesis and this will be discussed in the next section.

## Regulation of thyroid growth

The major regulation of thyroid growth is achieved through the production of TSH by the thyrotroph cells of the pituitary gland. Administration of a substance (a goitrogen) that inhibits one of the chain of events concerned with thyroid hormone synthesis – usually either an iodide pump inhibitor (e.g. perchlorate; Wyngaarden, Stanbury & Rapp, 1953), or a TPO inhibitor (e.g. thiouracil; Taurog, 1976), leads to a drop in thyroid hormone output. This in turn leads to an increase in TSH, and to thyroid follicular cell growth if the degree of reduction of $T_3$ and $T_4$ production is sufficiently great and sufficiently prolonged. Hypophysectomy abolishes the goitrogenic response, thus showing the key role of the pituitary (Jemec, 1980). This simple feedback regulation of thyroid growth conceals a much more complex system that is not yet fully understood.

When the intact animal is exposed to prolonged TSH elevation (whether induced by iodide deficiency or goitrogen exposure) thyroid growth results. This was originally assessed only by the weight increase of the gland and it was observed that the weight increase was not continuous but was initially rapid followed by a new steady state or plateau (Christov, 1975). Several tissue components contribute to the overall weight of the gland. Careful morphometric studies have, however, shown that although the relative amount of colloid declines, both follicular cell mass and follicular cell number increase with prolonged goitrogen treatment and reach a plateau after about six weeks exposure in the rat (Wynford-Thomas, Stringer & Williams, 1982a). Measurement of serum TSH in prolonged goitrogen treatment showed that this remained elevated throughout, and measurement of the functional response to TSH – in this case the iodide pump response – showed that this was unimpaired. The growth response measured as metaphase index, at first rose dramatically in response to the elevated TSH but after a few weeks dropped sharply to reach levels close to those found in untreated animals. These studies, therefore, showed that the growth and functional response of the thyroid to elevated TSH became uncoupled after a few weeks (Wynford-Thomas *et al.*, 1982b). Removal and reintroduction of the goitrogen led to a drop in TSH followed by a rapid rise to the former elevated levels. This second rise in TSH was not accompanied by a second peak in the metaphase index, showing that the change was not a simple down-regulation of TSH receptors or other reversible phenomenon but appeared to be a permanent change (Wynford-Thomas *et al.*, 1982c).

Incision of the thyroid isthmus was accompanied by mitotic activity in the adjacent follicular cells and this ability of the follicular cells was not impaired in long term goitrogen treated animals (Wynford-Thomas *et al.*, 1985). This shows that whatever mechanism limits the growth response of the follicular cell to TSH is not an inability to divide, as would be expected by simple senescence, as is seen in cultured fibroblasts (Hayflick, 1965), but is at least partly stimulus specific. Control of normal proliferation is recognized as being regulated by a mixture of stimulatory and inhibitory factors. The follicular cell growth restriction mechanism to TSH may, therefore, involve production of a factor which normally limits proliferation (a so-called anti-oncogene effect), either in a direct or indirect manner. If this growth restriction mechanism is lost, due to mutation in one cell during long-term goitrogen treatment, the resulting clone of cells will continue to divide in response to the elevation of TSH.

## Growth factor control of normal follicular cell proliferation

The proof that TSH is indeed the main mitogen for thyroid follicular cells was made difficult for many years by the problems encountered demonstrating that TSH was mitogenic for thyroid cells in culture (Westermark, Karlson & Walinder, 1979). More recently these problems have been shown to be the result of a requirement for other growth factors in the culture medium. Primary follicular cell cultures do not usually survive for more than a few days or weeks – presumably in part because of the anti-oncogene effect. Using a thyroid cell line which was immortal but retained TSH responsiveness, it was shown that the cells would grow in response to TSH in the presence, but not the absence, of a cocktail of five growth factors (Ambesi-Impiombata, Parks & Coon, 1980). Several groups have now shown that a dose-dependent growth response to TSH occurs in primary culture of follicular cells in synthetic medium if only one growth factor, either insulin at high concentrations or insulin-like growth factor 1 ($IGF_1$) at physiological concentrations, is present. This has been shown for rat (Smith *et al.*, 1986), man (Williams, Wynford-Thomas & Williams, 1987; Williams, Williams & Wynford-Thomas, 1988) and dog follicular cells (Roger, Servais & Dumont, 1983). Porcine thyroid cells, however, have not been shown to grow in response to TSH in culture, even in the presence of $IGF_1$ (Gartner & Greil, 1986).

It is likely that the *in vitro* requirement for $IGF_1$ to allow a growth response to TSH to occur is also an *in vivo* requirement, although this has not been shown directly. The source of the $IGF_1$ *in vivo* is also not known but it may be from thyroid epithelial cells from the thyroid stroma – certainly fibroblasts have been shown to be capable of producing $IGF_1$ in culture (Adams *et al.*, 1984). A positive feedback loop between follicular and stromal cells would permit the co-ordinated growth that is necessary – follicular growth must normally be accompanied by stromal growth to maintain structure. In its simplest model this would involve the TSH mediated production by the thyroid follicular cells of a substance stimulating the stromal cell to produce $IGF_1$; with TSH and $IGF_1$ being necessary for follicular cell growth, and possibly $IGF_1$ and the other intercellular growth factor being required for stromal cell growth. This model using three factors – TSH, an unknown and $IGF_1$ – is the simplest, but several other growth factors are known from *in vitro* studies to be produced by, or to influence follicular cell growth. These include $IGF_2$ (Maciel *et al.*, 1988), epidermal growth factor (EGF) and fibroblast growth factor (FGF), (Roger & Dumont, 1984). Interestingly, EGF stimulates follicular cell growth but inhibits follicular cell function (Roger & Dumont, 1984). As well as stimulatory factors, inhibitory factors may also occur and TGFβ has been shown to inhibit the growth stimulatory effect of both TSH (with $IGF_1$) and EGF (Grubeck-Loewenstein *et al.*, 1989).

There is also evidence for an autoregulatory effect related to the availability of iodide; the thyroid growth response to exogenous TSH in hypophysectomized rats has been shown to be greater in iodide deficient than in iodide replete rats (Bray, 1968). It has been suggested that this response may be due to an organic iodide compound which inhibits the follicular cell growth response to TSH (Becks, Eggo & Burrow, 1988).

The discussion of the control of physiological growth of the thyroid follicular cell has largely, and properly, centred on the role of TSH. However, follicular cell growth can occur in the absence of TSH as was shown for developmental thyroid growth by Jost (1953) and for the growth of thyroid autografts by Williams & Doniach (1963). The growth that follows direct injury can also occur in the TSH suppressed animal. Follicular cell growth has also been described following the refeeding of iodide to iodide deficient mice; this appears to be unrelated to TSH (Many *et al.*, 1983). It is associated with a sudden increase in thyroglobulin production and could follow rapid follicular distension.

## Thyroid carcinogenesis

The physiological mechanisms of control of the thyroid follicular cells are complex, and through control of function and growth maintain the effective level of thyroid hormone at an appropriate setting while also maintaining an ability to respond rapidly to any sudden demand. The mechanisms involved in thyroid carcinogenesis can only be understood against a background of how the normal control system operates and indeed how some of the complexity of the mechanisms of growth control may be related to the 'need' to limit the frequency with which cancers can develop – the more complex the system, in general, the more defects will be required to overcome the safeguards.

## Pathology of thyroid lesions

Before considering the mechanisms which are involved in thyroid tumourigenesis, it is necessary to consider briefly the patterns of human and experimental lesions. In man, benign thyroid tumours are common, while carcinomas are rare. The benign lesions are divided into nodules and adenomas, both with follicular architecture but with the typical nodule being an encapsulated lesion composed of colloid rich follicles lined by inactive flattened epithelium, while the typical adenoma is encapsulated and composed of more cellular follicles sometimes with trabecular or solid areas. While the two types of lesions are typically easily separable it is not uncommon to find lesions which are difficult to classify, particularly in nodular goitres from patients from iodide deficient areas.

Thyroid carcinomas derived from the follicular cell are divided into follicular and papillary carcinomas. These terms are unfortunate as they focus attention on the architecture of the lesion rather than the overall differences between these two separate biological entities. Follicular carcinomas are encapsulated, solitary lesions. They show invasion of veins and characteristically metastasize to bones. Papillary carcinomas are unencapsulated and multifocal. They show invasion of lymphatics and characteristically metastasize to the lymph nodes. Follicular carcinomas may show a follicular, trabecular or solid structure. Papillary carcinomas commonly show a mixture of papillary and follicular architecture – rarely they may show an entirely follicular structure. Papillary carcinomas also characteristically show crowded, irregular, often grooved nuclei which may show cytoplasmic inclusions and may appear pale on light microscopic examination (Hedinger, Williams & Sobin, 1988). It is of particular interest that follicular carcinomas are more common in iodide deficient areas while papillary carcinomas are more common in areas with a high iodide intake (Williams et al., 1977).

The rare undifferentiated (anaplastic) carcinoma of the thyroid is an exceptionally rapidly growing malignant tumour which is composed of extremely pleomorphic spindle and giant cells. It shows no evidence of papillary or follicular differentiation, except for areas of surviving papillary or follicular carcinoma from which it may have arisen.

In experimental animals the same pattern of tumours may be seen except that the distinction between papillary and follicular tumours is much less clear-cut. It must be remembered that most experimental tumours are induced by mechanisms involving a high level of TSH stimulation and that the majority of such tumours are purely follicular in structure. One exception is in experimental tumours of the guinea-pig where most lesions show a papillary structure (Williams E.D., unpub. obs.).

## Animal models of thyroid carcinogenesis

The models of thyroid carcinogenesis followed in most experimental studies use prolonged goitrogen treatment alone or use radiation with or without subsequent goitrogen treatment. Radiation obviously has a mutagenic effect but the mutagenic effect alone is not by itself, carcinogenic, as has been shown by the lack of tumour formation if radiation is given to hypophysectomized rats (Nadler, Mandavia & Goldberg, 1970), or if radiation is followed by prolonged TSH suppression with thyroid hormone (Doniach, 1974). Carcinogenic doses of radiation given to rats are followed by a rise in TSH resulting from the destructive effects of radiation on the gland. Increasing the dose of radiation increases the destructive effect until all cells are eventually destroyed or rendered incapable of division. The dose effect curve of radiation alone in thyroid carcinogenesis is, therefore, bell-shaped, with the peak carcinogenic dose resulting from a balance between the effects of the increasing dose in increasing the number of appropriate mutations and the effect of the increasing dose in increasing the damage to the thyroid. The latter effect leads to an increase in TSH levels but the consequence of this, in increasing tumour numbers, is counteracted at higher doses through loss of cells with the potential to divide. The key role of TSH stimulation in these experimental models of thyroid carcinogenesis is paralleled in follicular tumours in man. The link of benign follicular tumours and of follicular carcinoma to iodide deficiency suggests the importance of TSH in their genesis and more direct evidence is provided in patients with dyshormonogenesis. Here a congenital defect in one of the steps in the formation of thyroid hormone leads, in the absence of treatment, to a life-long increase in TSH. Untreated patients usually present with nodular goitre in their teens or early adult life and are found to have numerous benign tumours, both nodules and adenomas. While carcinoma is uncommon, when it does occur it is almost always follicular in type (Vickery, 1981).

## Pathobiology of thyroid tumours

It seems likely that both in humans and other animals there is a sequential progression to increasing malignancy with follicular adenoma giving rise to follicular carcinoma, and follicular carcinoma to anaplastic carcinoma. The evidence that a proportion of follicular adenomas progress to follicular carcinomas is based on the age incidence and on the morphology of the lesions. Follicular carcinomas and adenomas can in general only be distinguished morphologically by the presence of invasion in the former. In addition, it is common to see foci of a less differentiated tumour within more differentiated adenomas. The evidence that both follicular and papillary carcinomas can progress to anaplastic carcinoma is based on the regular finding of foci of either papillary or follicular carcinoma within anaplastic carcinomas. As the differentiated carcinomas are slow growing while the anaplastic carcinoma is very rapidly growing, the conclusion that the anaplastic carcinoma is derived from a pre-existing more differentiated carcinoma seems clear (Ibanez *et al.*, 1966). The age incidence of the tumours concerned is consistent with this. Interestingly, papillary carcinomas apparently arise directly from follicular epithelium.

The stepwise progression from normal follicular cell to follicular adenoma, to follicular carcinoma, to anaplastic carcinoma, supports the clonal progression theory of malignancy. In this, tumours arise as a result of one or more mutations in a single cell which gives rise to a clone of cells, one cell of which then generates a sub-clone, which through a further mutation acquires an additional growth advantage.

This sequential development of malignancy ignores the nodule. It may precede an adenoma but this is not clear. To investigate this and to study the clonality of thyroid adenomas we have developed an approach using a system to identify clonality, based on the histochemical identification of glucose-6-phosphate dehydrogenase (G6PD) in female mice heterozygous for G6PD deficiency. As the enzyme is X-linked, and as in female mammals only one X-chromosome is expressed in each somatic cell Lyon, 1972), the technique shows that the female heterozygote is composed of a mixture of cells of high and of low enzyme activity (Thomas, Williams & Williams, 1988). As the pattern of suppression of the X-chromosome (paternal or maternal) is inherited at the cellular level, histochemistry of tumours induced in these animals can be used to demonstrate their clonality. Benign thyroid follicular lesions showed two patterns of clonality which correlated with their morphology – nodules showed polyclonal epithelium, while the adenomas showed monoclonal epithelium (Thomas, Williams & Williams, 1989). It seems likely that this conclusion will apply to human thyroid tumours also.

In the stepwise development of spontaneous human thyroid follicular carcinoma, a number of defects must be acquired, but three events are pre-requisite. The cells must lose their growth limitation, they must acquire TSH independent growth and they must acquire invasiveness. Normally it is likely that this is the order of events. We have investigated the clonality and the ability to regress of adenomas and carcinomas induced by high dose radiation and prolonged goitrogen treatment. Both adenomas and carcinomas were shown to be monoclonal. However, when the goitrogen treatment was withdrawn these tumours regressed – even the carcinomas with clear-cut vascular invasion (Thomas *et al.*, 1991). This finding we interpret as showing that when thyroid tumours are induced by prolonged blocking doses of goitrogen the high TSH removes any selective advantage that may have been conferred by the development of TSH independent growth. As TSH independent growth does not occur, malignancy develops as a result of one less step than is found in the spontaneous tumour. This explanation accounts for the much greater frequency of experimental tumours when the regime includes any agent that induces a high level of TSH.

A second mechanism may also be important. We know that translocation is an important mechanism in carcinogenesis and we suggest that translocation of an oncogene to a TSH dependent promoter may be a significant mechanism in thyroid carcinogenesis, and one which is more likely to occur and to be effective in persistently TSH stimulated cells. This would also account for the regression that occurs when TSH stimulation is withdrawn in the absence of the development of any TSH independent growth.

These are theories, but the practical importance of these observations, and the subsequent discussion, is that regression of the lesion on withdrawal of a growth stimulus should not be taken as proof that the lesion is not a tumour. A non-mutagenic agent that interferes with any aspect of thyroid hormone synthesis or metabolism that leads to an increased TSH level will increase the frequency of thyroid tumour production. Administration of a mutagen followed by a goitrogen will also increase the frequency of thyroid tumour production, and as we have shown these tumours will regress when the goitrogen is withdrawn. Regression, therefore, not only does not prove that the lesion is not a tumour, it also does not prove that the agent given was not mutagenic.

The discussion on the control of normal thyroid growth pointed out that growth factors other than TSH are involved; these growth factors are also likely to be important in carcinogenesis. Work in our department has shown that follicular cells from human thyroid adenomas will, unlike normal follicular cells, grow in culture in response to TSH without added $IGF_1$ (Williams *et al.*, 1988). Later studies showed that this was due to autocrine production of $IGF_1$ by the follicular adenoma cells themselves (Williams *et al.*, 1989). The production of $IGF_1$ by stromal cells is possibly required for normal thyroid follicular cell growth; it may also be a limiting factor in early neoplastic growth. This limitation could be overcome by the development of autocrine production of $IGF_1$. It is likely that other examples of the subversion of the role of normal stimulating or inhibiting growth factors in neoplasia will be found in the future.

The changes in growth control stem from mutations or epimutations and the nature of these has also been investigated. Mutations in the ras gene have been shown to be common in human follicular tumours, possibly less so in papillary carcinoma. Interestingly, the ras mutation seems to occur in the microfollicular adenoma rather than the macrofollicular adenoma and then occurs with roughly equal frequency in differentiated follicular carcinomas and in anaplastic carcinomas. Mutations of all three ras genes (Harvey, Kirsten and N) are found, and there is a surprisingly frequent occurrence of gly to arg mutations at position 61 (Lemoine *et al.*, 1989). Papillary carcinomas show a relatively low frequency of ras mutation but a proportion show a newly described oncogene, ptc, derived from translocation of the related ret oncogene (Fusco *et al.*, 1987). The exact role of these mutations in the neoplastic process is not known. The ras gene is one of the more frequent oncogenes to show mutations in human epithelial tumours. It is known to be a G protein and it is likely, therefore, that the mutation leads to it being constitutively active. It is not, however, known with which receptor the ras G protein is associated (Sigal, 1988).

## Summary

The mechanisms of carcinogenesis in the thyroid, therefore, are both genotoxic and non-genotoxic, and frequently the two are combined. We can now begin to see the way in which the sequential changes in the genome that lead to development of thyroid carcinoma interact with changes in the growth control mechanisms, allowing the successive clones of tumour cells to increase their growth rate and acquire independence from negative growth control. The molecular basis of many of these changes remains to be discovered. From the point of view of the toxicologist, perhaps the most important fact is the role that TSH plays in increasing the incidence of thyroid tumours. Any substance that leads to a significant rise in the level of TSH can be predicted to produce an increase in thyroid neoplasia. Addition of a mutagen to the growth stimulation causes more thyroid tumours, including carcinomas, but these tumours may still be capable of regression after the growth stimulus is withdrawn. The development of thyroid tumours following the administration of a drug which interferes with thyroid hormone metabolism does not prove that the drug is mutagenic. The regression of such tumours when the drug is withdrawn does not prove that it is not mutagenic. Such regression does however show that the lesion has not developed autonomous growth. We conclude that the development of thyroid tumours following administration of a substance that has been shown to interfere with thyroid hormone synthesis or metabolism cannot on its own be used as evidence that the substance is carcinogenic in the conventional sense of the term.

## References

Adams, S.O., Kapadia, M., Mills, B. & Daughaday, W.H. (1984). Release of insulin-like growth factors and binding protein activity into serum-free medium of cultured human fibroblasts. *Endocrinol.*, **115**, 520–6.

Alexander, N.M. & Burrow, G.N. (1970). Thyroxine biosynthesis in human goitrous cretinism. *J. Clin. Endocrinol. Metab.*, **30**, 308–15.

Ambesi-Impiombato, F.S., Parks, L.A.M. & Coon, H.G. (1980).

Culture of hormone-dependent functional epithelial cells from rat thyroids. *PNAS USA*, **77**, 3455–9.

Bastomsky, C.H. (1984). Thyroid iodide transport. In *Handbook of Physiology*, vol III *Endocrinology*, ed. R.O. Greep & E.B. Astwood, pp. 81–9. Washington DC: American Physiological Society.

Becks, G.P., Eggo, M.C. & Burrow, G.N. (1988). Organic iodide inhibits deoxyribonucleic acid synthesis and growth in FRTL-5 thyroid cells. *Endocrinol.*, **123**, 545–51.

Bray, G.A. (1968). Increased sensitivity of the thyroid in iodine-depleted rats to the goitrogenic effects of thyrotropin. *J. Clin. Invest.*, **47**, 1640–7.

Christov, K. (1975). Thyroid cell proliferation in rats and induction of tumours by X-rays. *Cancer Res.*, **35**, 1256–62.

Doniach, I. (1974). Carcinogenic effect of 100, 200, 250 and 500 rad X-rays on the rat thyroid gland. *Br. J. Cancer*, **30**, 487–95.

Fusco, A., Grieco, M., Santoro, M., Berlingieri, M.T., Pilotti, S., Pierotti, M.A., Della Porta, G. Vecchio, G. (1987). A new oncogene in human thyroid papillary carcinomas and their lymph-nodal metastases. *Nature*, **328**, 170–2.

Gartner, R. & Griel, W. (1986). The mitogenic activity of IGF1, insulin and EGF on isolated porcine thyroid follicles under negative control of TSH and cAMP. *Ann. Endocrinol.*, **47**, 66A.

Grubeck-Loewenstein, B., Buchan, G., Sadeghi, R., Kissonerghis, M., Londei, M., Turner, M., Pirich, K., Roka, R., Niederle, B., Kassal, H., Waldhausal, W. & Feldman, M. (1989). Transforming growth factor β regulates thyroid growth. *J. Clin. Invest.*, **83**, 764–70.

Halmi, N.S. (1986). Anatomy and histochemistry. In *The Thyroid*, ed. S.H. Ingbar & L.E. Braverman, pp. 24–42. Philadelphia: J.P. Lippincort Co.

Hayflick, L. (1965). The limited *in vitro* lifetime of human diploid strains. *Exp. Cell Res.*, **37**, 614–46.

Hedinger, Ch., Williams, E.D., Sobin, L.H. (1988). *Histological Typing of Thyroid Tumours*, 2nd edn, *WHO International Histological Classification of Tumours*. Berlin: Springer-Verlag.

Ibanez, M.C., Russell, W.O., Albores-Saavedra, J., Lampertico, P., White, E.C. & Clark, R.L. (1966). Thyroid carcinoma – biological behaviour and mortality. *Cancer*, **19**, 1039–52.

Jemec, B. (1980). Studies on the goitrogenic and tumorigenic effect of two goitrogens in combination with hypophysectomy or thyroid hormone treatment. *Cancer*, **45**, 2138–48.

Jost, A. (1953) Sur le développement de la gland thyroide chez le foetus de lapin decapité. *Arch. Anta. Micro. Morph. Exp.*, **42**, 168.

Lazarus, J.H. (1986). *Endocrine and Metabolic Effects of Lithium*. New York: Plenum Medical Book Company.

Lemoine, N.R., Mayall, E.S., Wyllie, F.S., Williams, E.D., Goyns, M., Stringer, B. & Wynford-Thomas, D. (1989). High frequency of ras oncogene activation in all stages of human thyroid tumorigenesis. *Oncogene*, **4**, 159–64.

Lyon, M.F. (1972). X-chromosome inactivation and developmental patterns in mammals. *Biol. Rev.*, **57**, 1–35.

Maciel, R.M.B., Moses, A.C., Villone, G., Tramontano, D. & Ingbar, S.H. (1988). Demonstration of the production and physiological role of insulin-like growth factor II in rat thyroid follicular cells in culture. *J. Clin. Invest.*, **82**, 1546–53.

Many, M.C., Denef, J.P., Gathy, P. & Haumont, S. (1983). Morphological and functional changes during thyroid hyperplasia and involution in C3H mice: evidence for folliculogenesis during involution. *Endocrinology*, **112**, 1292–302.

Nadler, N.J., Mandavia, M., Goldberg, M. (1970). The effect of hypophysectomy on the experimental production of rat thyroid neoplasia. *Cancer Res.*, **30**, 1909–11.

Nisula, B.C. & Talisadourus, G.S. (1980). Thyroid function in gestational fibroblastic neoplasia. Evidence that the thyrotrophic activity of chorionic gonadotrophin mediates the thyrotoxicosis of choriocarcinoma. *Am. J. Obstet. Gynaecol.*, **138**, 77–5.

Reed Larsen, P. (1982). Thyroid-pituitary interaction. *N. Eng. J. Med.*, **306**, 23–32.

Refetoff, S. & Reed Larsen, P. (1989). Transport, cellular uptake and metabolism of thyroid hormones. In *Endocrinology*, ed. L. De Groot, vol I, pp. 541–61. Philadelphia: WB Saunders & Co.

Roger, P.P. & Dumont, J.E. (1984). Factors controlling proliferation and differentiation of canine thyroid cells cultured in reduced serum conditions: effects of thyrotrophin, cyclic AMP and growth factors. *Mol. Cell Endocrinol.*, **36**, 79–93.

Roger, P.P., Servais, P. & Dumont, J.E. (1983). Stimulation by thyrotropin and cyclic AMP of the proliferation of quiescent canine thyroid cells cultured in a defined medium containing insulin. *FEBS Letters*, **157**, 323–9.

Salvatore, G., Stanbury, J. B. & Rall, J. E. (1980). Inherited defects of thyroid hormone biosynthesis. In *Comprehensive Endocrinology: The Thyroid Gland*, ed. M. De Visscher, pp. 443–87. New York: Raven Press.

Sigal I.S. (1988). The ras oncogene: a structure and some function. *Nature*, **332**, 485–6.

Smith, P., Wynford-Thomas, D., Stringer, B.M.J. & Williams, E.D. (1986). Growth factor control of rat thyroid follicular cell proliferation. *Endocrinology*, **119**, 1439–45.

Stanbury, J.B. & Chapman, E.M. (1960). Congenital hypothyroidism with goitre: absence of an iodide-concentrating mechanism. *Lancet*, **i**, 1162–5.

Stanbury, J.B. & Hedge, A.N. (1950). A study of a family of goitrous cretins. *J. Clin. Endocrinol.*, **10**, 1741–58.

Stanbury, J.B. & Morris, M.L. (1958). Deiodination of diiodotyrosine by cell-free systems. *J. Biol. Chem.*, **233**, 106–8.

Taurog, A. (1976). The mechanism of action of the thiourylene anti-thyroid drugs. *Endocrinology*, **98**, 1031–46.

Thomas, G.A., Williams, D. & Williams, E.D. (1988). The demonstration of tissue chonality by X-linked enzyme histochemistry. *J. Pathol.*, **155**, 101–8.

Thomas, G.A., Williams, D. & Williams, E.D. (1989). The clonal origin of thyroid nodules and adenomas. *Am. J. Pathol.*, **134**, 141–7.

Thomas, G.A., Williams, D. & Williams, E.D. (1991). Reversibility of the malignant phenotype in monocloncal thyroid in the mouse. *Br. J. Cancer*, **63**, 213–16.

van Herle, A.J., Vassart, G. & Dumont, J.E. (1979). Control of thyroglobulin synthesis and secretion. *N. Eng. J. Med.*, **301**, 239–49.

Vickery, A.L. (1981). The diagnosis of malignancy in dyshormono-genetic goitre. *Clinics. Endocrinol. Metabl.*, **10**, 317–35.

Westermark, B., Karlson, F.A. & Walinder, D. (1979). Thyrotropin is not a growth factor for human thyroid cell in culture. *PNAS USA*, **76**, 2022–6.

Williams, D.W., Williams, E.D. & Wynford- Thomas, D. (1988). Loss of dependence on IGF-1 for proliferation of human thyroid adenoma cells. *Br. J. Cancer*, **57**, 535–9.

Williams, D.W., Williams, E.D. & Wynford-Thomas, D. (1989). Evidence for autocrine production of IGF-1 in human thyroid adenomas. *Mol. Cell. Endocrinol.*, **61**, 139–43.

Williams, D.W., Wynford-Thomas, D. & Williams, E.D. (1987) Control of human thyroid follicular cell proliferation in suspension and monolayer culture. *Mol. Cell. Endocrinol.*, **31**, 33–40.

Williams, E.D. & Doniach, I. (1963). Thyroid autografts in hypophysec-tomised and thyroxine treated rats. *J. Endocrinol.*, **26**, 479–88.

Williams, E.D., Doniach, I., Bjarnasan, O. & Michie, W. (1977). Thyroid cancer in an iodide rich area. *Cancer*, **39**, 215–22.

Wynford-Thomas, D., Stringer, B.M.J., Harach, H.R. & Williams, E.D. (1985). Mitotic response in goitrous and normal rat thyroid: implications for thyroid growth control. *Cell Tissue Kinet.*, **18**, 467–73.

Wynford-Thomas, D., Stringer, B.M.J. & Williams, E.D. (1982a). Goitrogen induced thyroid growth in the rat: a quantitative morpho-metric study. *J. Endocrinol.*, **94**, 131–40.

Wynford-Thomas, D., Stringer, B.M.J. & Williams, E.D. (1982b). Dissociation of growth and function in the rat thyroid during prolonged goitrogen administration. *Acta Endocrinol.*, **101**, 210–16.

Wynford-Thomas, D., Stringer, B.M.J. & Williams, E.D. (1982c) Desensitisation of rat thyroid to the growth stimulating action of TSH during prolonged goitrogen administration. *Acta Endocrinol.*, **101**, 562–9.

Wyngaarden, J.B., Stanbury, J.B. & Rapp, B. (1953). The effect of iodide, perchlorate thiocyanate and nitrate administration upon the iodide concentrating mechanism of the rat thyroid. *Endocrinology*, **52**, 568–74.

CHRISTOPHER K. ATTERWILL,
CHRISTINE JONES AND CAROL G. BROWN

# 6    Thyroid gland II – Mechanisms of species-dependent thyroid toxicity, hyperplasia and neoplasia induced by xenobiotics

## Introduction

Thyroid function can be perturbed by agents affecting a number of processes involved in the thyroid endocrine homeostatic system (Fig. 6.1). These agents can affect function directly by interacting with thyroid cell receptors or their intracellular transduction mechanisms (see Fig. 6.7). Alternatively thyroid function may be altered indirectly by agents affecting thyroid hormone metabolism – this event being followed by the release of thyrotrophic factors, or by xenobiotic-mediated alterations in the release of these factors themselves from the hypothalamus or pituitary gland (see also review by Cavalieri & Pitt-Rivers, 1981).

### Control of thyroid function

For ease of understanding of the following sections it is necessary to consider in detail the control of mammalian thyroid follicular function as shown schematically in Fig. 6.1, together with the points at which agents may perturb function. The most common classes of agent affecting function are shown at loci A–E.

The various control mechanisms and factors influencing hormone synthesis, distribution and metabolism can be summarized as follows: thyroid hormone ($T_3$ & $T_4$) synthesis and secretion from the thyroid gland are controlled by thyroid stimulating hormone (TSH) released from the pituitary gland. This in turn is under control by hypothalamic thyrotrophin releasing hormone (TRH) and circulating levels of the thyroid hormones.

Thyroid hormones exist in the circulation in the free (free $T_4$ ($FT_4$) and free $T_3$ ($FT_3$)) and protein-bound forms (approx. 99% of total $T_4$–$TT_4$ and total $T_3$–$TT_3$) and it is the $FT_3$ hormone produced by deiodination from $T_4$ which has both a physiological action on $T_3$ nuclear receptors in target tissues and influences pituitary TSH output.

Protein-binding of the hormone in the circulation takes place on

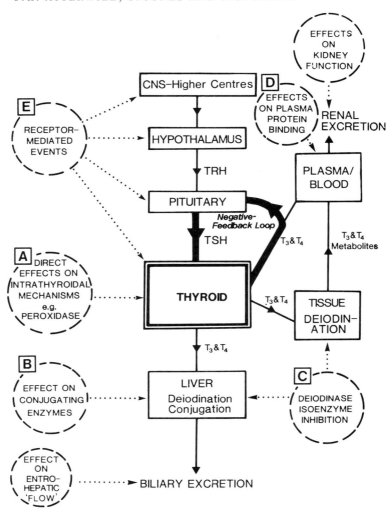

Fig. 6.1. Drugs and thyroid function.

several moieties, the profiles of which vary between different species. The major proteins are thyroglobulin (TBG), thyroid binding prealbumin (TBPA) and albumin. Free and bound $T_3$ and $T_4$ are in dynamic equilibrium in the circulation and because of differences in affinity for the binding proteins there is more $T_3$ in the unbound form (approx. 0.4% of total) than $T_4$ (approx. 0.04% of total).

Thyroid hormone synthesis takes place at the apical membrane of the polarized follicular epithelial cells and depends on TSH-stimulated active iodide uptake under the influence of many extracellular and intracellular factors and signals (see Fig. 6.4). Iodide is oxidized by peroxidase enzymes which mediate the incorporation of iodine into the tyrosyl residues of the colloidal glycoprotein, thyroglobulin. Colloid-bound thyroid hormone is stored in the follicular lumen and is released into the circulation by lysosomal action on the colloidal complex following endocytosis of colloid droplets into the cells.

Metabolism of $FT_3$ and $FT_4$ is achieved by three routes (see Fig. 6.5). The two major ones are deiodination and conjugation (glucuronidation and sulphation) and a minor one is deamination/decarboxylation. Bastomsky (1973) studied the excretion of $T_4$ in the Gunn rat, a strain genetically deficient in several glucuronyl-transferases (including $T_4$-glucuronyltransferase) and concluded that that rate-limiting step in the biliary excretion of $T_4$ is the formation of the glucuronic acid conjugate. Hepatic conjugation, either sulphation (preferring $FT_3$) or glucuronidation (preferring $FT_4$) yields a more water-soluble product which is excreted in the bile. Deiodination can occur at several sites – the ones of major importance from the clearance aspect being liver and kidney whilst pituitary deiodination is essential for controlling responsiveness to circulating $FT_4$ levels. The deiodinases exist as three isozymes: Type I ($5^1$-D; localized in liver, kidney, thyroid and central nervous system (CNS) tissue; and is propylthiouracil (PTU) sensitive); Type II ($5^1$-D; localized exclusively in the CNS, brown adipose tissue, and pituitary; PTU-insensitive); and Type III (5-D, CNS; PTU insensitive) and have different affinities for $T_4$, different maturational patterns and different compensatory responses to hypothyroidism (see Kohrle, Brabant & Hesch, 1987).

The initial thyroid responses to increasing TSH levels are follicular cell hypertrophy, loss of colloid and vascular dilatation. In conventional animal toxicology studies performed for regulatory authorities one of the first indices of thyrotoxicity, therefore, is the observation of altered thyroid histopathology primarily as follicular cell hypertrophy and/or diffuse hyperplasia, often leading to focal hyperplasia, thyroid adenomas and adenocarcinomas in longer-term toxicity studies.

## Thyroid follicular cell hyperplasia and neoplasia

Thyroid neoplasia (see Fig. 6.2) develops predictably in experimental species exposed to any procedure inducing prolonged and excessive TSH secretion, for example, the administration of chemical goitrogens, chronic iodine deficiency or subtotal thyroidectomy, although humans and mouse appear to be more resistant to TSH-induced thyroid neoplasia

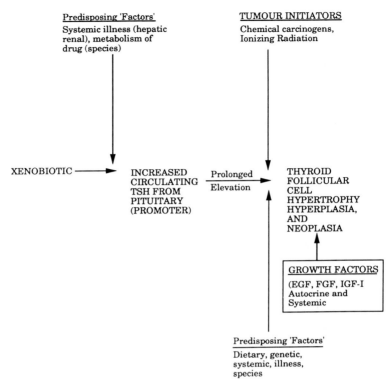

Fig. 6.2. Factors influencing the development of thyroid neoplasia.

than rat. The number of cytogenetic abnormalities within the thyroid epithelium increases with duration of excess TSH exposure, with follicular cell hyperplasia potentially leading to neoplasia. The histopathological sequence of events is as follows (see Zbinden, 1987): following hypertrophy of the follicular epithelial cells focal hyperplasias appear in the gland which are distinct areas of papillary growth with enlarged epithelia. As these foci continue to grow they form nodules partly surrounded by collagenous fibres. These lesions are transition states between focal hyperplasias and adenomas. Adenomas are larger nodules that compress the surrounding tissue and have a distinct capsule. Follicular microcarcinomas (characterized by irregular gland-like structures, basophilia and nuclear crowding) may appear in some nodules. Larger carcinomas usually retain a follicular structure but sometimes consist of solid sheets of polymorphous cells (Zbinden, 1987).

Two consecutive processes are thought to occur in the development of tumours; firstly, initiation which occurs quickly and is irreversible and secondly, promotion which occurs slowly and is reversible (and for which cell proliferation may be a necessary but not sufficient condition). Initiators may be ionizing radiation, chemical/biological agents or genetic factors, with TSH acting as promoting agent. Spontaneous thyroid follicular cell tumours arise from unknown aetiologies and factors such as age-induced changes in the cell membrane, growth factor and signal-transduction mechanisms may be involved. Small subpopulations of hyper-reactive epithelial cells retaining the high replication rate of the foetal stage have been identified (Smeds *et al.*, 1987; Peter *et al.*, 1982) which may enter clonal expansion following only slight elevations in TSH (such as those in handled or stressed animals) or other growth factors, leading to spontaneous nodular goitres (see Zbinden, 1987).

Many experimental studies have confirmed the key role of TSH as a stimulator of thyroid growth. In a rat thyroid cell line (FRTL-5) TSH-stimulated growth of the cells was found to be associated with a marked increase in c-fos and c-myc oncogene expression (Colletta, Cirafici & Vecchio, 1986). Another example of the tumour promoting capacity of TSH is given from studies where rats are given carcinogens such as N-methyl-N-nitrosourea (MNU) and then given phenobarbital or put on an iodine deficient diet. These treatments cause an early and increased incidence of thyroid follicular lesions and tumour formation (Oshima & Ward, 1984; Hiasa *et al.*, 1982). The duration of exposure to high circulating TSH concentrations is also important in that intermittent administration of chemical goitrogens with TSH 'normalization' does not appear to lead to follicular neoplasias.

An elaborate series of studies (see Fig. 6.3) have shown that a sustained elevation of serum TSH in the rat leads to three phases of thyroid growth: (1) a phase of rapid growth lasting one to two months, followed by (2) a plateau phase of three to six months (growth desensitizing mechanism (GDM) limiting epithelial cell mitotic response), followed eventually by (3) appearance of multiple follicular cell tumours (loss of GDM; see Wynford-Thomas, Stringer & Williams, 1982; Stringer, Wynford-Thomas & Williams, 1985; Smith *et al.*, 1986). The reversibility of TSH-induced thyroid focal hyperplasia will evidently depend, therefore, on the stage during these 'timed' cellular changes in the first six months (see Fig. 6.3) at which the TSH stimulus is withdrawn. Once the GDM is non-operative reversibility is not possible.

Tumour progression seems to occur by a multi-stage process involving clonal 'expansion' and naturally occurring clones of cells have been demonstrated with high intrinsic proliferation potential in the mouse thyroid gland (Smeds *et al.*, 1987) perhaps helping to explain the focal nature of hyperplastic and neoplastic lesions. The loss of a GDM within

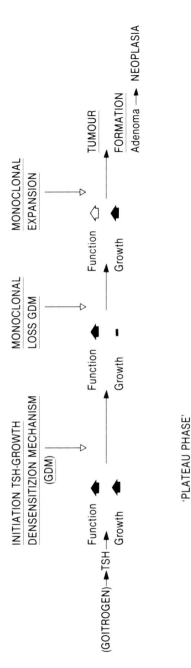

∘ International Survey – Good correlation between goitrogen-induced thyroid function block and tumour-induction potential. No correlation with inherent drug genotoxic potential.

Fig. 6.3. Thyroid growth control. (Wynford-Thomas *et al.*, 1982; Williams *et al.*, 1987.)

the follicular cells appear to be accompanied by an altered dependence or sensitivity to certain growth factors as well as the possible loss of an anti-oncogene which limits the follicular cell's growth response to TSH. For example, the growth of normal cultured human thyroid cells requires TSH and insulin-like growth factor 1 ($IGF_1$) in combination, whereas cells from adenomatous tissue *in vitro* proliferate in response to either TSH or IGF independently (Williams, Wynford-Thomas & Williams, 1987). This is due to the acquisition of autocrine production of $IGF_1$ by the tumour cells themselves. This work is described in detail in chapter 5 by Thomas & Williams (see also Thomas & Williams, 1991).

There is, therefore, good evidence that sustained TSH drive to the thyroid gland can lead to a de-regulation of thyroid function. When investigating xenobiotic or drug-induced thyroid tumour formation, the mechanisms whereby TSH drive is increased can be understood by undertaking a series of experimental studies using *in vitro* and *in vivo* techniques. Having delineated the mechanism of the thyrotoxic effect it may then be possible to determine whether a particular drug or compound elicits a similar response in different species (including humans) and the dose-response relationship for this effect investigated.

## Classification of reported xenobiotic effects on thyroid function, follicular cell hyperplasia and neoplasia

Considered below are the types of thyroid hormonal and glandular changes associated with treatment with specific classes of pharmacological or toxicological drug treatment acting at the loci (A–F) shown in Fig. 6.1 and in Tables 6.1–6.6. For detailed and further reviews on this subject readers are referred to Cavalieri & Pitt-Rivers (1981) and Capen & Martin (1989). In these tables we have attempted to relate classes of agent with their reported ability to act as thyroid tumour promoters by virtue of TSH elevation. As previously stated the lesion and tumour-promoting potential of 'toxic' xenobiotics is determined both by the nature and number of sites at which it acts to perturb hormones of the thyroid axis. For example, the classical antithyroid agent PTU inhibits both $T_4$ synthesis and peripheral deiodinases and is a potent goitrogen, whereas the salicylates and diazepam which affect only plasma protein binding, a reversible process, are not.

### Class A: direct antithyroid agents
Classical antithyroid drugs such as the thioamide class (PTU, methimazole, etc.) directly prevent hormone synthesis by inhibiting the thyroid-peroxidase catalysed organification of iodide. This will lead to

sustained circulating $T_3$ and $T_4$ reductions which will consequently produce sustained elevations in circulating TSH. Thyroid follicular hypertrophy and hyperplasia follow, producing the classical goitre, cystic and cellular nodules, adenomas and other neoplasias after long-term exposure (see Table 6.1, for affected species and references). The early changes are usually reversible (see Todd, 1986) with remodelling of the gland to a normal structure following cessation of treatment, but this may depend upon the molecular desensitization (GDM) stages reached as described in Fig. 6.3.

Species differences exist where thyroid enlargement and tumours are mainly seen in rodents. For example, it has been shown that rats are more sensitive than squirrel monkeys to the antithyroid effects of PTU and sulfamonomethoxine (Takayama et al., 1986) and more sensitive to salicylazosulfapyridine than mice (Kari, Kutzman & Thompson, 1987). Sulphamethaxozole induces thyroid nodules in rats at doses as low as 50 mg/kg body-weight given for one year whereas in rhesus monkeys the drug caused no such changes even at 300 mg/kg (Swarm et al., 1973). Another example of species specificity occurs in the case of aminotriazole where rats have been shown to be exquisitely sensitive to this compound whereas in golden hamsters and mice no tumour induction is seen. These species differences may be due to several factors including differences in the half-life of the thyroid hormones between rodent and primates (12–24 hours rat vs. 5–9 days human) and differences in the responsiveness of thyroid cells to TSH. For example, in cell cultures in vitro TSH does not induce proliferation of porcine, ovine or human follicular cells but does stimulate the growth of cells from rat and dog thyroid glands (Westermark, Karlsson & Westermark, 1985).

Due to the chronic $T_3/T_4$ deficit following anti-thyroid drugs secondary hypothyroidism will be seen with these agents. Some of this class of drug do have additional effects and therefore act at multiple sites. For example, PTU can both inhibit peripheral thyroid hormone deiodination and affect thyroid hormone clearance.

### Class B: drugs affecting liver thyroid hormone conjugating enzymes

The induction of hepatic microsomal P450 enzymes not only alters the metabolism of xenobiotics but also alters the metabolism of various hormones including cortisol (Werk et al., 1971), testosterone (Levin, Welch & Conney, 1974), oestrogens (Bolt, Bolt & Kappus, 1977) and thyroxine (Taurog, 1955). Drugs which induce the conjugating enzyme uridine diphosphate glucuronyltransferase (UDP-GT), lead to increased clearance of $T_4$ and/or $T_3$ from the circulation with increased biliary

Table 6.1. *Class: A. Effect: direct antithyroid effect*

| Agent | Trade name | Pharmacological class | Changes in (species) | Notes | TSH/* tumour | Reference |
|---|---|---|---|---|---|---|
| Carbimazole Methimazole | Neomercazole | Anti-thyroid | Rat, man | Prevent organification of iodide. Low doses also prevent coupling of DIT T$_4$ | T<br>T,H(rat)<br><br>T<br>T,H(rat) | Redmond & Ruffery (1981)<br>Bowman & Rand (1980)<br>Bowman & Rand (1980)<br>Bowman & Rand (1980)<br>Wynford-Thomas et al., (1982) |
| Iodothiouracil Methylthiouracil Propylthiouracil Aminotriazole | | | | | | |
| Perchlorate Fluoroborate Nitrate Permanganate Pertechnetate | | | Rat, man | Compete for iodide pump | | Bowman & Rand (1980) |
| Iodine (high doses) | | | Man | ↓ thyroid hormone output in hyperthyroidism | T | Bowman & Rand (1980) |
| Thiocyanate | | | Rat | Prevents iodide uptake | | Wenzel (1981) |
| Iodine (deficiency) | | | Rat, man | Goitre → tumours. Potentials, effect of many tumour promoters | T,H | Axelrod & Leblond (1955)<br>Doniach & Williams (1962) |
| Partial thyroidectomy | | | Rat | Induces thyroid tumours | H | Doniach & Williams (1962) |
| Aminosalicyclic acid | | Antitubercular | Man | Goitre and hypothyroidism occur with long term treatment | | Bowman & Rand (1980) |
| Phenylbutazone | Butazolidin, Butacote, Butazone | NAZID | | Inhibition of thyroid hormone synthesis | | Bowman & Rand (1980) |
| Aminoglutethimide | Orimetin | Inhibitor of adrenal cortex activity, and anticonvulsant and anticancer agent | | Inhibits organification of iodine | | Bowman & Rand (1980) |

Table 6.1. (*Cont.*)

| Agent | Trade name | Pharmacological class | Changes in (species) | Notes | TSH/* tumour | Reference |
|---|---|---|---|---|---|---|
| Carbutamide | | Sulphonylurea Oral hypoglycaemic | | ↓ I uptake, thyroid enlargement | | Hershman & Konerding (1968) |
| Goitrin – contained in plants of the genus *Brassica* (e.g. cabbage, turnip, mustard, rape | | | Rat, rabbit | Hypothyroidism, thyroid tumours | H | Griesbach *et al.*, (1945) |
| Polybrominated biphenyl congeners | | | Rat | Inhibition of peroxidase organification of iodide | | Akoso *et al.*, (1982) |
| Erythrosine BS | | Colouring agent | Rat | | T, H | Capen & Martin (1982) |
| Cobalt salts, e.g. dicobalt edetate | Kelocyanor | Antidote to cyanide poisoning | | | | |
| Dimercaprol | | Antidote to heavy metal poisoning | | | | |
| Resorcinol | | | | | | |
| Somatostatin | | | Man | | | Wenzel (1981) |
| Prostaglandins | | | Man | | | Wenzel (1981) |
| Clomiphene | Clomid, Serophene | Oestrogen antagonist | Man | | T | Wenzel (1981) |
| Iodized oil | | | Man | | | Wenzel (1981) |
| Cotrimoxazole | Bactrim, Septrin, Cotrimox, Fectrim, Chemotrim, Comox, Laratrim | Antimicrobial | Man, rat | Peroxidase inhibition | | Wenzel (1981) |
| Co-trifamole | | Antimicrobial | Man | organification of iodine | | Wenzel (1981) |

| Drug | Trade names | Drug class | Species | Effect/Mechanism | Reference |
|---|---|---|---|---|---|
| Trimethoprim | Ipral, Monotrim, Syraprim, Tiempe, Trimopan, Unitrim Trimogal | Antimicrobial | | | |
| Amiodarone | Cordarone X | Anti-arrythmic | | ↓ $^{125}$I uptake | Cavalieri & Pitt-Rivers (1981) |
| Lithium | Liskonum, Camcolit, Priadel, Phasal | Antipsychotic | | Inhibit thyroid hormone synthesis | Berens et al., (1970) |
| Na nitroprusside | Nipride | Hypotensive agent | | Inhibit iodide uptake | Wenzel (1981) |
| Acetazolamide | Diamox | Carbonic anhydrase inhibitor (diuretic) | | Inhibit iodide uptake | |
| Propranolol | Inderal, Angilol, Apsolol, Bedranol, Berkolol, Sloprolol | β-adrenoceptor antagonist | Rat | ↓ thyroglobulin synthesis | Monaco et al., (1982) |

* T denotes elevated TSH conc. reported (mechanism of increase and thyroid status of subjects not always documented); H denotes thyroid hyperplasia or neoplasia reported

Table 6.2. Class: B. Effect: liver conjugating enzymes

| Agent | Trade name | Pharmacological class | Changes in (species) | Notes | TSH/* tumour | Reference |
|---|---|---|---|---|---|---|
| Phenytoin | Epanutin | Anticonvulsant | Rat | ↑ liver uptake of $T_4$ ↑ glucuronide formation | | Mendoza et al. (1966) |
| Phenobarbitone | Luminal, Parabal, Phenobarbitone Spansule | Hypnotic, Anticonvulsant | Rat, man | ↑ faecal $T_4$ excretion (may be due to ↑ bile flow) | T,H | Goldstein & Taurog (1968) McClain (1989) |
| Thiobarbitone Pentobarbitone Allobarbitone | Nembutal | Hypnotic Hypnotic | Rat | ? | | Langer et al. (1976) |
| Carbamazepine Primidone | Tegretol | Anticonvulsant | | ↑ conjugation ↑ conjugation | | Wenzel (1981) Wenzel (1981) |
| Methylphenidate | Ritalin | Sympathomimetic CNS stimulant | Rat | 'increased peripheral catabolism' of $T_4$ | | Greely et al. (1980) |
| 3-methylcholanthrene | | | Rat | ↑ UDP-glucuronyl transferase | ?T,H | |
| 3,4-benzpyrene Polychlorinated biphenyls (PCBs) | | | Rat Rat | ↑ UDP-glucuronyl transferase ↑ UDP-glucuronyl transferase | | Cavalieri & Pitt-Rivers (1981) |
| 7,12-dimethylbenz[a] anthracene (DMBA) | | | Rat | | ?T,H | Reuber & Glover (1969) |
| Dichlorodiphenyl–trichloroethane (DDT) | | | Rat | Slight ↑ biliary $T_4$ excretion (due to ↑ bile flow and some ↑ glucuronidation) | | Cavalieri & Pitt-Rivers (1981) |
| Butyl-4-hydroxy-3,5-diiodobenzoate (BHDB) | | | Rat | ↑ conjugation and biliary excretion | | Cavalieri & Pitt-Rivers (1981) |

| Compound | Synonyms | Activity/class | Species | Mechanism | T/H | Reference |
|---|---|---|---|---|---|---|
| SKF 525-A (Proadifen) | | Inhibitor of hepatic drug metabolism | Rat (in vivo) | ↑ faecal clearance of $T_4$ (due to displacement from plasma proteins) | | Cavalieri & Pitt-Rivers (1981) |
| β-Naphthoflavone | | P450 enzyme inducer | Rat | ↓ $T_3T_4$ microsomal enzymes ↑ | T,H | Johnson, (1990) |
| 2,3,7,8-tetrachloro-dibenzo-p-dioxin (TCDD) | | | Rat | ↑ UDP-glucuronyl transferase (p-nitrophenyl type) | T,H | Lucier et al. (1975) |
| Polybrominated biphenyls (PBB) | | | Rat, man | ↑ UDP-glucuronyl transferase | T,H(rat) | Akoso et al. (1982) |
| SC-37211 | | Antimicrobial | Rat | ↑ UDP-glucuronyl transferase | ?T,H | Comer et al. (1985) |
| Rifampicin | Rifadin, Rimactane | Antibiotic | Man | ↑ conjugation | | Ohnhaus & Studer (1983) |
| 2,4 dinitrophenol | | | Monkey (in vitro) | ↓ sulphation of 3.3'-$T_2$ and 3'-$T_1$ | | Cavalieri & Pitt-Rivers (1981) |
| Clofibrate | Atromid-S | Antihyperlipidaemic | Rat | ↑ biliary clearance of $T_4$ | | Cavalieri & Pitt-Rivers (1981) |
| Prophylthiouracil | | Antithyroid | Rat | ↑ biliary clearance of $T_4$ | | Cavalieri & Pitt-Rivers (1981) |
| Grisefulvin | Fucin, Grisovin | Antifungal | Rat | | H | Rustia & Shubik (1978) |

* T denotes elevated TSH conc. reported (mechanisms of increase and thyroid status of subjects not always documented); H denotes thyroid hyperplasia or neoplasia reported

Table 6.3. Class: C. Effect: affect deiodinases

| Agent | Trade name | Pharmacological class | Changes in (species) | Notes | TSH/* tumour | Reference |
|---|---|---|---|---|---|---|
| Omeprazole | | $H^+K^+$ ATPase inhibitor | Rat | $\downarrow$ 5'-deiodination | | Ekman et al. (1985) |
| Amiodarone | Cordarone | Anti-arrythmic | Rat, man, rabbit | $\downarrow$ 5'-deiodination | T | Cavalieri & Pitt-Rivers (1981) |
| Propylthiouracil | | Antithyroid | Rat, man | $\downarrow$ 5'-deiodination | T | Cavalieri & Pitt-Rivers (1981) |
| Ranitidine | Zantac | $H_2$-receptor antagonist | Man | $\uparrow$ 5'-deiodination | | Hine et al. (1984) |
| BHDB | | | Rat | $\downarrow$ deiodination, secondary to $\uparrow$ conjugation | | Cavalieri & Pitt-Rivers (1981) |
| Proadifen (SKF 525-A) | | | Rat | In vivo – $\uparrow$ deiodination secondary to displacement from plasma proteins. In vitro – $\downarrow$ oxygen-dependent deiodination | | Nakamura et al. (1981) |
| Propranolol Pindolol Metoprolol Nadolol | Inderal, etc. Visken Betaloc, Lopresor Corgard | $\beta$-adrenoceptor antagonist | Rat, man | Competitive inhibition of type 1 5'-deiodinase | | Reeves et al. (1985) Shulkin et al. (1984) Heymar et al. (1980) |

| | | | | | | |
|---|---|---|---|---|---|---|
| Iopanoate | Colepax, Telepaque, Bilijodon Na | X-ray contrast media | Man, rat | ↓ 5′-deiodination (types I and II) | T | Cavalieri & Pitt-Rivers (1981) |
| Ipodate | Orografin, Biloptin | | | | T | Cavalieri & Pitt-Rivers (1981) |
| Iobenzamic acid | Osbil | | | | T | |
| Tyropanoic acid | Bilopaque, Lumopaque | | | | T | |
| 2,4 dinitrophenol | | | Rat | ↑ 5′-deiodination | | Cavalieri & Pitt-Rivers (1981) |
| | | | Monkey liver (in vitro) | ↓ 5′-deiodination | | Hillier (1974) |
| Glucocorticoids | | | Man, rat | ↓ 5′-deiodinase, ↔ or ↑ 5-deiodinase | T | Cavalieri & Pitt-Rivers (1981) |
| Oestrogens | | | Rat | Transient ↑ in $T_4$-deiodination rate | | Cavalieri & Pitt-Rivers (1981) |
| Sodium salicylate | | | Rat | Competitive inhibition of 5′-deiodinase in liver and kidney | | Cavalieri & Pitt-Rivers (1981) |
| Clofibrate | Atromid-S | Antihyperlipidaemic | Rat | ↓ deiodination of $T_4$ | | Cavalieri & Pitt-Rivers (1981) |
| Phenobarbitone | Luminal, Parabal, Phenobarbitone Spansule | Hypnotic, anticonvulsant | Rat | ↑ deiodination of $T_4$ | | Cavalieri & Pitt-Rivers (1981) |

Table 6.3. (*Cont.*)

| Agent | Trade name | Pharmacological class | Changes in (species) | Notes | TSH/* tumour | Reference |
|---|---|---|---|---|---|---|
| Quinidine | Kinidin, Quinicardine, Kiditard | Anti-arrythmic | Rat | ↓ $T_4$-$T_3$ conversion in isolated renal tubules | | Cavalieri & Pitt-Rivers (1981) |
| Lithium | Liskonum, Camcolit, Priadel, Phasal | Antipsychotic | Rat | ↓ deiodination | | Cavalieri & Pitt-Rivers (1981) |
| Noradrenaline | | α-adrenoceptor agonist | Rat | ↑ type II 5′-deiodination | | Silva & Larsen (1983) |
| Phentolamine | Rogitine | α-adrenoceptor antagonist | Rat | Antagonises noradrenaline-induced ↑ in type II 5′-deiodination | | Silva & Larsen (1983) |
| Methylphenidate | Ritalin | Sympathomimetic CNS stimulant | Rat | ↑ peripheral catabolism of $T_3$ and $T_4$ | | Greely *et al.* (1980) |
| Carbon tetrachloride | | | Rat | ↓ 5′-deiodination | | |
| Amphetamine | Dexedrine | CNS stimulant | Rat | ↓ 5′-deiodination | | Engler & Burger (1984) |
| Growth hormone | | | Man | ↑ 5′-deiodination | | Wenzel (1981) |
| Cimetidine | Tagamet | $H_2$-receptor antagonist | Man | ↓ 5′-deiodination | | |

* T denotes elevated TSH conc. reported (mechanism of increase and thyroid status of subjects not always documented); H denotes thyroid hyperplasia or neoplasia reported

Table 6.4. Class: D. Effect: alterations in thyroid hormone binding to plasma proteins

| Agent | Trade name | Pharmacological class | Changes in (species) | Notes | TSH/* tumour | Reference |
|---|---|---|---|---|---|---|
| Oestrogens | | | Man, monkey | ↑ TBG | | Cavalieri & Pitt-Rivers (1981) |
| Androgens | | | Man | ↓ TBG | | Cavalieri & Pitt-Rivers (1981) |
| Glucocorticoids | | | Man | ↓ TBG, ↑ TBPA, No change in net binding. Also changes in cellular binding | T | Cavalieri & Pitt-Rivers (1981) |
| Anabolic steroids | | | Man | ↓ TBG, ↑ TBPA, Overall ↓ in plasma binding | | Cavalieri & Pitt-Rivers (1981) |
| L-asparaginase | | | Man | ↓ TBG | | Cavalieri & Pitt-Rivers (1981) |
| Diamorphine | | Narcotic analgesic | Man | ↑ TBG | | Wenzel (1981) |
| Methadone | Physeptone | Narcotic analgesic | Man | ↑ TBG | | Wenzel (1981) |
| 5-Fluorouracil | Efudix | Cytostatic | Man | ↑ TBG | | Wenzel (1981) |
| Salicylates | | NSAID | Man. rat | ↓ binding to TBG, TBPA | | Cavalieri & Pitt-Rivers (1981) |
| Fenclofenac | | NSAID | Man | ↓ binding to plasma proteins | | Cavalieri & Pitt-Rivers (1981) |

Table 6.4. (*Cont.*)

| Agent | Trade name | Pharmacological class | Changes in (species) | Notes | TSH/* tumour | Reference |
|---|---|---|---|---|---|---|
| Penicillin G | Crystapen | Antibiotic | Man, rat | ↓ binding, mainly to TBPA | | Cavalieri & Pitt-Rivers (1981) |
| Clofibrate | Atromid-S | Antihyperlipidaemic | Man, rat | ↑ TBG in man; ↓ plasma protein binding in rat | | Wenzel (1981); Cavalieri & Pitt-Rivers (1981) |
| Halofenate | | Antihyperlipidaemic | Man | ↓ binding to TBG | | Wenzel (1981) |
| Carbutamide | | Sulphonylurea oral hypoglycaemics | | | | |
| Tolbutamide | Rastinon, Glyconon, Pramidex | | Man, rat | | | |
| Chlorpromide | Diabenese, Glymese, Melitase | | Man, rat | ↓ binding to plasma proteins | | Cavalieri & Pitt-Rivers (1981) |
| Acetohexamide | Dimelor | | Man, rat | | | |
| Chlordiazepoxide | Librium, Tropium, Valium, Alupram, | Anxiolytic | Man | ↓ binding to plasma proteins *in vitro* | | Cavalieri & Pitt-Rivers (1981) |
| Diazepam | Arensine, Diazemuls, Evacalm, Solis, Stesolid, Tensium, Valrelease | Anxiolytic | Man | | | |
| Heparin | | Anticoagulant | Man | ↓ binding to plasma proteins | | Cavalieri & Pitt-Rivers (1981) |
| Phenylbutazone | Butazolidin, Butacote, Butazone | NSAID | Man | ↓ binding to plasma proteins | | Wenzel (1981) |

| | | | | | |
|---|---|---|---|---|---|
| Fatty acids | | | Man, *in vitro* | ↓ binding to plasma proteins | Wenzel (1981) |
| Orphenadrine | Disipal, Biorphen | Spasmolytic | Man, *in vitro* | ↓ binding to plasma proteins | Wenzel (1981) |
| Phenytoin | Epanutin | Anticonvulsant | Man, rat | ↓ binding to plasma proteins | Wenzel (1981) |
| Proadifen (SKF-525A) | | | | ↓ binding to plasma proteins | Cavalieri & Pitt-Rivers (1981) |
| Propranolol | Inderal, Angilol, Apsolol, Bedranol, Berkolol, Sloprolol | β-adrenoceptor antagonist | | ↓ binding to plasma proteins | Jurney *et al.* (1983) |
| Dicoumarol | | Anticoagulant | Man | ↓ binding to plasma proteins | Bowman & Rand (1980) |
| PCBs | | | Rat | ↓ binding to plasma proteins | Cavalieri & Pitt-Rivers (1981) |
| BHDB | | | Rat | ↓ binding to plasma proteins | Cavalieri & Pitt-Rivers (1981) |
| 2, 2 bis(chlorophenyl 4-chlorophenyl)-1, 1-dichloroethane (o, p'-DDD) | | Anti-adrenal tumour | Man | ↓ binding to TBG | Cavalieri & Pitt-Rivers (1981) |
| 2, 4 dinitrophenol | | | Rats, human serum *in vitro* | ↓ binding to TBPA | Cavalieri & Pitt-Rivers (1981) |
| Frusemide | Lasix, Aluzine, Diuresal, Dryptal, Frusetic, Frusid | Diuretic | | ↓ binding to plasma proteins | Stockigt *et al.* (1984) |

* T denotes elevated TSH conc. reported (mechanisms of increase and thyroid status of subjects not always documented); H denotes thyroid hyperplasia or neoplasia reported

Table 6.5. *Class E. Effect: receptor mediated*

| Agent | Trade name | Pharmacological class | Changes in (species) | Notes | TSH/* tumour | Reference |
|---|---|---|---|---|---|---|
| Dopamine | | | Man | ↓ basal and TRH-stimulated TSH conc. | | Wenzel (1981) |
| Bromocriptine | Parlodel | Dopamine agonist | Man | ↓ TSH conc. | | Wenzel (1981) |
| Peribidil | | Dopamine agonist | Man | ↓ TSH conc. | | Wenzel (1981) |
| Apomorphine | | Dopamine agonist | Man | ↓ TSH conc. | | Wenzel (1981) |
| Lisurde | | Dopamine agonist | Man | ↓ TSH conc. | | Wenzel (1981) |
| Pyridoxine | | Coenzyme for dopamine synthesis | Man | ↓ TSH conc. | | Wenzel (1981) |
| Fusaric acid | | Dopamine hydroxylase inhibitor | Man | ↓ TSH conc. | | Wenzel (1981) |
| L-Dopa | | Dopamine precursor | Man | ↓ basal and TRH-stimulated TSH conc. | | Wenzel (1981) |
| Phentolamine | Rogitine | α–adrenoceptor antagonist | Man | ↓ TRH-stimulated TSH conc. | | Wenzel (1981) |
| Thioridazine | Melleril | Antipsychotic - adrenoceptor antagonist | Man | ↓ TRH-stimulated TSH conc. | | Wenzel (1981) |
| Metergoline | | 5-HT-antagonist | Man | ↓ TSH conc. | | Wenzel (1981) |

| | | | | | |
|---|---|---|---|---|---|
| Cyproheptadine | Periactin | 5-HT-antagonist | Man | ↓ TRH-stimulated TSH conc. | Wenzel (1981) |
| Methysergide | Deseril | 5-HT-antagonist | Man | ↓ TRH-stimulated TSH conc. | Wenzel (1981) |
| Morphine [Leucine]-enkephalin Diamorphine Dermorphin | | Opioids | Man | ↑ or ↓ TRH-stimulated TSH release | Wenzel (1981) Devilla & Williams (1982) |
| Clofibrate | Atromid-S | Antihyperlipidaemic | Man | ↓ TSH conc. | Wenzel (1981) |
| Fenclofenac | | NSAID | Man | Transient ↓ in basal and TRH-stimulated TSH release | Wenzel (1981) |
| Glucocorticoids | | | Man | ↓ TRH-stimulated TSH release | Wenzel (1981) |
| D-thyroxine | Choloxin | Antihyperlipidaemic | Man | ↓ basal and TRH-stimulated TSH conc. | Wenzel (1981) |
| Etiroxate-HCl | | | Man | ↓ basal and TRH-stimulated TSH conc. | Wenzel (1981) |
| 3, 5-dimethyl-3'-isopropyl-L-thyronine (DIMIT) | | | Man | ↓ and TRH-stimulated TSH conc. | Wenzel (1981) |
| Oestrogens | | | Man | ↑ basal and TRH-stimulated T TSH conc. | Wenzel (1981) |
| Clomiphene | Clomid, Serophene | | Man | ↑ basal and TRH-stimulated T TSH conc. | Wenzel (1981) |

Table 6.5. (*Cont.*)

| Agent | Trade name | Pharmacological class | Changes in (species) | Notes | TSH/* tumour | Reference |
|---|---|---|---|---|---|---|
| Iodine | | | Man | ↑ basal and TRH-stimulated TSH conc. (secondary to thyroid hormone output) | T | Wenzel (1981) |
| Amiodarone | Cordarone X | Anti-arrythmic | Man | ↑ basal and TRH-stimulated TSH conc. | T | Wenzel (1981) |
| Metoclopramide | Maxolon | Antiemetic dopamine antagonist | Man | ↑ basal and TRH-stimulated TSH conc. | T | Wenzel (1981) |
| Domperidone | Motilium | Antiemetic dopamine antagonist | Man | ↑ TSH conc. | T | Wenzel (1981) |
| Sulpiride | Dolmatil | Dopamine antagonist | Man | ↑ basal and TRH-stimulated TSH conc. | T | Wenzel (1981) |
| Benserazide | | Decarboxylase inhibitor | Man | ↑ TSH conc. | T | Wenzel (1981) |
| Monoiodotyrosine | | | Man | ↑ TSH conc. | T | Wenzel (1981) |
| Pimozide | Orap | Antipsychotic | Man | ↑ or ↓ TSH conc. | T | Wenzel (1981) |
| Chlorpromazine | Largactil, Chloractil, Dozine | Antipsychotic | Man | ↑ basal and TRH-stimulated TSH conc. | T | Wenzel (1981) |
| Biperidine | | Antipsychotic | Man | ↑ basal and TRH-stimulated TSH conc. | T | Wenzel (1981) |

| Drug | Proprietary names | Class | Species | Effect | T* | Reference |
|---|---|---|---|---|---|---|
| Haloperidol | Seranace, Haldol, Dozic, Fortunan | Antipsychotic | Man | ↑ basal and TRH-stimulated TSH conc. | T | Wenzel (1981) |
| Cimetidine | Tagamet | $H_2$-receptor antagonist | Man | ↑ TRH-stimulated TSH conc. | | Wenzel (1981) |
| Somatostatin | | | Man | Transient ↓ in basal and TRH-stimulated TSH release | | Wenzel (1981) |
| Spironolactone | Aldactone, Diatensec, Laractone, Spiretic, Spiroctan, Spirolone | Aldosterone antagonist diuretic | Man | ↑ TRH-stimulated TSH conc. | T | Wenzel (1981) |
| Theophylline | Nuelin, Lasma, Provent, Slo-Phyllin, Theodur, Theograd, Uniphyllin | Bronchodilator | Man | ↑ TRH-stimulated TSH conc. | T | Wenzel (1981) |
| Growth hormone | | | Man | ↓ TRH-stimulated TSH conc. due to ↑ 5'-deiodination | | Wenzel (1981) |
| Salicylates | | | Man | ↓ TRH-stimulated TSH conc. due to $T_4$ displacement from plasma protein binding sites | | Wenzel (1981) |
| Amphetamine | Dexedrine | CNS stimulant | Man | ↑ TSH secretion | T | Engler & Burger (1984) |
| Cannabis | | | Man | ↓ $T_4$ due to central effect | | Wenzel (1981) |
| Phenytoin | Epanutin | Anticonvulsant | Rat | Acts as thyroid hormone agonist at pituitary level | | Cavalieri & Pitt-Rivers (1981) |

* T denotes elevated TSH conc. reported (mechanism of increase and thyroid status of subjects not always documented).

Table 6.6. *Class E. Effect: miscellaneous*

| Agent | Trade name | Pharmacological class | Changes in (species) | Notes | TSH/* tumour | Reference |
|---|---|---|---|---|---|---|
| N-bis (2-hydroxypropyl) nitrosamine | | | Rat | Causes thyroid tumours Phenobarbitone and barbitone act as promoters | H | Hiasa *et al.* (1982) |
| N-methyl N-Nitrosourea | | | Rat | Induces thyroid tumours Iodine deficient diet acts as promoter ↑ pituitary thyrotrophs seen | H | Ohshima & Ward (1984) |
| 4, 4′-Oxydianiline | | | Rat | Induces thyroid tumours Increased pituitary thyrotrophs seen Hypothyroidism + TSH tumourigenesis, or direct effect on follicular cells? | H | Murthy *et al.* (1985) |
| 4, 4′-thiodianiline 4, 4′-methylene-bis (N, N-dimethyl)- benzeramine 4, 4′-methylenedianiline | | | | also produce thyroid tumours | H H H | Murthy *et al.* (1985) |
| 2, 4-diaminoanisol | | Hair dye component | Rat | Induces thyroid tumours | H | |
| N-Nitrosomethylurea | | | Rat | Induces thyroid tumours Phenobarbitone acts as promoter | H | Tsuda *et al.* (1983) |
| ZAMI-1305 | | β-adrenoceptor antagonist | Rat, (females only) | Induces thyroid hyperplasia directly related to preneoplastic and neoplastic changes in the liver | H | Zavenella *et al.* (1983) |
| Thiazides | | Diuretics | Man | ↑ Serum $T_3$ due to shift in distribution volume | | Wenzel (1981) |

| Insulin | | | Man | ↑ Serum $T_4$ due to release from the liver | Wenzel (1981) |
| Halothane | Fluothane | Inhalational anaesthetic | Man | ↑ Serum $T_4$ due to release from liver | Wenzel (1981) |
| Colestipol | Colestid | Antihyperlipidaemic | Man | ↓ Serum $T_3$ due to reduced reabsorption | Wenzel (1981) |
| Phenothiazines | | Antipsychotics | Man | ↓ Serum $T_4$ – mechanism unknown | Wenzel (1981) |

* H denotes thyroid hyperplasia or neoplasia reported

excretion of the $T_4$ glucuronide-conjugate. This route is one of the major $T_4$ elimination routes in animals and humans. Different UDP-GT isoenzymes for $T_3$ and $T_4$ exist and there are species and sex differences in function. Although elevations in circulating TSH arise from the reduced negative feedback by $T_4$ (and/or $T_3$), species and sex differences in this type of response are likely to be due to the factors mentioned above.

Since this is an 'indirect' tumour-promoting effect via TSH elevation, and thyroid hormone synthesis by the thyroid gland is not usually inhibited (PTU is an exception), such marked and continuous elevations in TSH are not likely to occur relative to that noted with Class A agents. Examples of agents affecting these enzymes are phenobarbital (Oppenheimer, Bernstein & Surks, 1968) B-Naphthoflavone (Johnson, 1990) and the Searle imidazole-containing, antimicrobial compound, SC 37211 (Comer et al., 1985). These compounds cause hepatocellular and thyroid follicular cell hypertrophy and are associated with increased hepatic microsomal enzyme induction and/or UDP-GT activity. Phenobarbital and barbitone have been clearly demonstrated as thyroid tumour-promoting agents in rats treated with an initial sub-effective dose of the initiator N-bis-(2-hydroxypropyl) nitrosamine (DHPN) which can act quite specifically on the thyroid gland alone causing tumourigenesis (Hiasa et al., 1982). The incidence of thyroid tumours increases with duration of phenobarbital treatment (Hiasa et al., 1984) and the promoting effect appears to be much greater in male than in female rats (Hiasa et al., 1985; McClain, 1989). Tsuda et al. (1983) and Diwan et al. (1985) have also shown that phenobarbital will enhance thyroid tumours after initiation with N-nitroso urea (NNu). This tumourogenic effect of phenobarbital can be reversed by co-administration of $T_4$ proving that tumour promotion is via elevated circulating TSH levels (McClain, 1989).

### Class C: deiodinase inhibitors

Compounds affecting the deiodination of thyroid hormones are generally, if not exclusively, inhibitory on these enzymes. An exception to this being $T_3$ treatment itself (for review see Kohrle et al., 1987). The level of enzymatic control of thyroid hormone levels by the deiodinases is affected by such factors as kidney and liver disease, systemic illness, thyroid status and development. Therefore, it follows that the changes in thyroid hormones produced by drugs inhibiting deiodinase will also be magnified by such factors. Inhibition of 5'-deiodinase (which converts $T_4$ to $T_3$, and reverse $T_3$ ($rT_3$) to further deiodinated metabolites) alters circulating thyroid hormone concentrations. The pattern of changes produced is reduced circulating $T_3$, increased TSH, increased $rT_3$ and normal or elevated $T_4$. Hypothyroidism may be seen clinically, for example with

Amiodarone (see Boronski *et al.*, 1985). This drug has been shown to double serum TSH concentrations in humans.

If the pituitary deiodinase isoenzyme is not affected by a deiodinase inhibiting agent then reflex increased $T_4$ levels will inhibit further TSH output (and lower thyroidal $T_4$ production), and thus sustained elevations in TSH may not occur. Exceptions to this would be circumstances where the compound has an additional direct effect on thyroid function. In some cases a $5'$-deiodinase inhibitor such as propranolol is actually used clinically to reverse hypothroidism by preventing excessive circulating $T_3$.

Detailed studies by Capen & Martin (1989) on FD & C Red No. 3 (Erythrosine), which is used as a colour additive in foods, cosmetics and pharmaceuticals, have revealed actions on the thyroid via deiodinase inhibition. Carcinogenicity studies showed that male, but not female, Sprague-Dawley rats fed a 4% concentration of Red No. 3 in the diet developed follicular adenomas but no other body tumours which was not due to any genotoxic properties of the compound. Lowered circulating $T_3$ plasma levels, increased $T_4$ levels, and increased $rT_3$ levels suggested an inhibitory influence of the dye on $5^1$-deiodinase of the liver and kidney (decreased $T_4$ conversion to $T_3$) with no effect on 5-deiodinase (net increase in $T_4$ to $rT_3$ conversion with decreased $rT_3$ breakdown by $5^1$-deiodinase). The increased TSH levels together with the thyroid pathological changes indicate, therefore, an epigenetic mode of action for this compound via inhibited metabolising enzymes and increased TSH drive to the thyroid follicles (Capen & Martin, 1989).

### Class D: compounds drugs affecting the plasma protein binding of thyroid hormones

Since the concentrations of free thyroid hormones are in equilibrium with hormone bound to plasma proteins any perturbation in this equilibrium will initially result in alterations in concentrations of free thyroid hormone in the circulation. This will be followed by transient alterations in circulating TSH (increase or decrease) and thyroid hormone clearance. However, these transient effects lead to a new equilibrium and complete adjustment in terms of circulating thyroid hormones and TSH usually occurs. Exceptions to this would be compounds which also affect deiodinating capacity, for example thyromimetics, or those influencing liver thyroid hormone metabolizing systems – e.g. phenytoin. Other situations such as liver failure (site of TBG clearance) or nutritional status (certain amino acids such as tryptophan required for binding proteins) will influence these xenobiotic-induced thyroid effects. Some drugs known to affect the plasma protein binding of thyroid hormone have also recently been shown to inhibit $T_3$ transport and binding by hepatocytes, and thus hormone metabolism (see Topliss, Kolliniatis & Stockigt, 1987), but their 'potency ranking' in this respect is not identical to the effects on plasma binding proteins.

### Class E: drugs acting at receptors involved in the hypothalamic-pituitary-thyroid axis (Table 6.5)

Certain neurotransmitters have been implicated in controlling TRH output and TSH output at the hypothalamic and pituitary levels, respectively. These include hypothalamic adrenoceptors, dopaminergic receptors and histamine receptors. In this context certain drugs have been reported clinically to alter TSH output and/or the TSH response to a new TRH challenge. For example, dopamine antagonists such as metoclopramide and domperidone increase pituitary TSH as the thyrotroph dopamine receptor is of the inhibitory type. The α-adrenergic blocking drug phentolamine has been reported to decrease the TSH response to a TRH challenge. The effect of histamine antagonists on TSH release is unclear although histamine receptors do exist in the hypothalamus and pituitary gland. There have been reports of increased TSH responses to a TRH challenge in humans following cimetidine treatment.

### Dietary factors: effect of iodine and dietary goitrogens on thyroid function

A dietary supply of iodine of around 150 μg/day is required for normal thyroid hormone synthesis. This intake varies geographically. For example a typical daily dietary intake of iodine in the USA is now about 500 μg and iodine deficiency is still found in developing countries and in some regions of Europe. Prolonged deficiency of iodine intake leads in some cases to goitrous hypothyroidism. Furthermore, mental retardation can occur in the newborn if iodine deficiency takes place during pregnancy. The major dietary sources of iodine are water, iodated bread and iodinated salt. Excessive iodine intake (of the level of 2 mg/day) induces transient alterations of thyroid function. This occurs through the 'Wolff-Chaikoff' block where, beyond a critical dose level, progressively larger doses of iodine lead to the generation of smaller quantities of organified iodine within the thyroid gland. Qualitative alterations in intrathyroidal iodine metabolism through this block are similar to those produced by the classic antithyroid agents. However, the normal human thyroid can escape from the Wolff-Chaikoff block since iodide myxoedema does not ordinarily develop. In a small percentage of patients the adaptive response may be inadequate and clinical effects may ensue.

In some subjects, probably those already affected by subclinical thyroid

Table 6.7. *Medications containing iodine*

| Radiographic contrast agents: | Iopanoic acid |
| | Ipodate sodium |
| | Tyropanoate sodium |
| | Ioglycamic acid |
| | Ditrizoate sodium |
| | Lipiodol |
| Benzofurane derivatives: | Aminodarone |
| | Benziodarone |
| Phenazone derivative: | Iodoantipyrine |
| Hydroxyquinoline derivative: | Iodochlorhydroxyquinoline |
| Iodophores: | Povidone-iodine |

disease, excessive amounts of iodine can induce either hyperthyroidism, known as the Jodbasedow effect, or hypothyroidism as already mentioned. Other sites for iodine to affect thyroid hormone metabolism have been examined but appear to be refractory to change (see Cavalieri & Pitt-Rivers, 1981). There is evidence, however, that iodine can enhance immunological responses. An increased frequency of lymphocytic thyroiditis has been noted in certain goitres, which parallels the increase in iodine intake in the particular area of survey. Furthermore, recent animal studies in thyroiditis, predisposed strains of chickens and rats have shown an increase in antibody production, and of lymphocytic thyroiditis in iodine treated animals (Bagchi *et al.*, 1985). Another example is the drug Amiodarone (which contains 38% iodine) which may not only directly affect thyroid function in an adverse fashion but may be responsible for the development of antithyroid antibodies in patients receiving this drug (Monteiro *et al.*, 1986).

Because of the wide variety of medications containing iodine (see Table 6.7), the effects of iodine deficiency and excess on thyroid glandular function warrant serious consideration alongside the better classified effects on drugs on thyroid function. This is because, additionally, iodine is an important constituent of the thyroid hormone synthetic 'machinery'.

## Experimental examples of xenobiotic induced thyroid dysfunction

We now present a number of detailed experimental 'case-histories' in the following sections providing an overview of the thyroid effects produced in rats by several classes of agents (Figs. 6.4 a–d) studied in our laboratories and producing different effects on the pituitary-thyroid-liver axis. In addition, we describe how an understanding of thyroid auto-regulatory systems can lead to a better design of therapeutic agents, and delineation of exact sites of action of drugs and dietary components on thyroid activity.

## Effects of D- and L-triiodothyronine ($T_3$) on pituitary TSH secretion and peripheral deiodinase activity in the rat

Thyroid hormones (see Fig. 6.4) are important as potential therapeutic agents since they could be of therapeutic use in hypercholesterolaemia and as adjuncts to antidepressant therapy, but only at high does which also increase oxygen consumption and heart rate, and decrease pituitary TSH release. In the search for selective analogues, the most useful separations of hypolipidaemic from metabolic, pituitary-thyroid sup-pression and cardiac effects have been achieved with D-$T_4$ and $T_3$. A comparison of the pharmacological and toxicological characteristics of the isomers of thyroid hormones may help to define the requirements for specificity of thyromimetic effects coupled with minimal toxicity. A com-parative study has been carried out, therefore, on the ability of D- and L-$T_3$ to suppress pituitary-thyroid function in male rats. Pharmacological effects were assessed by measuring serum $T_4$ and TSH concentrations and TSH output from isolated superfused pituitary glands (see Jones *et al.*, 1986). 5'-deiodinase enzyme activity, important homeostatically and tox-icologically as a means of removal of thyroid hormones, was also measured in liver and kidney homogenates (Jones *et al.*, 1987).

Both D- and L-$T_3$ induced a dose-related decrease in serum TSH and $T_4$ and in TSH secretion from the isolated superfused pituitary gland. D-$T_3$ had between one and 10% of the activity of L-$T_3$. In contrast, the increase in 5'-deiodinase activity (as a homeostatic reflex mechanism to clear the high levels of hormone from the systemic circulation) in the liver and kidney did not appear to discriminate between the D- and L-isomers, as both were equally effective in activating the clearance mechanism (Jones *et al.*, 1987). These observations indicate that separation of the therapeutic effect of a compound from other unwanted side-effects such

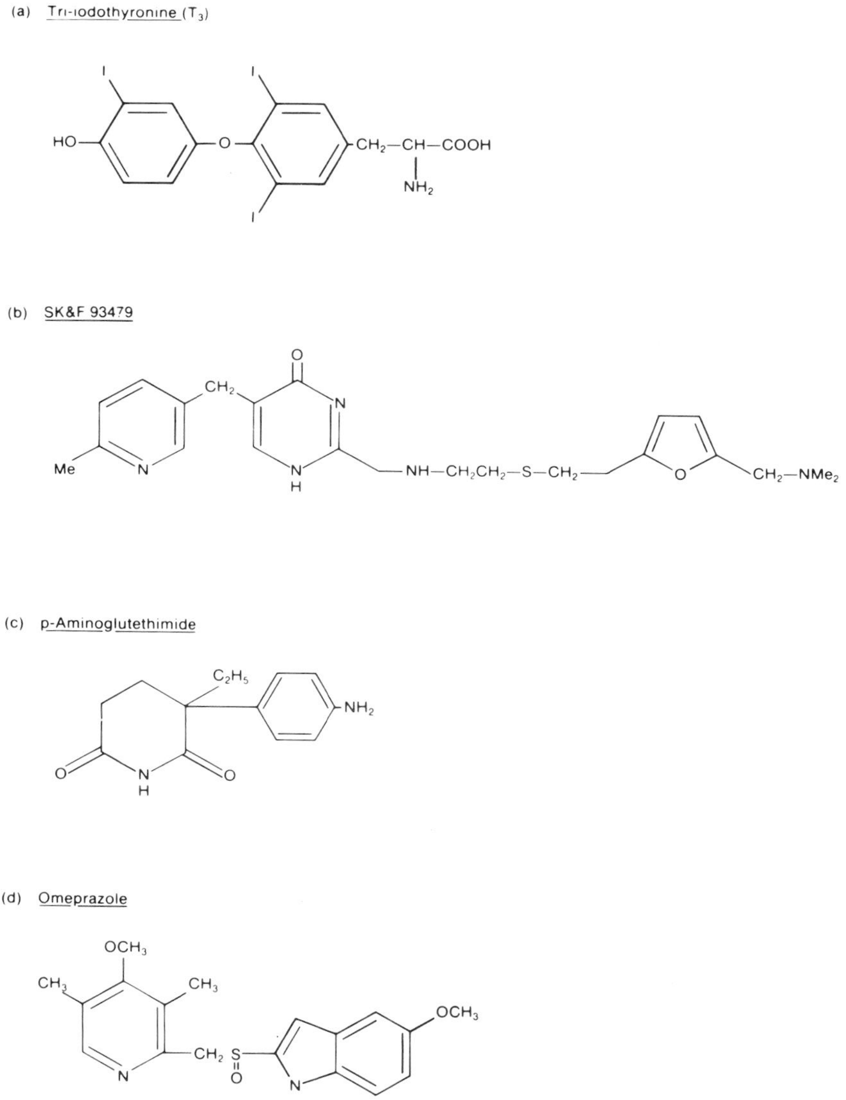

(a) Tri-iodothyronine (T₃)

(b) SK&F 93479

(c) p-Aminoglutethimide

(d) Omeprazole

Fig. 6.4. Structures of compounds studied.

as those on the pituitary-thyroid axis may be achieved by a study of the differential activity of its enantiomers on target tissues both *in vivo* and *in vitro*. In the case of the thyromimetic agents the data imply that in toxicological terms, D-enantiomers will suppress pituitary function less than the

L form but will be cleared as effectively from the circulation, thus giving a much reduced potential for unwanted side-effects.

## Mechanistic studies of the effects of toxic doses of the histamine antagonists Lupitidine (SK&F 93479) and Temelastine (SK&F 93944) on the thyroid gland in different species

There have been a number of reports on the toxicological effects of histamine $H_2$ antagonists, including ranitidine and cimetidine, on thyroid function, although no clear picture has emerged as to their primary mechanism of action (Pasquali *et al.*, 1981; Hugues *et al.*, 1982). Thyroid lesions have been observed in rats treated with very high doses of an isocytosine $H_2$ antagonist SK&F 93479 (Fig. 6.4b) with pathological investigation revealing increased thyroid activity in short-term studies (colloid depletion, follicular cell hyperplasia and hypertrophy – 21 days treatment 500 mg/kg and 1000 mg/kg both sexes – no effect at 200 mg/kg). Long-term administration to rats gave rise to thyroid follicular hyper-plastic foci, adenomas and adenocarcinomas (1000 mg/kg daily for two years, both sexes). Some studies in dog 200 mg/kg daily for 12 months and mouse (1000 mg/kg daily for 30 days) suggested a species-specificity for the lesion as no histopathological changes were seen.

A series of investigative studies was set up to delineate the mechanism of toxicological action of SK&F 93479 on thyroid function in the rat (see Brown *et al.*, 1987). Oral administration of high doses of SK&F 93479 to rats (up to 1000 mg/kg/day) for 10 days resulted in alterations in thyroid morphology indicative of increased activity of the thyroid gland. Measurement of thyroidal $^{125}I$ incorporation substantiated these findings. Treatment with SK&F 93479 resulted in a dose-dependent increase in thyroidal iodide incorporation that was apparent after a single dose of the compound. The effect was reversible after seven days dosing. The increased incorporation of $^{125}I$ into the thyroid gland was apparently dependent on TSH since both hypophysectomy and pretreatment with thyroxine ($T_4$) markedly reduced thyroidal $^{125}I$ uptake.

In an assessment of possible effects on the hypothalamic-pituitary sites it was found that hypothalamic TRH and pituitary TSH concentrations were not altered by SK&F 93479 treatment and in TRH challenge experiments circulating TSH concentrations were not altered from controls. These data suggest unaltered hypothalamic-pituitary sensitivity by treatment with SK&F 93479. Direct effects on thyroid follicular cell function were also discounted as SK&F 93479 had no effects on radioiodide disposition in either cultured rat (FRTL-5 cell line) or porcine thyrocytes (see Brown, Fowler & Atterwill, 1986). Having eliminated various loci for effects on the thyroid axis, the question of altered thyroid hormone metabolism was examined. Circulating $T_4$ and TSH levels were altered in SK&F 93479-treated rats. Generally, $T_4$ levels were reduced six hours after dosing and this was followed by elevated TSH levels at 24 hours after dosing. $T_3$ levels were unaltered by SK&F 93479 treatment. To account for the rapid falls in circulating $T_4$ the effect of SK&F 93479-treatment on $T_4$ clearance was measured by examining the elimination of radioactivity from the circulation of rats previously injected with $^{125}I$-$T_4$. One oral dose of 1000 mg/kg SK&F 93479 was found to be associated with markedly increased $T_4$ clearance.

These results suggest that SK&F 93479 affects thyroid follicular activity indirectly by a primary effect on $T_4$ clearance. Reductions in circulating $T_4$ lead to increased TSH levels and subsequent stimulation of thyroid activity.

These changes were similar to those previously observed in rats by Oppenheimer *et al.* (1968) using phenobarbital. A number of other compounds including the polychlorinated biphenyls (PCBs), 2,3,7,8-tetra-chloro-dibenzo-p-dioxin, the Searle imidazole antimicrobial agent SC-37211, and more recently L-649,923 (a leukotriene $D_4$ antagonist) and Diproteverine (a calcium antagonist) appear to produce similar thyroid lesions to those produced by SK&F 93479 in rats (Bastomsky, 1974, 1977; Collins *et al.*, 1977; Comer *et al.*, 1985; Flack *et al.*, 1989; Saunders *et al.*, 1988) with concomitant increases in liver weight, centrilobular hepatocellular hypertrophy, microsomal enzyme induction and increases in $T_4$ clearance. These effects were sometimes attributed to UDP-GT enzyme induction with increased biliary clearance of $T_4$. However, the changes induced by SK&F 93479, unlike those after phenobarbital treatment, do not appear to correlate temporally with either enhanced UDP-GT, B-glucuronidase or altered deiodinase activities (Brown *et al.*, 1988) and a sub-class of this type of agent with effects on hepatocellular $T_4$ binding and/or uptake remains a possibility.

It was subsequently found that another SK&F isocytosine histamine $H_2$ antagonist Temelastine (SK&F 93944 – which is pharmacologically unrelated to Lupitidine) causes TSH-driven thyroid lesions similar to Lupitidine. A species comparison in dog, mouse and rat confirms that these lesions occur only in the rat, although the follicular stimulation is greater than that caused by Lupitidine as measured by net thyroid radio-iodide accumulation (Atterwill *et al.*, 1989b). *In vitro* studies with Temelastine using cultured rat hepatocytes suggest that the rapidly increased $T_4$ clearance *in vivo* (occurring within a few hours after one dose of compound) caused by these compounds is due in fact to an enhanced hepatocellular $T_4$ uptake (Atterwill *et al.*, 1989b). Transport-mediated, active $T_4$ uptake by the hepatocyte is an important prerequisite for both nuclear hormonally-mediated events, and the metabolism and excretion of $T_4$ (Fig. 6.5; Krenning *et al.*, 1982; Blondeau, 1986). Thus a class of xenobiotics acting very rapidly on thyroxine clearance, as distinct from another class acting through sub-acute induction of liver microsomal enzymes, may do so by an action of the membrane-located $T_4$ transporter in the hepatocyte. Much further investigation of this phenomenon is now needed.

## Thyrotoxicity of the anticonvulsant and aromatase inhibitor aminoglutethimide

Aminoglutethimide (AG; Fig. 6.4c) was first introduced as an anticonvulsant drug in 1960, but had to be withdrawn from clinical use following reports of goitrous hypothyroidism in children. *In vivo* studies in rats have indicated that AG treatment increases thyroid weight and reduces both thyroid iodide uptake and production of thyroxine and diiodotyrosine suggestive of a direct antithyroid effect. The direct thyroid inhibitory mechanism of action of AG has now been confirmed by examining its effect in an *in vitro* model for the detection of potentially thyrotoxic compounds. The effects of para-AG on iodide metabolism by thyroid cells in culture have been compared with structurally related compounds, meta-AG, glutethimide, nitroglutethimide, and acetyl-aminoglutethimide.

Porcine thyrocytes were obtained as described in Brown *et al.* (1986). After three days in culture the effects of compounds on iodide metabolism were assessed, also as described in Brown *et al.* (1986). Para-AG and meta-AG inhibited $^{125}$I-organification in a concentration dependent manner both with an IC50 of 20 μM with no effect on $^{125}$I-uptake (see Fig. 6.6). Glutethimide, nitroglutethimide and acetyl-aminoglutethimide had no effect on either parameter. These results confirm that the *in vivo* effect of AG on the thyroid gland is due to a direct inhibition of thyroid iodide organification and furthermore, that this effect appears dependent upon the presence of a free amino group in the phenyl ring of the molecule. In addition, the potential of this *in vitro* system for the detection of drug induced antithyroid effects and structure–activity relationships is demonstrated.

As we have seen in the previous sections referring to the different classes of agent inducing thyroid lesions it is extremely important to compare a number of parameters of thyroid function both *in vivo* and *in vitro* in order to delineate the mechanisms of toxicity.

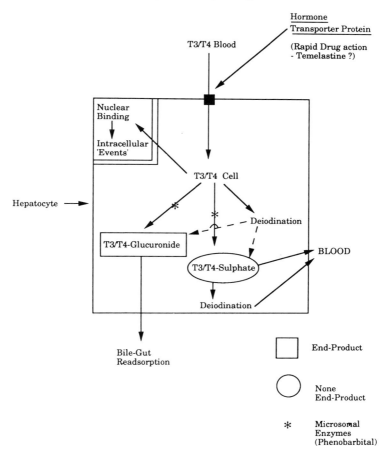

Fig. 6.5. Hepatic events leading to hormone elimination.

## Effects of omeprazole on rat thyroid function

The above-mentioned approach is exemplified in the case of omeprazole (Fig. 6.4d). Toxicological studies on this compound, a $K^+$, $H^+$-ATPase inhibitor, in rats (400–1200 µmol/kg/day) have shown changes in thyroid hormone metabolism with no pathological effect (Ekmann *et al.*, 1985). Omeprazole could have direct effects on the thyroid gland in view of the reported $K^+$, $H^+$-ATPase immunoreactivity in thyroid tissue (Saccomani *et al.*, 1979). In order to fully evaluate the mechanism of the changes produced by omeprazole its effects on a number of thyroid parameters were studied.

SK&F Wistar rats were dosed with omeprazole (414–500 mg/kg *p.o.*) for 7–14 days. Following administration of omeprazole at 500 mg/kg *p.o.* for 14 days, there were reductions (ranging between 20–52%) in plasma total $T_3$ and $T_4$ concentrations on days 1, 3, 7 and 14, both 6 hours and 24 hours following drug administration compared to controls. Serum TSH concentrations were increased in male rats after 14 days (24 hours post dose) where a 60% increase against controls was observed. Despite these changes in hormone levels the accumulation of $^{125}I$ by the rat thyroid gland and its organification *in vivo*, as measured by the perchlorate-discharge test (Atterwill *et al.*, 1987), were unaltered by omeprazole. *In vitro* studies with cultured porcine thyrocytes revealed that omeprazole did inhibit TSH-stimulated $^{125}I$ organification by the cells (see Figs 6.6 and 6.8) but only at high concentrations IC50=2.8 µM and 1.5 µM, respectively). In agreement with the results of Ekmann *et al.* (1985) treatment of male rats with the same dose of (414 mg/kg) omeprazole for 7 days caused a 55% decrease in liver 5'-deiodinase activity (control=147 ± 9; treated=66 ± 7 pg $T_3$/mg protein/10 min; $P<0.05$, n=6), but female liver enzyme activity was unaltered. $T_4$ clearance measured following the elimination of $^{125}I$-$T_4$ (10 µCi/kg) was, however, unaltered following one dose of 500 mg/kg omeprazole. These data support the findings of Ekmann *et al.* (1985) where omeprazole appears to inhibit peripheral 5'-deiodinase activity and decrease plasma $T_3$ concentrations. However, in view of the observed reductions in circulating $T_4$ it may also be a weak, and direct inhibitor of thyroidal hormone biosynthesis as supported by its *in vitro* action in cultured thyrocytes. Despite these actions no effect on radio-iodide disposition in the rat thyroid gland *in vivo* could be detected, indicating that the small rises in serum TSH are probably not sufficient to markedly affect this aspect of thyroid follicular cell function.

## Further studies on xenobiotics acting directly on the thyroid gland using cultured cells

*In vitro* toxicological studies with primary cultures of porcine thyrocytes of various xenobiotics (see also Brown, 1987; Reader, 1987; Atterwill & Fowler, 1990) have similarly provided evidence for excellent *in vitro/in vivo* correlations of potency. Using the *in vivo* Perchlorate Discharge Test in rats it has been demonstrated that neither histamine $H_2$ antagonist, SK&F 93479 nor omeprazole (Atterwill *et al.*, 1989a) inhibit iodide organification, whereas the thyrotoxic anticonvulsant drug Aminoglutethimide does so with a similar potency to antithyroid drugs such as Methimazole and Propylthiouracil (see Brown, 1987). A similar inhibitor potency profile is exhibited *in vitro* using the porcine thyrocytes

Table 6.8. *Comparison of xenobiotic potential for inhibition of iodide organification by the thyroid* in vivo *and* in vitro

| Compound | Order of inhibitory potency in: | |
|---|---|---|
| | (a) Rat perchlorate discharge test *in vivo* | (b) Iodide organification – pocrine thyrocytes ($IC_{50} = \mu M$) |
| SK&F 93479 | No effect | No effect |
| Omeprazole | No effect | > 100 |
| Noxythiolin | No effect | 9.0 |
| Aminoglutethimide | 25% 'Discharge' | 20 |
| Propylthiouracil | 60% 'Discharge' | 0.6–1.5 |

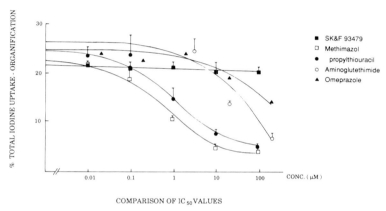

COMPARISON OF $IC_{50}$ VALUES

Fig. 6.6. Effects of different compounds on iodine organification by porcine thyrocytes.

(Table 6.8). In the case of Aminoglutethimide the studies further showed that only relatively small compound structural differences can lead to markedly differing thyroid effects as discussed in the above sections.

The rat FRTL-5 cell line is able to accumulate but not organify iodide and form follicular structures like the primary cultured porcine thyrocytes. However, they are particularly useful for studying the mechanisms of direct effects of agents on the various membrane transport processes and ion-pumps critical for TSH-activated epithelial cell function (see Figs 6.7 and 6.8). In this respect it has recently been demonstrated (Fowler *et al.*, 1989; Atterwill & Fowler, 1990) that exposure of rat thyroid FRTL-5 cells to TSH for 24 hours *in vitro* activates [125]I but not ouabain-sensitive [86]Rb transport in the cells, whereas after 27 hours and above there are

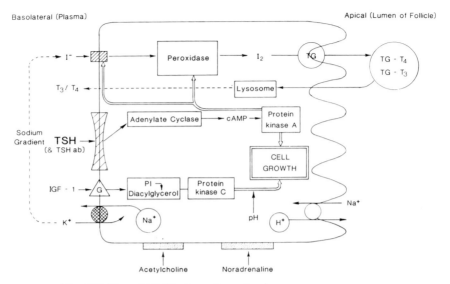

Fig. 6.7. Thyroid follicular cell mechanisms.

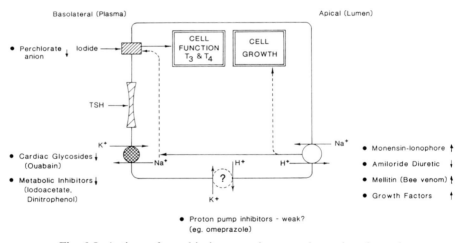

Fig. 6.8. Actions of xenobiotics on various membrane ion channels.

significant increases in the activity of both transporters. This is similar to results obtained *in vivo* in propylthiouracil-treated rats where, unlike the very early increases in *in vitro* iodide transport, activation of thyroidal Na+, K+-ATPase activity in rat thyroid membranes occurs only around 24–48 hours following rises in serum TSH. These data confirm the presence of a $Na^+$, $K^+$-ATPase in cultured rat FRTL-5 thyroid cells which is activated several hours later than iodide accumulation by TSH, and presumably helps to maintain the $Na^+$ gradients necessary for iodide transport (Fig. 6.8). It was further shown that this $Na^+$ pump is sensitive to drugs such as the cardiac glycoside, ouabain, as well as other agents affecting intracellular $Na^+$ ion concentrations such as monensin and the diuretic, amiloride (Fowler *et al.*, 1989; Atterwill & Fowler, 1990).

## Conclusions

Knowledge of the mechanism and species specificity of the induction of both thyroid lesions and tumours by the toxicological effects of chemicals, drugs and dietary constituents such as iodine, is important and rapidly expanding, as the list of active agents and investigative techniques increases. The application of cell culture techniques has enabled studies of the mechanism and potency of drug and dietary agents with direct effects at different levels of the hypothalamic-pituitary-thyroid-liver axis and also their species-specificity. In some cases studies on human tissues have been possible. It has also become possible to use *in vitro* models of endocrine tissues such as the thyroid as 'prescreens' for ranking the organ-specific toxicological potency of drug development candidates. The influx of endocrinology and cell biology information into areas such as the control of thyroid hormone metabolism and the role of growth factors in the control of thyroid follicular cell growth and differentiation leads to a much better understanding of these toxicological events at the molecular level, and their likely relevance to humans.

With regard to the expanding list of hepatic microsomal enzyme inducers causing thyroid gland tumour promotion by an epigenetic mechanism involving 'indirect' elevation of plasma TSH levels, human studies indicate that these compounds do not alter thyroid function until a certain critical degree of enzyme induction occurs. An induction sufficient to increase antipyrine clearance by about 60% appears to be required before steady static hormone levels are altered (McClain, 1989). Williams & Weisberger (1985) have categorized chemicals into genotoxic and epigenetic categories. It is clear that there must be a limitation on the exposure to direct-acting carcinogens although there is still controversy with respect to the relevance to human exposure conditions of xenobiotics acting through an epigenetic mechanism. Thus it is important to establish mechanisms of endocrine tumourigenesis for the purpose of risk-assessment in humans, especially in view of the high background incidence of certain tumours in toxicologically-used species, and the number of xenobiotics increasing tumour incidence when tested at high doses in carcinogenicity studies. Only by considering xenobiotics in a case-by-case mechanistic fashion will it be possible to significantly influence the high attrition rate for development compounds at the same time as limiting exposure to potentially harmful xenobiotics through rigorous safety testing.

## References

Akoso, B.T., Sleight, S.D., Nachreiner, R.F. & Aust., S.D. (1982). Effects of purified polybrominated biphenyl congeners on the thyroid and pituitary glands in rats. *J. Am. College Toxicol.*, **3**, 23–36.

Atterwill, C.K., Brown, C.G., Fowler, K.L. & Jones, C.A. (1989a). Studies on the effects of omeprazole on thyroid function in the rat. *J. Pharm. Pharmacol.*, **41** (10), 733–5.

Atterwill, C.K., Collins, P., Brown, G.G. & Harland, R.F. (1987). The perchlorate discharge test for examining thyroid function in rats. *J. Pharmacol. Methods*, **18**, 199–203.

Atterwill, C.K. & Fowler, K.F. (1990). A comparison of cultured rat FRTL-5 and porcine thyroid cells for predicting the thyroid toxicity of xenobiotics. *Toxicology In Vitro*, **4**, 369–74.

Atterwill, C.K., Poole, A., Jones, C., Jones, R. & Brown, C. (1989b). Mechanistic investigation of species-specific thyroid lesions induced by treatment with the histamine $H_1$ antagonist Temelastine (SK&F 93944) in rats. *Food Chem. Toxicol.*, **27** (10), 681–90.

Axelrod, A.A. & Leblond, C.P. (1955). Induction of thyroid tumours in rats by a low iodine diet. *Cancer*, **8**, 339–67.

Bagchi, N., Brown, T.R., Urdinivia, E., *et al.* (1985). Induction of autoimmune thyroiditis in chickens by dietary iodine. *Science*, **203**, 325–7.

Bastomsky, C.H. (1973). The biliary excretion of thyroxine and its glucuronic acid conjugate in normal and Gunn rats. *Endocrinology*, **92**, 35–40.

Bastomsky, C.H. (1974). Effects of a polychlorinated biphenyl mixture (Aroclor 1254) and DDT on biliary thyroxine excretion in rats. *Endocrinology*, **95**, 1150–5.

Bastomsky, C.H. (1977). Enhanced thyroxine metabolism and high uptake goiters in rats after a single dose of 2,3,7,8-tetrachloro dibenzo-p-dioxin. *Endocrinology*, **101**, 292–6.

Berens, S.C., Bernstein, R.P., Robbins, J. & Wolff, J. (1970). Antithyroid effects of lithium. *J. Clin. Invest.*, **49**, 357–67.

Blondeau, J.P. (1986). Saturable binding of thyroid hormone to isolated rat hepatocytes. *FEBS Lett.*, **204**, 41–7.

Bolt, H.M., Bolt, M. & Kappus, H. (1977). Interaction of rifampicin treatment with pharmacokinetics and metabolism of ethinyloestradiol in man. *Acta Endocrinol.*, **85**, 189–97.

Boronski, G.C., Garafano, D.D., Roase, L.I. *et al.* (1985). Effect of long-term amiodarone therapy on thyroid hormone levels and thyroid function. *Am. J. Med.*, **78**, 443–50.

Bowman, W.C. & Rand, M.J. (1980). *Textbook of Pharmacology*. Oxford: Blackwell.

Brown, C.G. (1987). Application of thyroid cell culture to the study of thyrotoxicity. In *In Vitro Methods in Toxicology*, ed. C.K. Atterwill & C.E. Steele, p. 165. Cambridge: Cambridge University Press.

Brown, C.G., Fowler, K., Atterwill, C.K. (1986). Assessment of thyrotoxicity using *in vitro* cell culture systems. *Food Chem. Toxicol.*, **24**, 557–36.

Brown, C.G., Harland, R.F., Major, I.R. & Atterwill, C.K. (1987). Effects of toxic doses of a novel histamine ($H_2$) antagonist on the rat thyroid gland. *Food. Chem. Toxicol.* **25**, 787–94.

Brown, C.G., Lee, D.M., Jones, C.A. & Atterwill, C.K. (1988). Comparison of the effects of SK&F 93479 and phenobarbitone (PB) treatment on thyroid toxicity and hepatic thyroid hormone metabolizing enzymes in the rat. *Arch. Toxicol.*

Capen, C. & Martin, S. (1989). The effects of xenobiotics on the structure and function of thyroid follicular and C cells. *Toxicol. Pathol.*, **17** (2), 266–93.

Cavalieri, R.R. & Pitt-Rivers, R. (1981). The effects of drugs on the distribution and metabolism of thyroid hormones. *Pharmacol. Rev.* **33**, 55–80.

Colletta, G., Cirafici, A.M. & Vecchio, G. (1986). Induction of the c-fos oncogene by thyrotropic hormone in rat thyroid cells in culture. *Science*, **233**, 458–60.

Collins, W.T., Capen, C.C., Kazza, L., Carter, C. & Dailey, R.E. (1977). Effect of polychlorinated biphenyl (PCB) on the thyroid gland: ultrastructural and biochemical investigations. *Am. J. Path.*, **89**, 119–36.

Comer, C.P., Chengelis, C.P., Levin, S. & Kotsonis, F.M. (1985). Changes in thyroidal function and liver UDP glucuronyltransferase activity in rats following administration of a novel imidazole (SC-372211). *Toxicol. Appl. Pharmacol.*, **80**, 427–36.

Devilla, L. & Williams, E.D. (1982). Morphine-induced TSH release in normal and hypothyroid subjects. *Neuroendocrinol.*, **40**, 303–8.

Diwan, B.A., Palmer, A.E., Oshima, M. & Rice, J.M. (1985). N-nitroso-N-methylurea initiation in multiple tissues for organ-specific tumour promotion in rats by phenobarbitone. *J. Natl. Cancer Inst.*, **75**, 1099–105.

Doniach, L. & Williams, E.D. (1962). The development of thyroid and pituitary tumours in the rat two years after partial thyroidectomy. *Br. J. Cancer*, **16**, 22–231.

Ekmann, L., Hansson, E., Havu, N., Carlsson, E. & Lundberg, C.

(1985). Toxicological studies on Omeprazole. *Scand. J. Gastroenterol.*, **20**, 53–69.

Engler, D. & Burger, A.G. (1984). The deiodination of the iodothyronines and of their derivatives in man. *End. Rev.*, **5**, 151–84.

Flack, J.D., Hakansson, S., Jeffrey, D.J., Kelvin, A.S., Maile, P.A., McCurrdo, A.S. & Perkin, C.I. (1989). Investigation of the effects of diproteverine on the thyroid of the rat. *Human Toxicol.*, **8**, 411.

Fowler, K.L., Collins, P., Brown, C.G. & Atterwill, C.K. (1989). Studies on the TSH-activated $Na^+$, $K^+$-ATPase and iodide transporter in cultured rat thyroid cells and the effects of drugs. *Toxicology In Vitro*, **4**, 31–6.

Goldstein, J.A. & Taurog, A. (1968). Enhanced biliary excretion of thyroxine glucuronide in rats pretreated with benzpyrene. *Biochem. Pharmacol.*, **17**, 1049–65.

Greely, G.H., Jahnke, G., Nicholson, G.F. & Kizer, J.S. (1980). Decreased serum 4, 5, 3-triiodothyronine and thyroxine levels accompanying acute and chronic ritalin treatment in developing rats. *Endocrinology*, **106**, 898–904.

Griesback, W.E., Kennedy, T.H. & Purves, H.D. (1945). Studies on experimental goitre. VI. Thyroid adenoma in rats on a Brassica seed diet. *Br. J. Exp. Pathol.*, **26**, 18–24.

Hershman, J.M. & Konerding, K. (1968). Effects of sulfonylurea drugs on the thyroid and serum protein binding of thyroxine in the rat. *Endocrinology*, **83**, 74–8.

Heymar, P., Larkins, R.G., Higginbotham, L. & Ng, K.W. (1980). D-propranolol and DL-propranolol both decrease conversion of L-thyroxine to L-triiodothyronine. *Br. Med. J.*, **2**, 24–5.

Hiasa, Y., Kitahori, Y., Konishi, N., Enoki, N. & Fujita, T. (1984). Promoting effect of phenobarbital on N-bis(2-hydroxypropyl) nitrosamine thyroid tumorigenesis in rats. Effect of varying duration of exposure to phenobarbital. *IARC, Sci Publ.*, **56**, 77–82.

Hiasa, Y., Kitahori, Y., Konishi, N., Shimoyana, T. & Lin, J.C. (1985). Sex differential and dose dependence of phenobarbitone promoting activity in N-bis (2-hydroxypropyl) nitrosamine initiated thyroid tumourigenesis in rats. *Cancer Res.*, **45**, 4087–90.

Hiasa, Y., Kitahori, Y., Oshima, M., Fujita, T., Yuasa, T., Konishi, N. & Miyashiro, A. (1982). Promoting effects of phenobarbital and barbital on development of thyroid tumours in rats treated with N-bis (2-hydroxypropyl) nitrosamine. *Carcinogenesis*, **3**, 1187–90.

Hillier, A.P. (1974). Antagonistic effects of dinitrophenol and cyanide on hepatic thyroxine deiodination. *Acta Endocrinol.*, **77**, 122–7.

Hine, K.R., Harrop, J.S., Hopton, M.R., Holmes, G.K.T. & Mathews, H. L. (1984). The effects of ranitidine on pituitary-thyroid function. *Br. J. Clin. Pharmac.*, **18**, 608–11.

Hugues, J.N, Perret, G., Sebanon, J. & Modigliani, E. (1982). Effects of cimetidine on thyroid hormones. *Clin. Endocrinol.*, **17**, 297.

Johnson, S. (1990). The effects of B-Naphthoflavone-induced hepatic microsomal enzymes on thyroid gland function. *Human Toxicol.*, **9** (5), 349.

Jones, C.A., Brown, C.G. & Atterwill, C.K. (1987). Thyroid toxicity and iodothyronine deiodination. *Arch. Toxicol. Suppl.*, **11**, 250–2.

Jones, C.A., Brown, C.G., Smith, K. & Atterwill, C.K. (1986). *In vitro* models of the hypothalamic-pituitary system for studying drug toxicity. *Food Chem. Toxicol.*, **24**, 811–12.

Jurney, T.H., Smallridge, R.C., Routledge, P.A., Shand, D.G. & Wartofsky, L. (1983). Propranolol decreases serum thyroxine as well as triodothyronine in rats: a protein-binding effect. *Endocrinology*, **112**, 727–32.

Kari, F., Kutzman, R. & Thompson, M. (1987). Repeated dose exposure of salicylazosulfapyridine to rats and mice. *The Toxicologist*, **1** (19), 47.

Korhle, J., Brabant, G. & Hesch, R.D. (1987). Metabolism of thyroid hormones. *Hormone Res.*, **26**, 58–78.

Krenning, E.P., Docter, R., Bernard, B., Visser, T. & Hennemann, G. (1982). Decreased transport of thyroxine ($T_4$), 3,3$^1$,5-triiodothyronine ($T_3$) and 3,3$^1$,5$^1$-triodothyronine (r$T_3$) into rat hepatocytes in primary culture due to a decrease of cellular ATP content and various drugs. *FEBS Letts.*, **140** (2), 229–33.

Langer, P., Kokesave, H. & Gschwendtova, K. (1976). Acute redistribution of thyroxine after administration of univalent anions, salicylate, theophylline and barbiturates in rats. *Acta Endocrinol.*, **81**, 516–24.

Levin, W., Welch, R.M. & Conney, A.H. (1974). Increased liver microsomal androgen metabolism by phenobarbital: correlation with decreased androgen action on the seminal vesicles of the rat. *J. Pharmacol. Exp. Ther.*, **188**, 287–92.

Lucier, G.W., McDaniel, O.S. & Hook, G.E.R. (1975). Nature of the enhancement of hepatic uridine diphosphate glucuronyl-transferase activity by 2,3,7,8-tetrachlorodibenzo-p-dioxin in rats. *Biochem. Pharmacol.*, **24**, 325–34.

Mendoza, D.M., Flock, E.V., Owen, C.A. & Paris, J. (1966). The effect of 5, 5$^1$-diphenylhydantoin on the metabolism of L-thyroxine-$^{131}$I in the rat. *Endocrinology*, **79**, 106–18.

McClain, R.M. (1989). The significance of hepatic microsomal enzyme induction and altered thyroid function in rats: implications for thyroid gland neoplasia. *Toxicol. Pathol.* **17** (2), 294–306.

Monaco, F., Pontecorvi, A., de Luca, M., de Pirro, R.D., Armiento, M. & Roche, J. (1982). Inhibition of the biosynthesis of thyroglobulin with propranolol in the rat. *C.R. Soc. Biol. (Paris)*, **176**, 607–12.

Monteiro, E., Galvao-Telex, A., Santos, M.L. *et al.* (1986). Antithyroid antibodies as an early marker for thyroid disease induced by amiodarone. *Br. Med. J.*, **292**, 227–8.

Murthy, A.S., Russfield, A.B. & Snow, G.J. (1985). Effect of 4, 4[1]-oxydianiline on the thyroid and pituitary glands of F344 rats: a morphologic study with the use of the immunoperoxidase method. *J. Natl. Cancer Inst.*, **74**, 203–8.

Nakamura, Y., Bellamy, G. & Green, W.L. (1981). Effects of an inhibitor of hepatic drug metabolism, 2-diethyl-aminoethyl-2, 2-diphenylvalerate HCl (SK&F 525-A), on thyroxine metabolism in the rat. *Endocrinology*, **108**, 1516–36.

Ohnhaus, E.E. & Studer, H. (1983). A link between liver microsomal enzyme activity and thyroid hormone metabolism in man. *Br. J. Clin. Pharmac.*, **15**, 71–6.

Oppenheimer, J.H., Bernstein, G. & Surks, M.I. (1968). Increased thyroxine turnover and thyroidal function after stimulation of hepatocellular binding of thyroxine by phenobarbital. *J. Clin. Invest.*, **47**, 1399–406.

Oshima, M. & Ward, J.M. (1984). Promotion of N-methyl-N-nitrosourea-induced thyroid tumours by iodine deficiency in F334/NCr rats. *J. Natl. Cancer Inst.*, **73**, 289–96.

Pasquali, R., Corinaldesi, R., Miglioli, M., Melchionda, N., Capelli, M. & Barbara, L. (1981). Effect of prolonged administration of ranitidine on pituitary and thyroid hormones, and their response to specific hypothalamic releasing factors. *Clin. Endocrinol.*, **15**, 457.

Peter, H.J., Studer, H., Forster, R. & Gerber, H. (1982). The pathogenesis of 'hot' and 'cold' follicles in multinodular goitres. *J. Clin. Endocrinol. Metab.*, **55**, 941–6.

Reader, S.J. (1987). Assessment of the biopotency of antithyroid drugs using porcine thyroid cells. *Biochem. Pharmacol.*, **36**, 1825–28.

Redmond, O. & Ruffers, A.R. (1981). Thyroid proliferation, body weight, TSH and thyroid hormones in chronic antithyroid (carbimazole) treatment in rats. *J. Anat.*, **133**, 37–47.

Reeves, R.R., From, G.L., Paul, W. & Leenen, F.H. (1985). Nadolol, propranolol, and thyroid hormones: evidence for a membrane-stabilizing action of propranolol. *Clin. Pharmacol. Ther.*, **37**, 157–65.

Reuber, M.D. & Glover, E.L. (1969). Thyroiditis in buffalo strain rats ingesting 7,12-dimethyl-benz(a)-anthracenel. *Experimentia*, **25**, 753.

Rustia, M. & Subik, P. (1978). Thyroid tumours in rats and hepatomas in mice after griseofulvin treatment. *Br. J. Cancer*, **38**, 237–49.

Saccomani, G., Helander, G., Crago, S., Chang, H.H., Daley, D. & Sachs, G. (1979). Characterization of gastric mucosal membranes: X. Immunological studies of gastric $K^+$, $H^+$-ATPase. *J. Cell. Biol.*, **83**, 271–83.

Saunders, J.E., Eigenberg, D.A., Bracht, L.J., Wang, W.R. & van Zweiten, M. J. (1988). Thyroid and liver trophic changes in rats secondary to liver microsomal enzyme induction caused by an experimental leukotriene antagonist (L-649,923). *Toxicol. Appl. Pharmacol.*, **95**, 378–87.

Shulkin, B.L., Peele, M.E. & Utiger, R.D. (1984). Beta-adrenergic antagonist inhibition of hepatic 3, 5, 3$^1$-triiodothyronine production. *Endocrinology*, **115**, 858–61.

Silva, J.E. & Larsen, P.P. (1983). Adrenergic activation of triiodothyronine production in brown adipose tissue. *Nature*, **305**, 712–13.

Smeds, S., Peters, H.J., Jortso, E., Gerber, H. & Studer, H. (1987). Naturally occurring clones of cells with high intrinsic proliferation potential within the follicular epithelium of mouse thyroids. *Cancer Res.*, **47**, 1646–51.

Smith, P., Wynford-Thomas, D., Stringer, B.M.J. & Williams, E.D. (1986). Growth factor control of rat thyroid follicular cell proliferation. *Endocrinology*, **119**, 1439–45.

Steinhoff, D., Weber, H., Mohr, M. & Boehme, K. (1983). Evaluation of Amitrole (Aminotriazole) for potential carcinogenicity in rats, mice and golden hamsters. *Toxicol. Appl. Pharmacol.*, **69**, 161–9.

Stockigt, J.R., Lim, C.F., Barlow, J.W., Stevens, V., Topliss, D.J. & Wynne, K.N. (1984). High concentrations of furosemide inhibit serum binding of thyroxine. *J. Clin. Endocrinol. Metab.*, **59**, 62–6.

Stringer, B.M.J., Wynford-Thomas, D. & Williams, E.D. (1985). *In vitro* evidence for an intracellular mechanism limiting the thyroid follicular cell growth response to thyrotropin. *Endocrinology*, **116**, 611–15.

Swarm, R.L., Roberts, G.K.S., Levy, A.C. & Hines, L.R. (1973). Observations of the thyroid gland in rats following the administration of sulfamethoxazole and trimethorpim. *Toxicol. Appl. Pharmacol.*, **24**, 351–63.

Takayama, S., Aihara, K., Onodera, T. & Akimoto, T. (1986). Antithyroid effects of Propylthiouracil and sulphamono-methoxine in rats and monkeys. *Toxicol. Appl. Pharmacol.*, **82**, 191–9.

Taurog, A. (1955). Conjugation and excretion of thyroid hormone. *Brookhaven Symp. Biol.*, **7**, 111–36.

Thomas, G.A. & Williams, E.D. (1991). Evidence for and possible mechanisms of non-genotoxic carcinogenesis in the rodent thyroid. *Mutation Res.*, **248**, 357–70.

Todd, G.C. (1986). Induction and reversibility of thyroid proliferative changes in rats given an antithyroid compound. *Vet. Pathol.*, **23**, 110.

Topliss, D.J., Kolliniatis, E. & Stockigt, J.R. (1987). Drug inhibition of rapid T$_3$ uptake by cultures rat hepatocytes. *Annals. Endocrinol.*, **48**, 123.

Tsuda, H., Fukushima, S., Imaida, K., Kurata, Y. & Ito, N. (1983). Organ-specific promoting effect of phenobarbital and saccharin in induction of thyroid, liver, and urinary bladder tumours in rats after initiation with N-nitrosomethylurea. *Cancer Res.*, **43**, 3292–6.

Wenzel, K.W. (1981). Pharmacological interference with *in vitro* tests of thyroid function. *Metabolism*, **30**, 717–32.

Werk, E.E. Jr., Thrasher, K., Sholiton, L.J., Olinger, C. & Choi, Y. (1971). Cortisol production in epileptic patients treated with diphenylhydantoin. *Clin. Pharmacol. Ther.*, **12**, 698–703.

Westermark, K., Karlsson, F.A. & Westermark, B. (1985). Thyrotropin modulates EGF receptor function in porcine thyroid follicle cells. *Mol. Cell. Endocrinol.*, **40**, 17–23.

Williams, D.W., Wynford-Thomas, D. & Williams, E.D. (1987). Human Thyroid adenomas show escape from IGF-1 dependence for growth. *Ann. Endocrinol.*, **48** (2), 11.

Williams, G.M. & Weisberger, J.H. (1985). Carcinogenicity testing of drugs. *Progr. Drug Res.*, **29**, 155–213.

Wynford-Thomas, D., Stringer, B.M.J. & Williams, E.D. (1982). Dissociations of growth and function in the rat thyroid during prolonged goitrogen administration. *Acta Endocrinol.*, **101**, 210–16.

Zavanella, T., Presta, M. & Ragnotti, G. (1983). Thyroid modifications in male and female rats treated with the hepatocarcinogen beta-blocker ZAMI 1305. *Cancer Lett.*, **19**, 293–9.

Zbinden, G. (1987). Assessment of hyperplastic and neoplastic lesions of the thyroid gland. *T.I.P.S.*, (Dec. 1987) **8**, 511–14.

CHARLES C. CAPEN

# 7    Pathophysiology and xenobiotic toxicity of parathyroid glands in animals

## Introduction

Calcium plays a key role in many fundamental biologic processes and also is an essential structural component of the skeleton. These processes include neuromuscular excitability, membrane permeability, muscle contraction, enzyme activity, hormone release, and blood coagulation. The precise control of calcium in extracellular fluids is vital to health. To maintain a constant concentration of calcium, despite marked variations in intake and excretion, endocrine control mechanisms have evolved that primarily consist of the interactions of three major hormones. Although the direct roles of parathyroid hormone (PTH), calcitonin (CT), and cholecalciferol (vitamin D) frequently are emphasized in the control of blood calcium (Fig. 7.1), other hormones such as adrenal corticosteroids, oestrogens, thyroxine, somatotropic hormone (STH) or growth hormone (GH), glucagon, prolactin, and telocalcin from the corpuscles of Stannius in fish contribute to the maintenance of calcium metabolism and skeletal homeostasis under certain conditions.

The total concentration of calcium in the blood of mammals is approximately 10 mg/dl (2.5 mmol/L) with some variation due to species, age, dietary intake of calcium, and analytical method used to quantitate blood levels. The total calcium in the blood is composed of protein-bound and diffusible fractions. Diffusible calcium consists of calcium complexed to anions such as phosphate and citrate, plus the biologically active free (ionic) calcium (Capen, 1989b).

## Basic endocrinology and control mechanisms

### Parathyroid hormone

#### Anatomy

The parathyroid glands in most animal species consist of two pairs of glands in the anterior cervical region. They are present in all air-breathing

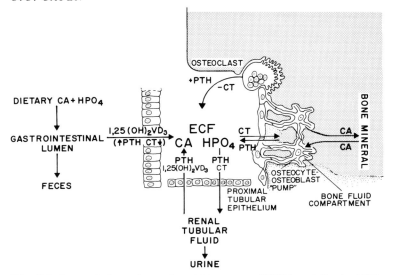

Fig. 7.1. Interrelation of parathyroid hormone (PTH), calcitonin (CT), and 1,25-dihydroxycholecalciferol (1,25 $(OH)_2VD_3$) in the hormonal regulation of calcium and phosphorus in extracellular fluids (ECF).

vertebrates having first appeared in amphibians coincidentally with the transition of life from an aquatic to a terrestrial environment. Embryologically, the parathyroids are of entodermal origin being derived from the pharyngeal pouch (III and IV).

For example, both pairs of the parathyroids (external and internal) are situated in close proximity to the thyroid gland in the dog and cat. The external parathyroid (III) in the dog is from 2 to 5 mm in length and is found in the loose connective tissue cranial and slightly lateral to the anterior pole of the thyroid. The internal parathyroid (IV) is smaller, flatter, and situated on the medial surface of the thyroid beneath the fibrous capsule. The blood supply of the two pairs of glands in the dog is separate from the external parathyroid being supplied by a branch from the cranial thyroid artery and the internal parathyroid by minute ramifications of the arterial supply to the thyroid.

### Functional cytology

#### Chief cells

The parathyroids contain a single basic type of secretory cell concerned with the elaboration of a single hormone. Parathyroids of animals and man are composed of chief cells in different stages of secretory activity and in transition to oxyphil cells in certain species (Fig. 7.2). Chief cells

## PARATHYROID GLAND CYTOLOGY

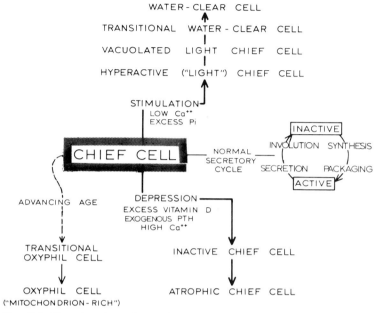

Fig. 7.2. Functional cytology of parathyroid glands under normal and pathologic conditions. (From Capen, 1989.)

interpreted to be in an inactive (resting or involuted) stage of their secretory cycle predominate in the parathyroid glands under normal conditions. Inactive chief cells are cuboidal and have uncomplicated interdigitations between contiguous cells. The relatively electron-transparent cytoplasm contains poorly developed organelles and infrequent secretory granules. The cytoplasm often has either numerous lipid bodies and lipofuscin granules or aggregations of glycogen particles. Chief cells in the active stage of the secretory cycle occur less frequently in the parathyroid glands of most species. The cytoplasm of active chief cells has an increased electron density due to the close proximity of organelles and secretory granules, increased density of the cytoplasmic matrix, and loss of glycogen particles and lipid bodies.

### Oxyphil cells
The second cell type in the parathyroid glands of certain animal species and human beings is the oxyphil cell (Fig. 7.2). They are absent in

parathyroids of the rat, chicken, and many species of lower animals. Oxyphil cells are observed either singly or in small groups interspersed between chief cells. They are larger than chief cells and their abundant cytoplasmic area is filled with numerous large, often bizarre-shaped, mitochondria. Glycogen particles and free ribosomes are interspersed between the mitochondria. Granular endoplasmic reticulum, Golgi apparatuses, and secretory granules are poorly developed in oxyphil cells of normal parathyroid glands, suggesting that oxyphil cells do not have an active function in the biosynthesis of parathyroid hormone. Oxyphil cells have been shown histochemically to have a higher oxidative and hydrolytic enzyme activity than chief cells associated with the marked increase in mitochondria.

Cells are observed with cytoplasmic characteristics intermediate between those of chief and oxyphil cells. These transitional oxyphil cells have numerous mitochondria but other organelles are present including rough endoplasmic reticulum, Golgi apparatuses, and secretory granules. The significance of oxyphil cells in the pathophysiology of the parathyroid glands has not been elucidated completely. They are not altered in response to either short-term hypocalcaemia or hypercalcaemia in animals but both oxyphil cells and transitional forms may be increased in response to long-term stimulation of human parathyroid glands. Therefore, oxyphil cells do not appear to be degenerate chief cells as previously suggested but rather are derived from chief cells as the result of ageing or some other metabolic derangement.

Biosynthesis by chief cells

A larger biosynthetic precursor molecule of parathyroid hormone is first synthesized on ribosomes of the rough endoplasmic reticulum in chief cells. Preproparathyroid hormone (pre-proPTH) is the initial translation product synthesized on ribosomes (Habener & Potts, 1979). It is composed of 115 amino acids and contains a hydrophobic signal or leader sequence of 25 amino acid residues that facilitates the penetration and subsequent vectorial discharge of the nascent peptide into the cisternal space of the rough endoplasmic reticulum (Kronenberg et al., 1986). Pre-proPTH is rapidly converted within 1 min or less of its synthesis to pro-parathyroid hormone (ProPTH) by the proteolytic cleavage of 25 amino acids from the $NH_2$-terminal end of the molecule (Habener, 1981). The intermediate precursor, proPTH, is composed of 90 amino acids and moves within membranous channels of the rough endoplasmic reticulum to the Golgi apparatus (Fig. 7.3). Enzymes within membranes of the Golgi apparatus cleave a hexapeptide from the $NH_2$-terminal (biologically active) end of the molecule forming active parathyroid hormone

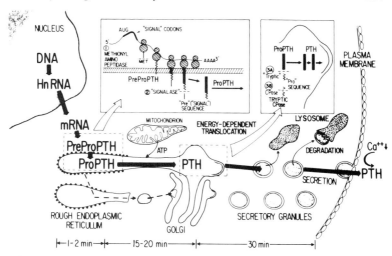

Fig. 7.3. Subcellular compartmentalization, transport and cleavage of precursors of parathyroid hormone (PTH). Pre-proparathyroid hormone (pre-proPTH) is the initial translation product from ribosomes of the rough endoplasmic reticulum, which is rapidly converted to parathyroid hormone (proPTH). The hydrophobic sequence on the amino-terminal end of the pre-proPTH facilitates penetration of the leading portion of the nascent peptide into the lumen of the endoplasmic reticulum. ProPTH is transported to the Golgi apparatus where it is converted enzymatically by a carboxypeptidase (CPase) to biologically active PTH. A major portion of the biosynthetic precursors and active PTH is degraded by lysosomal enzymes and is not secreted by chief cells under normal conditions. Parathyroid secretory protein (PSP) may be incorporated into secretory granules with PTH during intracellular storage and be released with PTH into the extracellular space. (From Habener & Potts, 1978, with permission.)

(Fig. 7.3). Active PTH is packaged into membrane-limited, macromolecular aggregates in the Golgi apparatus for subsequent storage in chief cells. Under certain conditions of increased demand (i.e. low calcium ion concentration in extracellular fluid compartment), PTH may be released directly from chief cells without being packaged into secretion granules by a process termed 'bypass secretion'.

Biologically active parathyroid hormone secreted by chief cells is a straight chain polypeptide consisting of 84 amino acid residues with a molecular weight of approximately 9500. Molecular fragments of PTH are formed in the peripheral circulation and in the liver. The immunoheterogeneity created by the multiple circulating fragments of PTH has caused significant problems in the development and application of highly specific radioimmunoassays to diagnostic problems in human patients and animals (Goltzman *et al.*, 1986).

### Control of secretion

Secretory cells in the parathyroid gland store small amounts of preformed hormone but are capable of responding to minor fluctuations in calcium concentration by rapidly altering the rate of hormonal secretion and more slowly by altering the rate of hormonal synthesis (Roth & Raisz, 1964). In contrast to most endocrine organs that are under complex controls involving both long and short feedback loops, the parathyroids have a unique feedback controlled by the concentration of calcium (and to a lesser extent magnesium) ion in serum. If the blood calcium is elevated by the intravenous infusion of calcium, there is a rapid and pronounced reduction in circulating levels of immunoreactive parathyroid hormone (iPTH) (Fig. 7.4). Conversely, if the blood calcium is lowered by EDTA (ethylenediaminetetraacetic acid), there is a brisk and substantial increase in iPTH levels (Fig. 7.4).

The concentration of blood phosphorus has no direct regulatory influence on the synthesis and secretion of PTH; however, several disease conditions with hyperphosphataemia in both animals and man are associated clinically with secondary hyperparathyroidism. An elevated blood phosphorus level may lead indirectly to parathyroid stimulation by virtue of its ability to lower blood calcium. If the blood phosphorus is elevated significantly by an infusion of phosphate and calcium administered simultaneously in amounts to prevent the accompanying reduction of blood calcium, plasma iPTH levels remain within the normal range (Fig. 7.4). Magnesium ion has an effect on parathyroid secretion rate similar to that of calcium, but its effect is not equipotent to that of calcium (Mayer & Hurst, 1978). The more potent effects of calcium ion in the control of PTH secretion, together with its preponderance over magnesium in the extracellular fluid, suggests a secondary role for magnesium ion in parathyroid control.

Calcium ion not only controls the rate of biosynthesis and secretion of PTH, but also other metabolic and intracellular degradative processes within chief cells (Chu *et al.*, 1973). An increase of calcium ions in extracellular fluids rapidly inhibits the uptake of amino acids by chief cells, synthesis of proPTH and conversion to PTH, and secretion of stored PTH. A shift in the percentage of flow of proPTH from the degradative pathway to the secretory route represents a key adaptive response of the parathyroid gland to a low calcium diet. Parathyroids from rats fed a low calcium (0.02%) diet convert approximately 40% of

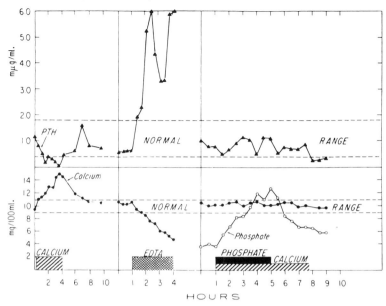

Fig. 7.4. Changes in plasma immunoreactive parathyroid hormone in response to hypercalcemia by calcium infusion, hypocalcemia produced by EDTA, and hyperphosphatemia with normocalcemia in a cow. (From Aurbach & Potts, 1964.)

proPTH to PTH compared to a 20% conversion in rats fed a control diet (normal calcium) (Chu *et al.*, 1973). During periods of long-term calcium restriction the enhanced synthesis and secretion of PTH would be accomplished by an increased capacity of the entire pathway in individual hypertrophied chief cells and through hyperplasia of active chief cells. Degradation of 'mature PTH' by lysosomal enzymes increases after prolonged exposure to a high calcium environment.

Recently synthesized and processed active PTH may be released directly in response to increased demand and bypass the storage pool of mature secretory granules in the cytoplasm of chief cells. Bypass secretion of parathyroid hormone can be stimulated only by a low circulating concentration of calcium ion (Fig. 7.5).

### Biologic actions

Parathyroid hormone is the principal hormone involved in the minute-to-minute fine regulation of blood calcium in mammals. It exerts its biologic actions by directly influencing the function of target cells primarily in bone and kidney, and indirectly in the intestine to maintain plasma cal-

BIOSYNTHESIS OF PARATHYROID HORMONE

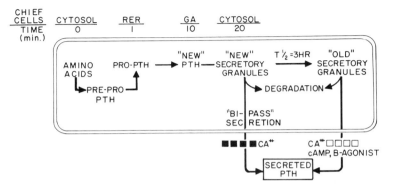

Fig. 7.5. Bypass secretion of parathyroid hormone (PTH) in response to increased demand signalled by decreased blood calcium ion concentration. Recently synthesized and processed active PTH (1-84) may be released directly and not enter the storage pool of mature ('old') secretory granules in the cytoplasm of chief cells. PTH from the storage pool can be mobilized by cyclic adenosine monophosphate (cAMP) and beta ($\beta$)-agonists (such as epinephrine, norepinephrine, and isoproterenol) as well as by lowered blood calcium ion, whereas secretion from the pool of recently synthesized PTH can be stimulated only by a decreased calcium ion concentration. RER=rough endoplasmic reticulum; GA=Golgi apparatus. (Redrawn from Cohn & MacGregor, 1981.)

cium at a level sufficient to ensure the optimal functioning of a wide variety of body cells. The action of PTH on bone is to mobilize calcium from skeletal reserves into extracellular fluids (Raisz & Kream, 1983). The administration of PTH causes an initial decline followed by a sustained increase in circulating levels of calcium. This transitory decrease in blood calcium is considered to be the result of a sequestration of calcium-phosphate in bone and soft tissues (Parsons & Robinson, 1971). The subsequent increase in blood calcium results from an interaction of PTH with osteoblasts and osteoclasts in bone, and increased tubular reabsorption of calcium in the kidney (Sutton & Dirks, 1978; High, Black & Capen, 1981).

*Bone*
Osteoclasts appear to be primarily responsible for the catabolic action of PTH on bone by increasing bone resorption (Chambers, 1980; Chambers *et al.*, 1984; Wong, 1986). PTH has been known for some time to stimu-

late an increased activity of preformed osteoclasts. This is interesting in light of recent findings which have failed to demonstrate specific receptors for PTH on osteoclasts; however, receptors were present on osteoblasts (Pliam, Nviredy & Arnaud, 1982; Silve *et al.*, 1982). Isolated osteoclasts do not respond to PTH without the concurrent presence of osteoblasts (McSheehy & Chambers, 1986). The mechanisms by which binding of PTH to osteoblasts results in stimulation of osteoblastic secretory products, which are capable of stimulating osteoclastic bone resorption, is not known but may include direct effects on the osteoblast and/or stimulation of osteoclastic secretory products which are capable of increasing osteoblastic bone resorption (Fig. 7.6) (Vaes, 1988). If the increase in PTH is sustained, the size of the active osteoclast pool in bone is increased by activation of osteoprogenitor cells in the endosteal bone-cell envelope.

The initial binding of PTH to osteoblasts lining bone surfaces appears to cause the cells to contract, thereby exposing the underlying mineral to osteoclasts (Fig. 7.6) (Rodan & Martin, 1981). The change in shape of osteoblasts associated with PTH may be critical to mediation of osteoclastic bone resorption stimulated by the hormone. Osteoblastic contraction is associated with microfilament disaggregation (Wong, 1986). The alteration in osteoblast shape exposes osteoid-covered bone matrix to osteoclasts; however, osteoclasts attach preferentially to mineralized bone matrix.

Osteoblasts secrete a latent collagenase and neutral proteases (such as plasminogen activator that can activate latent collagenase) which result in degradation of the osteoid matrix and exposes the underlying calcified matrix for osteoclastic bone resorption (Eeckhout *et al.*, 1988). Bone-resorbing hormones such as PTH, prostaglandin E2 (PG E2), and 1,25-dihydroxyvitamin D stimulate plasminogen activator activity in osteoblasts. A collagenase inhibitor (Cl-1, an analogue of collagen alpha chain sequence) can inhibit PTH-induced bone resorption (Delaisse *et al.*, 1985). Bone resorption products, particularly osteocalcin, can attract osteoclast precursors and enhance the resorption process.

Osteoblasts also may elaborate unidentified paracrine chemical mediators of osteoclastic bone resorption. None of the known bone-resorbing factors (PTH, PG E2, lymphokines, growth factors) have been shown to directly stimulate osteoclasts without the presence of osteoblasts (de Vernejoul *et al.*, 1988). The only substance that was found to stimulate bone resorption by isolated chicken osteoclasts in one investigation was murine splenic conditioned medium (de Vernejoul *et al.*, 1988). Bone resorption by isolated osteoclasts is inhibited by calcitonin and PG E2 which induce cAMP production in osteoclasts.

PARACINE CONTROL OF BONE RESORPTION

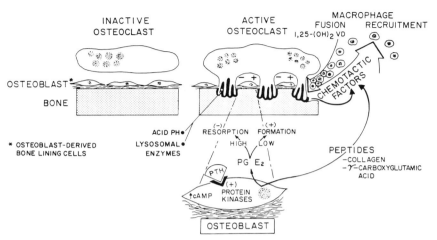

Fig. 7.6. Paracrine control of bone resorption. Specific receptors for parathyroid hormone are present on osteoblasts but not osteoclasts. In response to parathyroid hormone, osteoblasts contract, thereby exposing the underlying mineralized surface to osteoclasts and release soluble factors that increase osteoclastic activity.

PTH stimulation of osteoblasts results in induction of bone resorption due to osteoclast activation and increased osteoclast numbers. The plasma membrane of osteoclasts in intimate contact with the resorbing surfaces is modified to form a series of membranous projections referred to as the brush ('ruffled') border. The brush border of activated osteoclasts is isolated from the extracellular fluids by adjacent transitional ('sealing') zones, thereby localizing the lysosomal enzymes and acidic environment to the immediate area undergoing dissolution. PTH and other bone-resorbing agents increase proteolytic, lysosomal, and acid-producing enzymes in osteoclasts which include acid phosphatase, beta-glucuronidase, and carbonic anhydrase (Wong, 1986). Carbonic anhydrase is localized to the brush border and induces acidification of the brush border area.

Binding of PTH to specific isoreceptors on bone cells results in the activation of adenylate cyclase in the plasma membrane (Fig. 7.7). The adenylate cyclase catalyzes the conversion of ATP to cAMP in target cells. The accumulation of cAMP in target cells functions as an intracellular messenger of parathyroid hormone action in osteoblasts. Parathyroid hormone also induces an increase in cytoplasmic calcium and stimulates

**MECHANISM OF PARATHYROID HORMONE ACTION**

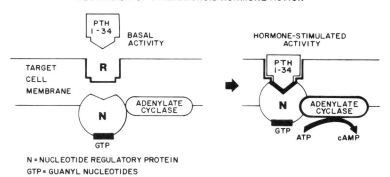

N = NUCLEOTIDE REGULATORY PROTEIN
GTP = GUANYL NUCLEOTIDES

Fig. 7.7. Mechanism of parathyroid hormone (PTH) action. The biologically active end of the hormone (PTH 1-34) binds to specific receptors
(R) on the surface of target cells. The receptor-hormone complex is
coupled to the catalytic subunit of adenylate cyclase in the cell membrane by a nucleotide regulatory (N)-protein. This results in the intracellular accumulation of cyclic adenosine monophosphate (cAMP),
which serves as the 'second messenger' for polypeptide hormones such
as PTH in target cells and results in expression of the biologic response
of the hormone.

phosphatidyl inositol turnover in osteoblasts; however, it has not been
determined which intracellular messenger is required for induction of
bone resorption by PTH-stimulation of osteoblasts (Donahue *et al.*, 1988;
Farndale *et al.*, 1988; Herrmann-Erlee *et al.*, 1988). The increase in
cytosolic calcium is partially dependent on cAMP accumulation. Calcium
concentration in the osteoblast also may be increased by the activation of
protein kinase C resulting in the production of inositol 1, 4, 5-trisphos-
phate and subsequent release of calcium from the endoplasmic reticulum
(Yamaguchi, Kleeman & Muallem, 1987).

*Kidney*
Parathyroid hormone has a rapid (within 5–10 min) and direct effect on
renal tubular function leading to decreased reabsorption of phosphate
and phosphaturia (Knox & Haramati, 1985). The site of PTH on blocking
tubular reabsorption of phosphate has been localized by micropuncture
methods to the proximal tubule of the nephron. Parathyroidectomy
decreases renal phosphate excretion. PTH binds to a receptor on the
basolateral aspect of renal epithelial cells. The hormone stimulates
adenylate cyclase, increases intracellular cAMP, and inhibits phosphate
reabsorption across the brush border through the actions of protein

kinases. PTH also increases the transport of calcium across the basolateral renal cell membrane and increases intracellular calcium which inhibits the formation of cAMP, thus decreasing the phosphaturic effects of PTH (Beck *et al.*, 1974; Knox & Haramati, 1985). PTH is capable of stimulating inositol 1, 4, 5-trisphosphate and diacylglycerol production in renal tubular cells (Hruska *et al.*, 1987). Therefore, regulation of phosphate transport by PTH may be mediated by two classes of receptors and transmembrane-signalling systems, one which activates adenylate cyclase and one which activates protein kinase C and increases intracellular calcium (Cole *et al.*, 1987).

Although the effects of PTH on the tubular reabsorption of phosphate have been considered to be of major importance, evidence has accumulated indicating that the ability of PTH to enhance the reabsorption of calcium is of considerable importance in the maintenance of calcium homeostasis. This effect of PTH upon tubular reabsorption of calcium appears to be due to a direct action on the distal convoluted tubule (Sutton & Dirks, 1978). The biochemical mechanism by which PTH enhances calcium reabsorption is unknown, but it is coupled to increases in intracellular cAMP (Hanai *et al.*, 1986). There are two calcium active transport systems in the basolateral membrane of renal cells, a high affinity calcium ATPase and a $Na^+/Ca^{++}$ exchanger.

The other important effect of PTH on the kidney is on the regulation of the conversion of 25-hydroxycholecalciferol to 1,25-dihydroxycholecalciferol and other metabolites of vitamin D (Brumbaugh, Hughes & Haussler, 1975). PTH has been shown to promote the absorption of calcium from the gastrointestinal tract in animals, under a variety of experimental conditions (Nemere & Norman, 1986). This effect is not as rapid as the action on the kidney and is not observed in vitamin D-deficient animals. The increase in intestinal calcium transport appears to be an indirect effect of PTH on absorptive cells by its action on stimulating synthesis of the biologically active metabolite of vitamin D by mitochondria in renal tubular epithelial cells (de Vernejoul *et al.*, 1988). The effects of PTH on the metabolism of 25-hydroxycholecalciferol appear to be mediated by cAMP and not dependent on calcium ion concentration (Henry, 1985). The active metabolites of vitamin D make bone cells more sensitive to the direct effects of PTH ('permissive effect') and greatly enhance the gastrointestinal absorption of calcium, thereby, amplifying the effect of PTH upon plasma calcium concentration.

The kidney is a major organ for the degradation of PTH. Biologically active PTH from the peritubular capillaries is degraded by specific proteases on the surface of renal tubular cells. In addition, both biologically active ($NH_2$-1-34) and inactive (34–84 COOH) fragments are degraded intracellularly by lysosomal enzymes within renal tubular cells (Hruska *et al.*, 1977).

## Parathyroid hormone-related protein

### Relationship to PTH

Parathyroid hormone-related protein (PTHrP) is a newly described hormone that is produced by multiple normal tissues and some malignant neoplasms (Orloff, Wu & Stewart, 1989b). The human PTHrP gene is present in a single copy and likely evolved from the PTH gene (Cole *et al.*, 1987; Goltzman, Hendy & Banville, 1989; Mangin *et al.*, 1989). The PTHrP gene is more complex than the PTH gene in that it contains at least two promoter regions and six exons compared to one promoter and three exons in the PTH gene (Simpson *et al.*, 1983; Goltzman *et al.*, 1989; Suva *et al.*, 1989). Alternate splicing of the exons that contain coding regions for C-terminal amino acids results in mature proteins that vary in their C-terminal regions. Human PTHrP is initially synthesized as a prepropeptide of 175, 177, or 209 amino acids. The 36 amino acid 'prepro' sequence is removed sequentially by proteases after the nascent protein penetrates into the endoplasmic reticulum and is processed to form a mature protein of 139, 141, or 173 amino acids. The first 139 amino acids of each form of PTHrP are identical.

The complete sequence for PTHrP is known at present only for the human and rat protein (Goltzman *et al.*, 1989; Yasuda *et al.*, 1989). The first 111 amino acids of the full length form of rat PTHrP (141 amino acids) has only two substitutions compared to human PTHrP (Yasuda *et al.*, 1989). This indicates that there has been stringent conservation of the structure of PTHrP between mammalian species during evolution. The canine form of PTHrP is likely to be similar to human PTHrP since antibodies and cDNA probes to human PTHrP have been used to identify PTHrP in normal tissues and tumours of dogs (Ikeda *et al.*, 1988a; Rosol *et al.*, 1990).

The first 13 N-terminal amino acids of PTHrP share 70% sequence homology with PTH. There is no further homology with PTH in the C-terminal region. The N-terminal sequence homology of PTHrP with PTH is important since it enables PTHrP to stimulate PTH receptors in bone and kidney cells (Nissenson, Diep & Strewler, 1988). The first seven amino acids of PTH are of critical importance for ligand-induced activation of intracellular secondary messengers after binding to PTH receptors. This is also true for PTHrP, since five of seven of the N-terminal amino acids of PTHrP are identical to PTH (Rabbani *et al.*, 1988). In contrast, amino acids 25–34 of PTH are biologically inactive but are of critical importance for the ability of PTH to bind to PTH receptors. There is no sequence homology of PTHrP to PTH in amino acids 25–34. This indicates that a nonhomologous region of PTHrP is able to bind to PTH receptors, whereas a homologous region of PTHrP is responsible for activating PTH receptors (Orloff *et al.*, 1989b).

PTH as discussed earlier in this chapter, is synthesized and secreted predominantly by chief cells in the parathyroid glands. By comparison, PTHrP was initially identified as a product of malignant tumours associated with humoral hypercalcaemia of malignancy (Ikeda *et al.*, 1988a; Mundy, 1988). It is now appreciated that PTHrP is produced under a variety of conditions by many normal tissues, including the parathyroid glands (especially foetal), adrenal glands (cortex and medulla), pancreas, thyroid gland, bone marrow, stomach mucosa, foetal liver, brain, lactating mammary gland, placenta, skin (keratinocytes), and lymphocytes (Rodda *et al.*, 1988; Orloff *et al.*, 1989b; Thiede, 1989). The function of PTHrP in many of the tissues where it is produced is not currently understood.

Biologic actions

PTHrP in the adult most likely functions as a paracrine regulatory substance in the tissues in which it is produced. Serum levels of PTHrP are low (<10 pg/ml) and difficult to measure by radioimmunoassay. It is probable that there are specific receptors for PTHrP; however, it has not been possible to differentiate biochemically between PTH and PTHrP receptors (Orloff *et al.*, 1989b). Most investigations have evaluated the actions of PTHrP in tissues or cells with well defined receptors for PTH, such as bone and kidney. PTHrP binds to PTH receptors with equal affinity as PTH (Nissenson *et al.*, 1988; Orloff *et al.*, 1989a) (Fig. 7.8). Parathyroid hormone activates at least three intracellular secondary messenger systems in bone and kidney cells, namely: (1) stimulation of adenylate cyclase to convert ATP to AMP, (2) stimulation of the hydrolysis of inositol phosphates to inositol 1, 4, 5-trisphosphate and diacylglycerol, and (3) increasing intracellular concentrations of calcium ion (Civitelli *et al.*, 1988; van Leeuwen *et al.*, 1988; Orloff *et al.*, 1989b).

PTHrP is equipotent to PTH in stimulating adenylate cyclase in bone cells; however, PTHrP is less potent than PTH in stimulating adenylate cyclase in renal membranes (Orloff *et al.*, 1989b). This suggests that there may be different subtypes of PTH receptors and that PTHrP is capable of activating the bone subtypes with greater efficiency compared to the renal subtypes. PTHrP also increases cytosolic calcium in bone cells with potency equal to that of PTH (Civitelli *et al.*, 1989).

PTHrP results in identical biologic effects in bone and kidney when compared to PTH. PTHrP stimulates bone resorption and increases the

**MECHANISM OF ACTION OF PTH-RELATED PROTEIN**

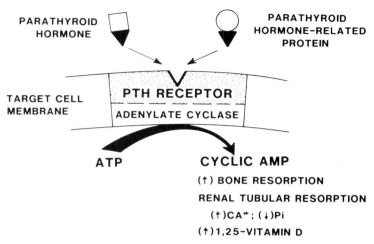

Fig. 7.8. Parathyroid hormone (PTH)-related protein produced by tumour cells appear to result in hypercalcemia by binding to PTH receptors in bone and kidney. The stimulation of increased bone resorption and renal tubular reabsorption of calcium results in the persistent elevation of blood calcium.

numbers of osteoclasts, increases in bone formation, and increases calcium reabsorption and phosphorus excretion by the kidney (Rosol, Capen & Horst, 1988; Yates *et al.*, 1988; Akatsu *et al.*, 1989; Ebeling *et al.*, 1989). Excessive bone resorption and increased calcium reabsorption by the kidney result in hypercalcaemia when PTHrP is present in the circulation in higher than normal levels. Hypercalciuria also occurs when serum levels of PTHrP are increased in spite of increased calcium reabsorption due to increased levels of filtered calcium (Rosol *et al.*, 1988). PTHrP increases nephrogenous cAMP levels due to the stimulation of adenylate cyclase in proximal and distal convoluted tubules (Ebeling *et al.*, 1989).

Relationship to humoral hypercalcaemia of malignancy
PTHrP was originally isolated from malignant neoplasms that were associated with humoral hypercalcaemia of malignancy (HHM) (Burtis *et al.*, 1987; Moseley *et al.*, 1987; Strewler *et al.*, 1987; Stewart *et al.*, 1988; Weir *et al.*, 1988b). Certain malignant tumours secrete PTHrP which induces hypercalcaemia by stimulating increased osteoclastic bone resorption and calcium reabsorption from the kidney (Rosol *et al.*, 1986b; Mundy, 1988; Broadus, 1988). These effects occur distant to the sites of the neoplasms

and represent an abnormal endocrine consequence of stimulation of PTH receptors in bone and kidney by increased serum levels of PTHrP (Budayr *et al.*, 1989a). Injection of antiserum to PTHrP is capable of normalizing serum calcium in experimental animals with HHM, indicating that circulating forms of PTHrP are likely to be responsible for inducing HHM (Kukreja *et al.*, 1988). It is also possible that tumours associated with HHM induce hypercalcaemia by producing additional factors capable of stimulating bone resorption, such as interleukin-1 and transforming growth factors (Merryman *et al.*, 1989; Mundy, 1989).

HHM occurs in humans and animals as well defined clinical syndromes associated with specific malignancies and sporadically with less common neoplasms (Rosol & Capen, 1988). Dogs develop HHM commonly with adenocarcinomas derived from apocrine glands of the anal sac and certain types of malignant lymphoma (Meuten *et al.*, 1983a; Meuten *et al.*, 1983b). A tumour-line derived from the apocrine adenocarcinoma and maintained in nude mice has been used to define the pathobiology of HHM as it occurs in the dog (Rosol *et al.*, 1986b). The canine apocrine adenocarcinoma is capable of stimulating bone resorption and adenylate cyclase in bone and kidney cells (Rosol, Capen & Minkin, 1986; Rosol, Capen & Brooks, 1987). Surgical removal of the adenocarcinoma resulted in a rapid return of serum calcium to normal levels (Rosol & Capen, 1988). The presence of PTHrP in the canine apocrine adenocarcinoma has been demonstrated by immunohistochemistry and immunoblotting using antiserum to human PTHrP. In addition, mRNA from the adenocarcinoma binds to a cDNA probe for human PTHrP (Rosol *et al.*, 1990). This suggests that the canine form of PTHrP is similar to human PTHrP and possibly acts by similar mechanisms as it does in human patients with HHM.

The canine adenocarcinoma also contains transforming growth factor α and β activities which may contribute to the systemic increase in bone resorption. However, these activities are not due to PTHrP, since the transforming growth factor activities can be separated completely from the PTHrP present in the neoplasm (Merryman *et al.*, 1989). Dogs with certain forms of malignant lymphoma and hypercalcaemia also may develop HHM due to autonomous production of PTHrP by the neoplastic lymphocytes. Dogs with such forms of lymphoma develop the characteristic syndrome of HHM (Weir *et al.*, 1988a) and the tumours contain mRNA for PTHrP which is not present in nonhypercalcaemic lymphomas (Ikeda *et al.*, 1988a). HHM also occurs sporadically in dogs, cats, and horses associated with various carcinomas, such as squamous cell carcinomas of the stomach in horses (Meuten *et al.*, 1978; Rosol & Capen, 1988; Klausner *et al.*, 1990).

Production of PTHrP by malignant tumours is possibly an exaggerated expression of a protein normally produced by the tissue of origin of the neoplasm. It is also possible that the expression of PTHrP by a tumour represents the aberrant expression by the cancer cells of a protein hormone not normally secreted by the cell of origin of the tumour.

Physiologic significance

PTHrP is produced by many normal tissues including keratinocytes of the skin, parathyroid glands (especially foetal and neoplastic parathyroid cells), lactating mammary gland, placenta, adrenal glands (cortex and medulla), pancreas, thyroid gland, bone marrow, stomach mucosa, foetal liver, brain, and lymphocytes (Donahue *et al.*, 1988; Ikeda *et al.*, 1988b; Rodda *et al.*, 1988; Orloff *et al.*, 1989b; Thiede, 1989). Its function and mechanism of action in most normal tissues is currently unknown, but it appears to function as a paracrine or autocrine regulator of calcium metabolism and cell differentiation.

Immunohistochemical staining has demonstrated strong reactivity for PTHrP in keratinocytes of the prickle cell layer and hair follicles in the skin of humans and dogs (Danks *et al.*, 1989; Hayman *et al.*, 1989; Rosol *et al.*, 1990). Keratinocytes also have been shown to secrete PTHrP into cell culture medium *in vitro* (Merendino *et al.*, 1986). The function of PTHrP in the skin is not known; however, PTHrP may act in an autocrine manner to decrease keratinocyte proliferation and enhance squamous differentiation (Holick, Nussbaum & Persons, 1988). Squamous cell carcinomas, areas of squamous differentiation in benign skin tumours, and hair follicle tumours consistently stain positive for PTHrP in human patients (Danks *et al.*, 1989; Hayman *et al.*, 1989). Interestingly, these tumours were not associated with the clinical syndrome of HHM (Danks *et al.*, 1989).

The production of PTHrP by a neoplasm does not necessarily result in hypercalcaemia in patients. It is likely that many skin tumours either synthesize but do not secrete PTHrP resulting in low levels of PTHrP or secrete PTHrP in a form that is not biologically active. In contrast, squamous cell carcinomas that are associated with HHM appear to induce hypercalcaemia by secreting an excessive amount of PTHrP into the systemic circulation (Stewart *et al.*, 1986). Dermal fibroblasts have also been reported to have PTH/PTHrP receptors (Pun, Arnaud & Nissenson, 1988). Since adenylate cyclase in dermal fibroblasts is more effectively stimulated by PTHrP than by PTH (Orloff *et al.*, 1989b) it is possible that PTHrP produced by keratinocytes interacts with dermal fibroblasts in a paracrine manner.

PTHrP is produced by foetal parathyroid glands and placentomes in sheep (Rodda *et al.*, 1988; Loveridge *et al.*, 1988). It has been demonstrated that PTHrP acts in an endocrine manner as a hormone in foetal sheep to maintain normal levels of serum calcium (Rodda *et al.*, 1988). PTHrP also facilitates calcium transport from the dam to the foetus across the placentomes (Rodda *et al.*, 1988). Parathyroid glands in adult animals produce low levels of PTHrP in the normal state; however, parathyroid adenomas may produce excessive amounts of PTHrP and contribute to the development of hypercalcaemia (Ikeda *et al.*, 1988b).

The mammary glands express PTHrP mRNA during lactation that is dependent on prolactin secretion from the pituitary gland (Thiede, 1989). The expression of PTHrP is rapidly terminated after weaning (Thiede & Rodan, 1988). It has been suggested that PTHrP may control calcium uptake by the mammary gland during lactation. Milk contains high levels of PTHrP, but it is not known whether PTHrP has any role in the neonate after consumption of milk during PTHrP (Budayr *et al.*, 1989b).

It has been speculated that PTHrP produced in the adrenal cortex and medulla may have a role in vascular regulation (Ikeda *et al.*, 1988b; Orloff *et al.*, 1989b). Relatively high concentrations of PTH and PTHrP are able to cause acute hypotension by stimulating relaxation of smooth muscle in arteries. This effect is most prominent in celiac, coronary, and renal vascular systems (Orloff *et al.*, 1989b). PTH and PTHrP also have positive inotropic and chronotropic effects on cardiac muscle (Nickols *et al.*, 1989).

Lymphocytes contain receptors for PTH/PTHrP but the role of PTHrP in the regulation of immune function is unknown (Yamamoto *et al.*, 1988). Human lymphocytes infected with human T-cell lymphotropic virus-I (HTLV-I) have been reported to produce and secrete PTHrP (Motokura *et al.*, 1988; Fukumoto *et al.*, 1989). Some patients with lymphoma caused by HTLV-I infection develop HHM possibly due to PTHrP production by the neoplastic lymphocytes (Motokura *et al.*, 1989). A similar situation may occur with a subset of canine patients with malignant lymphoma, since mRNA production for PTHrP has been identified in dogs with lymphoma and HHM (Ikeda *et al.*, 1988a; Weir *et al.*, 1988c).

In summary, PTHrP is produced by diverse tissues. It appears that in most instances PTHrP acts as an autocrine or paracrine factor to locally regulate cellular function. Exceptions to this rule may be the role of PTHrP in regulation of serum concentration of calcium in the foetus and cardiovascular regulation in the adult. The syndrome of HHM is due to the abnormal production and secretion of PTHrP by malignant tumours. This results in elevated circulating levels of biologically active PTHrP that stimulate PTH receptors in bone and kidney cells to induce hypercalcaemia. HHM of malignancy represents an abnormal endocrine role of PTHrP in the cancer patient. Normal circulating concentrations of PTHrP are very low (<2.5 p mol/L or 10 pg/ml) (Budayr *et al.*, 1989a). However, sensitive and specific radioimmunoassays for PTHrP are not yet readily available for most animal species. A better understanding of the endocrine function of PTHrP will be possible when PTHrP can be accurately measured in serum of experimental animals.

## Lesions of parathyroid gland

### Proliferative lesions of chief cells

Incidence

Proliferative lesions of the parathyroid gland include hyperplasia (diffuse and focal), adenomas, and carcinomas (Capen, 1989a; Capen, 1990). Neoplasms of the parathyroid glands are relatively uncommon in all species of laboratory and domestic animals (Capen, 1985b; Capen, 1989a), but occur in low incidence in rats, Syrian hamsters, dogs, and rarely mice. Parathyroid hyperplasia occurs much more frequently and may be primary or secondary. Primary parathyroid hyperplasia or parathyroid tumours may be functional (endocrinologically active) or nonfunctional depending on their ability to secrete PTH (Capen, 1988). Primary hyperparathyroidism is a disorder that results from excessive and autonomous secretion of PTH from adenomas or chief cell hyperplasia. Atrophy of the remaining normal parathyroid tissue is present with functional tumours and multinodular parathyroid hyperplasia.

Hyperplasia

*Focal*

Chief cell hyperplasia may affect the parathyroid in a distinctly focal or multifocal distribution (Capen, 1983). In focal parathyroid hyperplasia there are single or multiple nodules in one or both glands where there is an increased number of closely packed chief cells often with an expanded cytoplasmic area (Fig. 7.9). The focal area(s) of chief cell hyperplasia is (are) poorly demarcated and not encapsulated from adjacent parenchyma. Chief cells within the nodules have a relatively uniform composition with a high cytoplasm:nuclear ratio and a more hyperchromatic nucleus than adjacent normal chief cells. There may be slight compression of adjacent chief cells around larger focal areas of hyperplasia. Focal chief cell hyperplasia often is difficult to separate from a chief cell adenoma using only morphologic criteria. The presence of multiple nodules of varying sizes and uniform cellularity in one or both

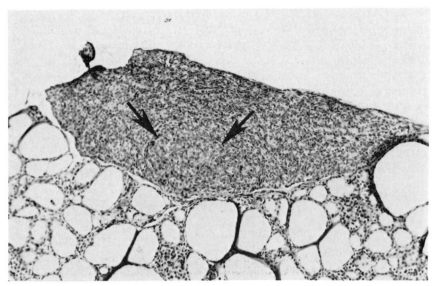

Fig. 7.9. Food hyperplasia (arrows) of chief cells in parathyroid glands of a rat. The focal areas of increased cellularity are poorly demarcated and not encapsulated from adjacent parathyroid parenchyma. (From Capen, 1989, with permission.)

parathyroids with minimal compression and no encapsulation is more compatible with an interpretation of focal hyperplasia than chief cell adenoma.

*Diffuse*

Parathyroid hyperplasia such as seen with chronic renal failure and long-term dietary imbalances results in a uniform enlargement of all parathyroid glands. In rats with chronic renal failure, diffusely hyperplastic parathyroid glands may be detected macroscopically as 1–2 mm nodules projecting from the surface of each thyroid lobe (Capen, 1989a). The uniform enlargement of parathyroid glands in diffuse hyperplasia is due to both hypertrophy and hyperplasia of chief cells. There is not a peripheral rim of compressed atrophic parathyroid parenchyma as around a functional adenoma, but rather a uniform population of hyperplastic chief cells extending to the capsule of the gland (Fig. 7.10). The chief cells are closely packed together often with indistinct cell boundaries. The expanded cytoplasmic area of chronically stimulated chief cells is lightly eosinophilic with occasional distinct vacuoles. A more prominent fibrovascular stroma in some diffusely hyperplastic

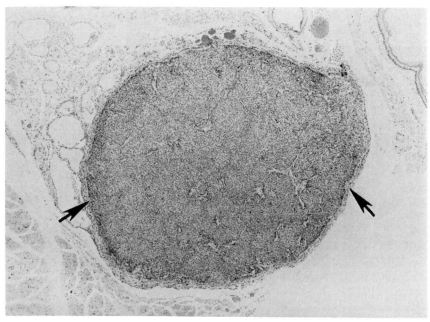

Fig. 7.10. Diffuse hyperplasia of chief cells with enlargement of parathyroid gland in an F344 rat. There is a uniform increase in cellularity due to hypertrophy and hyperplasia of chief cells. Arrows indicate parathyroid capsule. (From Capen, 1989, with permission.)

parathyroids may result in a lobulated appearance (Fig. 7.10). In other hyperplastic parathyroids the chief cells form distinct acinus-like structures in the gland.

### Adenoma

Parathyroid adenomas in rats vary from microscopic in size to unilateral nodules several millimetres in diameter located in the cervical region by the thyroids or infrequently in the thoracic cavity near the base of the heart (Capen, 1989a; Capen, 1990). Parathyroid neoplasms in the precardiac mediastinum are derived from ectopic parathyroid tissue displaced into the thorax with the expanding thymus during embryonic development. Tumours of parathyroid chief cells do not appear to be a sequela of long-standing secondary hyperparathyroidism of either renal or nutritional origin. The unaffected parathyroid glands may be atrophic if the adenoma is functional, normal if the adenoma is nonfunctional, or enlarged if there is concomitant hyperplasia. In functional adenomas the normal mechanism by which PTH secretion is controlled by the concentration of blood calcium is lost and hormone secretion is excessive in spite of an increased level of blood calcium.

Adenomas are solitary nodules that are sharply demarcated from adjacent parathyroid parenchyma (Fig. 7.11). Since the adenoma compresses the rim of surrounding parathyroid to varying degrees depending upon its size, there may be a partial fibrous capsule either from compression of existing stroma or proliferation of fibrous connective tissue (Fig. 7.11).

Adenomas are usually nonfunctional in rats but may be functional in dogs, cats, and humans (Capen, 1990). Chief cells in nonfunctional adenomas are cuboidal or polyhedral and arranged either in a diffuse sheet, lobules, or acini with or without lumens. Nuclei are round-to-oval, often vesicular, and mitotic figures may be present; however, they are usually infrequent. Chief cells from functional adenomas often are closely packed into small groups by fine connective tissue septae. The chief cells are cuboidal and the cytoplasm stains lightly eosinophilic. The cytoplasmic area varies from normal size to an expanded area. There is a much lower density of cells in functional parathyroid adenoma compared to the adjacent rim with atrophic chief cells. Occasional oxyphil cells, water-clear cells, and transitional forms may be distributed throughout the adenoma.

Some parathyroid adenomas in the rat become cystic. The cystadenomas contain solid areas of tumour cells and large cystic areas lined by neoplastic chief cells. The cysts contain a densely eosinophilic proteinaceous fluid. As the cystic spaces enlarge the tumour cells lining the cysts become flattened. Interspersed between the cysts are solid islands of tumour cells.

Chief cells comprising functional parathyroid adenomas ultrastructurally are in the actively synthesizing stage of the secretory cycle. Multiple large lamellar arrays of rough endoplasmic reticulum and clusters of free ribosomes are present in the cytoplasm. Few mature secretory granules are present in autonomous chief cells, suggesting that the rate of PTH secretion is faster than synthesis and storage.

Larger parathyroid adenomas, such as those that are detected macroscopically, often nearly incorporate the entire affected gland. A narrow rim of compressed parenchyma may be detected at one side of the gland or the affected parathyroid may be completely incorporated by the adenoma. Chief cells in this rim often are compressed and atrophic due to pressure and the persistent hypercalcaemia. Peripherally situated follicles in the adjacent thyroid lobe may be compressed to a limited extent by larger parathyroid adenomas. The parathyroid glands that do not contain a functional adenoma also undergo trophic atrophy in response to the hypercalcaemia and become smaller. Atrophic parathyroids, particularly

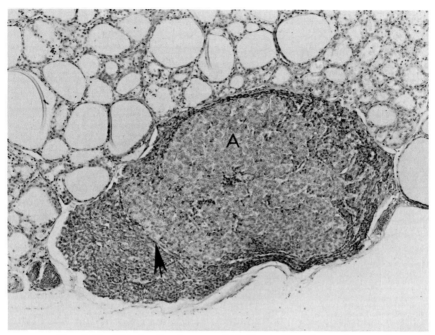

Fig. 7.11. Chief cell adenoma (A) illustrating sharp demarcation and partial encapsulation (arrow) from adjacent parathyroid in Fisher rat. Chief cells in the adenoma have a larger cytoplasmic area than those in the compressed rim of the parathyroid gland. (From Capen, 1989, with permission.)

in certain species, have an interstitial infiltration of fat which replaces the normal parenchyma. Multiple white foci may be seen macroscopically in the thyroids of animals with functional parathyroid tumours. These represent areas of C-cell hyperplasia in response to the long-term hypercalcaemia.

### Carcinoma

Chief cell carcinomas are encountered rarely in laboratory rats and domestic animals (Capen, 1990). Carcinomas result in a macroscopically detectable enlargement usually of one gland. Parathyroid carcinomas often are more fixed in position than chief cell adenomas due to invasion of either the adjacent thyroid lobe or adjacent cervical skeletal muscle. Some of the enlargement may be due to central necrosis and haemorrhage in the carcinoma.

The malignant chief cells either are arranged in solid sheets subdivided into lobules by a fibrovascular stroma, palisade along blood sinusoids, or form acinar structures. There is usually complete incorporation of the affected gland and evidence of invasion through the parathyroid capsule. Evidence of vascular invasion and formation of tumour cell emboli are observed infrequently. Malignant chief cells may be more pleomorphic than those comprising adenomas but mitotic figures are infrequent. The cytoplasmic area stains lightly eosinophilic and boundaries of adjacent chief cells are indistinct.

## Parathyroid cysts

Embryologically, parathyroids are of entodermal origin being derived from the III and IV pharyngeal pouches in close association with primordia of the thymus (Fig. 7.12). Parathyroid (Kürsteiner's) cysts develop from a persistence and dilatation of remnants of the duct that connects the parathyroid and thymic primordia during embryonic development (Fig. 7.12). The cyst fluid has been reported to contain higher levels of immunoreactive PTH (1–84 intact molecule and 39–84 COOH fragments) than serum (Ayer *et al.*, 1989). The lining cells stain for PTH by immunohistochemistry. Similar cysts may be present in the anterior mediastinum when remnants of the embryonic duct are displaced with the caudal migration of the thymus.

Small cysts are observed frequently within the parenchyma of the parathyroid or in the immediate vicinity of the glands in rats, dogs, and occasionally in other animal species (Capen, 1983). Parathyroid cysts usually are multiloculated, lined by a cuboidal to columnar (often partially ciliated) epithelium, and contain a densely eosinophilic proteinic material. The lining epithelial cells have an electron-dense cytoplasm and numerous microvilli projecting into the lumen of the cyst, but they have poorly developed synthetic and secretory organelles.

Parathyroid cysts are distinct from midline cysts derived from remnants of the thyroglossal duct. The latter are lined by multilayered thyroido-genic epithelium that often has colloid-containing follicles. They usually are located near the midline from the base of the tongue caudally into the mediastinum.

## Multinucleated syncytial cells

Parathyroid glands of dogs and rats occasionally develop a unique multinucleated syncytial giant cell (Capen, 1983; Meuten *et al.*, 1984). Syncytial cells often are more numerous near the periphery of the

**EMBRYOLOGY OF THYROID AND PARATHYROID GLANDS**

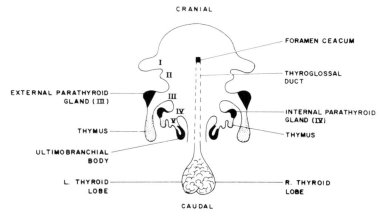

Fig. 7.12. Embryology of thyroid and parathyroid glands.

parathyroid gland (Fig. 7.13) but this is variable between animals and considerable numbers can be present in the more central portions of the gland. The number of syncytial cells often varies considerably between parathyroids in the same animal but may account for up to one-half of the parenchyma of the gland. They appear to form by the fusion of the cytoplasmic area of adjacent chief cells.

The cytoplasm of syncytial cells is densely eosinophilic and homogenous, and the plasma membranes between adjacent cells often are indistinct (Fig. 7.14). The nuclei are smaller, more hyperchromatic and oval, than those in adjacent chief cells. The electron-dense cytoplasm of syncytial cells often has organelles with early degenerative changes. Membrane-limited secretory granules are observed infrequently in the cytoplasm. Plasma membranes of chief cells forming the syncytial cell are disrupted and incomplete, resulting in coalescence of the cytoplasmic area of adjacent cells. Adjacent chief cells are well-fixed with distinct plasma membranes (Fig. 7.14). The mechanism by which syncytial cells form is uncertain but it does not appear to be related to improper fixation of the parathyroid. Syncytial cells have been observed following either immersion fixation or perfusion of the gland with glutaraldehyde fixatives of varying concentrations and direct fixation in osmium tetroxide. They usually do not occur in numbers sufficient to interfere with parathyroid function (Meuten *et al.*, 1984).

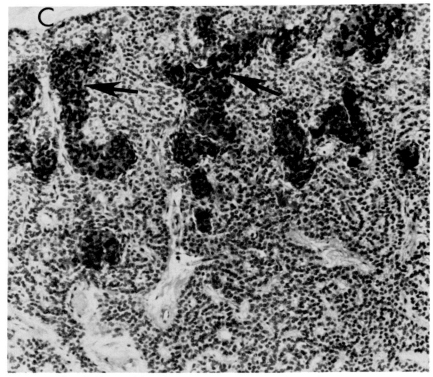

Fig. 7.13. Multinucleated syncytial cells (arrow) near periphery of
canine parathyroid gland. The syncytial cells are sharply demarcated
from adjacent normal chief cells. C=capsule of parathyroid.

## Suppression of chief cells

### High calcium diets
To investigate the mechanisms by which high calcium prepartal diets
predispose to the development of profound hypocalcaemia at parturition,
adult cows were fed a high calcium diet (150 g/day or 6 times recommended quantity) with normal phosphorus (25 g/day) content for 50 days
prepartum (Black, Capen & Arhaud, 1973). The serum calcium increased
after 10 days (11.8 mg/100 ml) and remained elevated above values in
controls fed a balanced diet with recommended amounts of calcium (25 g)
and phosphorus. However, the ability to respond to the hypocalcaemic
challenge associated with parturition and the initiation of lactation was
less in animals fed the high calcium diet and the decrease in serum
calcium at parturition was greater than in controls.

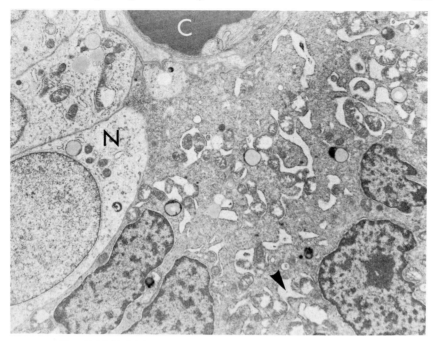

Fig. 7.14. Multinucleated syncytial cell (right) and adjacent inactive chief cells (left). The large cytoplasmic area of syncytial cell is formed by fusion of adjacent chief cells following disruption of plasma membranes. The multiple nuclei are smaller and more electron-dense than in normal chief cells (N) (left) and have condensed chromatin. Mitochondria are swollen with disruption of cristae in syncytial cells, and profiles of endoplasmic reticulum are distended (arrowhead). C=capillary. ×4,900.

Plasma immunoreactive PTH did not significantly increase prepartum in animals fed the high calcium diet and decreased from 1240 pg/ml at parturition to 735 pg/ml at 48 hours postpartum (Black *et al.*, 1973). Control cows fed the balanced diet with only the recommended amount of calcium had consistently higher immunoreactive PTH levels prepartum which increased from 2970 pg/ml at parturition to 7880 pg/ml at 48 hours postpartum. Chief cells in the inactive stage of the secretory cycle predominated in parathyroids of animals fed the high calcium diet. The cytoplasm contained numerous lipid bodies, dispersed individual profiles of endoplasmic reticulum, small Golgi apparatuses, occasional lipofuscin granules but infrequent secretion granules.

Atrophic chief cells were present frequently in parathyroids of cows fed high calcium diets (Fig. 7.15). They were irregular in outline, had an

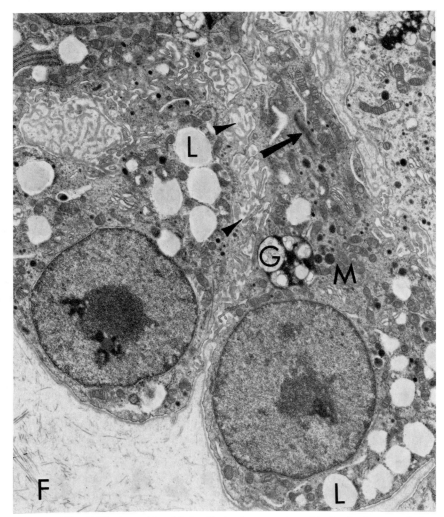

Fig. 7.15. Atrophic chief cells in the parathyroid gland of a cow fed a high calcium diet prepartum. The cells are irregularly shaped and separated by widened intercellular spaces with cytoplasmic processes (arrowheads). The electron-dense cytoplasm contains many lipid bodies (L), large lipofuscin granules (G), and occasional secretory granules. Cytoplasmic organelles other than mitochondria (M) are poorly developed. Note the condensation of microfilaments (arrow) in the cytoplasm of an atrophic chief cell. The widened perivascular space contains many collagen fibers (F). ×9,300. (From Black, Capen & Arnaud, 1973, with permission.)

electron-dense cytoplasm, and were shrunken from adjacent chief cells. Secretory organelles were poorly developed and storage granules were infrequent. Active chief cells with lamellar arrays of endoplasmic reticulum, large Golgi apparatuses, and many secretion granules predominated in parathyroids of control parturient animals (Black *et al.*, 1973).

### Vitamin D

Ultrastructural changes in secretory activity of parathyroid glands in response to persistent hypercalcaemia have been investigated in cows given $30 \times 10^6$ of vitamin $D_2$ (irradiated ergosterol) daily for intervals of 3 to 30 days (Capen, Cole & Hibbs, 1968). The parathyroid glands had ultrastructural alterations suggesting suppression of parathyroid hormone synthesis and secretion (Capen, Koestner & Cole, 1965). Hypercalcaemia did not appear to affect the entire population of chief cells uniformly. After 3 to 7 days of vitamin D the blood calcium was increased to 12.3 mg/100 ml. The parathyroid glands contained chief cells primarily in the inactive stage of the secretory cycle as well as occasional atrophic and active chief cells.

The most striking initial alteration in response to hypercalcaemia was an accumulation of numerous secretory granules within some chief cells. These cells appeared to have entered a phase of active hormonal synthesis prior to or during the development of hypercalcaemia. They completed the secretory cycle and returned to the inactive stage, but the products of synthesis accumulated as increased numbers of granules. Secretory granules were present throughout the cytoplasm but often in large aggregates near the plasma membrane.

The changes in the parathyroid glands in response to hypercalcaemia of longer duration (10 to 30 days) were similar but became progressively more severe. Inactive chief cells predominated in the parathyroid glands but atrophic cells became more numerous. Atrophic chief cells were more electron-dense and smaller than inactive chief cells. The nucleus was irregularly shrunken and the cytoplasmic matrix was dense and contained lipofuscin and lipid bodies, ribosomes, a small Golgi apparatus, and often many secretory granules. The intercellular spaces were widened between adjacent atrophic chief cells. Cells with characteristics intermediate between inactive and atrophic chief cells were observed, suggesting that the latter are derived from inactive chief cells.

Chronic hypercalcaemia appeared to inhibit but not prevent chief cells from entering the active stage of the secretory cycle. Occasional chief cells were observed with lamellar aggregations of endoplasmic reticulum and clusters of ribosomes, suggesting active hormonal synthesis, in cells with many peripherally situated storage granules. The number of secretory granules in chief cells decreased progressively from the 10th to the 30th day of hypercalcaemic suppression. Multivesicular bodies, distended peripheral Golgi cisternae, and swollen prosecretory granules were observed near Golgi apparatuses. The increased lysosomal bodies, sometimes partially surrounding a secretory granule, together with the presence of partially degraded granules within autographic vacuoles suggests a mechanism by which chief cells degrade their secretory product in response to chronic hypercalcaemia.

### *Solanum malacoxylon* (1,25-[OH]$_2$-Vitamin D containing plant) intoxication

Livestock grazing on calcinogenic plants develop a progressive debilitating disease with widespread soft tissue mineralization that has been recognized world-wide. *Cestrum diurnum* (day-blooming jessamine) in Florida and the southern USA and *Trisetum flavescens* in the Bavarian and Austrian Alps cause calcinosis in horses, cattle, and sheep (Dirksen *et al.*, 1975; Krook *et al.*, 1975; Wasserman, Corradino & Krook, 1975). *Solanum malacoxylon* found in Argentina and Brazil produces the disease (Enteque Seco or Espichamento in cattle) which is characterized by the development of hypercalcaemia, hyperphosphataemia, and widespread soft tissue mineralization (Carillo & Woker, 1967; Döbereiner *et al.*, 1971).

The leaves of these calcinogenic plants contain a substance(s) possessing vitamin D-like biological activity (Wasserman, 1975). The dried leaves of *S. malacoxylon* have been shown to contain a steroid-glycoside conjugate in which the steroidal component is identical with 1$\alpha$, 25-dihydroxycholecalciferol (1$\alpha$, 25[OH]$_2$D$_3$) (Haussler *et al.*, 1976; Wasserman *et al.*, 1976). This active principle in *S. malacoxylon* stimulates intestinal calcium absorption and enhances calcium-binding protein synthesis both under normal conditions (Corradino & Wasserman, 1974) and conditions in which the conversion of 25-hydroxycholecalciferol to 1$\alpha$, 25-(OH)$_2$D$_3$ is blocked by high dietary levels of strontium or by nephrectomy. The active principle of *S. malacoxylon* interacts with the intestinal receptor system for 1$\alpha$,25(OH)$_2$D$_3$ and decreases the steady state levels of renal 25-hydroxycholecalciferol-1$\alpha$-hydroxylase (Proscal *et al.*, 1976).

Other evidence for the potent vitamin D-like action of *S. malacoxylon* comes from studies on experimental *S. malacoxylon* intoxication of cattle. After ingestion of the dried leaves of *S. malacoxylon* there is a rapid rise in serum calcium levels accompanied by an increase in serum inorganic phosphorus. Chronic *S. malacoxylon* intoxication in cattle results in widespread mineralization of the cardiovascular system, lung, kidney, and other organs (Döbereiner, Done & Beltran, 1975).

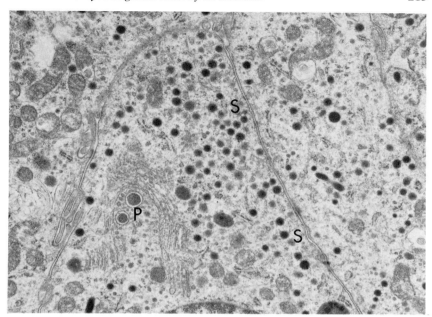

Fig. 7.16. Suppression of parathyroid chief cell by feeding *Solanum malacoxylon* (1,25-[OH]₂-Vitamin D containing plant) for 1 day. Numerous PTH-containing secretory granules (S) are present near the plasma membrane and large prosecretory granules (P) are present near the Golgi apparatus. ×20,400. (From Collins *et al.*, 1977, with permission.)

Experimental intoxication of cattle with pharmacological levels of the parent vitamin D compound results in similar lesions and changes in levels of serum electrolytes (Capen, Cole & Hibbs, 1968).

After feeding *S. malacoxylon*, parathyroid chief cells initially accumulated secretory granules and later underwent involution and atrophy (Collins *et al.*, 1977). There was an accumulation of mature secretory granules near the plasma membrane of chief cells after feeding leaves (0.4 g/kg) of *S. malacoxylon* for only one day (Fig. 7.16). Golgi apparatuses were moderate in size and associated with a few large prosecretory granules. Individual profiles and small lamellar arrays of rough endoplasmic reticulum were present in the cytoplasm. The plasma membranes were straight and had occasional uncomplicated interdigitations with adjacent chief cells.

Chief cells of cattle fed *S. malacoxylon* leaves for six (0.067 g/kg/day) and 32 (0.029 g/kg/day) days appeared to be predominately in the inactive stage of the secretory cycle. The cytoplasmic area was diminished and the nucleus was more irregular. Secretory granules were reduced compared to animals fed *S. malacoxylon* for one day, but there were increased numbers of lysosomal and lipofuscin bodies. Mitochondria were numerous but the rough endoplasmic reticulum was dispersed into small individual profiles. The intercellular spaces between adjacent inactive chief cells were widened and traversed by numerous interdigitating cytoplasmic processes (Collins *et al.*, 1977).

### 1,25-$(OH)_2$ vitamin D alone and in combination with 24R,25-$(OH)_2$-vitamin D

The active metabolites of vitamin D have a direct effect on the parathyroid gland, in addition to their well known effect on the intestine and bone. Parathyroid glands selectively localize and contain specific cytoplasmic and nuclear receptors for 1,25-$(OH)_2D_3$ (Henry & Norman, 1975; Brumbaugh *et al.*, 1975). Henry, Taylor & Norman (1977) reported a significant regression in parathyroid weight of vitamin D deficient ($-D$) chicks by either 1,25-$(OH)_2D_3$ or vitamin $D_3$ ($+D$); however, lower doses of 1,25-$(OH)_2D_3$ (1.3 nM) required 24R,25-$(OH)_2D_3$ (3.9 nM) to produce a similar decrease in parathyroid gland weight and DNA content.

The fine structural alterations in chief cells associated with the regression of parathyroid gland weight produced by vitamin $D_3$ and its metabolites (alone or in combination) has been investigated in $-D$ chicks (Table 7.1) (Henry *et al.*, 1977). Hyperactive chief cells predominated in $-D$ chicks and had an expanded cytoplasmic area containing extensive arrays of rough endoplasmic reticulum with dilated cisternae, few mature secretory granules, and prominent Golgi apparatuses with prosecretory granules (Fig. 7.17). Plasma membranes of adjacent cells were intricately interdigitated (Capen, Henry & Norman, 1977).

Inactive and atrophic chief cells predominated in $-D$ chicks administered 1,25-$(OH)_2D_3$ (3.9 or 5.2 nM per day for 5 or 7 days) (Fig. 7.18). The cytoplasmic area of inactive chief cells was markedly diminished. Numerous lysosomal bodies, prosecretory granules, and prominent microtubules were associated with the Golgi apparatus in chief cells suppressed by 1,25-$(OH)_2D_3$. Atrophic chief cells were irregularly shrunken with widened intercellular spaces, were not electron-dense, and had vacuolated mitochondria and poorly developed secretory organelles.

Chief cells in $-D$ chicks receiving lower doses (1.3 nM) of 1,25-$(OH)_2D_3$ for 5 or 7 days remained predominately in the active stage of the secretory cycle. Inactive and atrophic chief cells were much less frequent than in chicks receiving higher dose of 1,25-$(OH)_2D_3$. Inactive chief cells predominated in parathyroid glands of $-D$ chicks given vitamin $D_3$ (100 international units) and atrophic chief cells were present frequently in chicks receiving vitamin $D_3$ for 5 to 7 days. Numerous lysosomal bodies

Table 7.1. *Effect of vitamin D and metabolites (alone and in combination) on parathyroid (PTG) weight and serum calcium in vitamin D-deficient chicks*

| Steroid | nM/Day | Days | N | Serum Ca (mg/dl) | *Relative PTG weight (%) |
|---------|--------|------|---|------------------|--------------------------|
| $-D_3$ | 0 | 7 | 10 | 5.9 ± 1.2 | 100 |
| $+D_3$ | 6.5 | 2 | 3 | 7.5 ± 0.8 | 74 |
|  | 6.5 | 5 | 2 | 7.6 ± 0.2 | 64 |
|  | 6.5 | 7 | 8 | 8.0 ± 0.6 | 58 |
| 1, 25– $(OH)_2D_3$ | 1.3 | 7 | 6 | 7.6 ± 0.6 | 97 |
| 1, 25– $(OH)_2D_3$ | 3.9 | 2 | 5 | 7.3 ± 0.5 | 76 |
|  | 3.9 | 5 | 3 | 7.4 ± 0.4 | 57 |
|  | 3.9 | 7 | 3 | 7.8 ± 1.1 | 73 |
| 1, 25– $(OH)_2D_3$ | 5.2 | 2 | 3 | 8.3 ± 0.2 | 64 |
|  | 5.2 | 5 | 3 | 7.7 ± 0.3 | 44 |
|  | 5.2 | 7 | 5 | 7.8 ± 0.4 | 48 |
| 24R, 25– $(OH)_2D_3$ | 5.2 | 7 | 3 | 7.2 ± 0.9 | 87 |
| 1, 25– $(OH)_2D_3$ | 1.3 | 2 | 4 | 6.8 ± 0.7 | 124 |
| 24R, 25– $(OH)_2D_3$ | 3.9 | 5 | 2 | 7.6 ± 0.6 | 46 |
|  |  | 7 | 4 | 7.9 ± 0.5 | 58 |

\* *Treated weight*
  Untreated weight × 100
$-D_2$ = vitamin D deficient; $+D_3$ = vitamin $D_3$ replete
1, 25– $(OH)_2D_3$ = 1, 25-dihydroxycholecalciferol
24R, 25– $(OH)_2D_3$ = 24R, 25-dihydroxycholecalciferol
(From: Henry, H. L., Capen C. C. & Norman, A. W., unpublished data.)

were present in close proximity to or fused with secretory granules in chicks administered vitamin $D_3$ for shorter intervals (2 days).

Severe parathyroid suppression was evident in chicks given 1,25-$(OH)_2D_3$ (1.3 nM) and 24R, 25-$(OH)_2D_3$ (3.9 nM) simultaneously for 5 to 7 days. Inactive chief cells predominated with occasional atrophic chief cells. The inactive chief cells had increased lipid and lysosomal bodies with prominent clusters of microfilaments (Fig. 7.19). The significant decrease in parathyroid gland weight following administration of vitamin $D_3$ or its metabolites to $-D$ chicks was associated with a rapid involution of hyperactive chief cells to a population of inactive and atrophic chief cells with a striking reduction in cytoplasmic area and profound suppression of synthetic and secretory organelles.

Aluminium
Evidence for a direct effect of aluminium on the parathyroid was suggested from studies of patients with chronic renal failure treated by

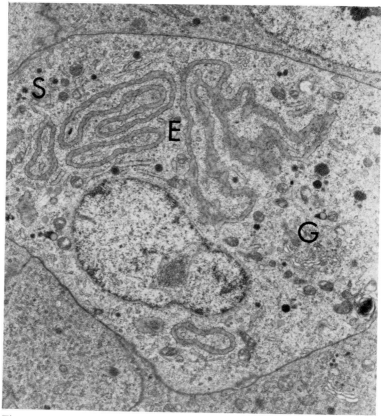

Fig. 7.17. Hyperactive chief cell from vitamin D-deficient chick. The expanded cytoplasmic area contains extensive profiles of endoplasmic reticulum (E), large Golgi apparatus (G) but few mature secretory granules (S).

haemodialysis with aluminium-containing fluids or orally administered drugs containing aluminium. These patients often had normal or minimal elevations of immunoreactive parathyroid hormone (iPTH), little histologic evidence of osteitis fibrosa in bone, and a depressed parathyroid response to acute hypocalcaemia (Bourdeau *et al.*, 1987). Studies by Morrissey *et al.* (1983) have reported that an increase in aluminium concentration *in vitro* over a range of 0.5 to 2.0 mM in a low calcium medium (0.5 mM) progressively inhibited the secretion of iPTH. At 2.0 mM aluminium iPTH secretion was inhibited by 68% while high medium calcium (2.0 mM) without aluminium maximally inhibited iPTH secretion

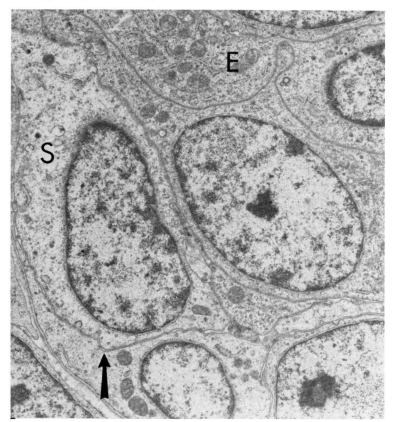

Fig. 7.18. Inactive chief cells in parathyroid gland of chick administered 1,25-$(OH)_2$-Vitamin D (5.2 nM) for 5 days. The diminished cytoplasmic area contains dispersed profiles of endoplasmic reticulum (E) and few secretory granules (S). Plasma membranes of adjacent chief cells are straight (arrow).

only 39%. The inhibitiion of PTH secretion by aluminium does not appear to be due to an irreversible toxic effect since normal secretion was restored when parathyroid cells were returned to 0.5 mM calcium medium without aluminium. The incorporation of [$^3$H] leucine into total cell protein, parathyroid secretory protein, proparathyroid hormone or PTH was not affected by aluminium; however, the secretion of radiolabelled protein by dispersed parathyroid cells was inhibited by aluminium (Morrissey *et al.*, 1983).

Bourdeau *et al.* (1986) using porcine parathyroid slices demonstrated

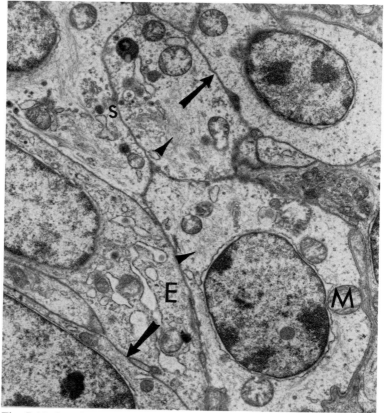

Fig. 7.19. Inactive chief cells in parathyroid gland of a chick suppressed by 1,25-(OH)$_2$-Vitamin D (1.3 nM) and 24R,25-(OH)$_2$-Vitamin D (3.9 nM) daily for 5 days. There are scattered mitochondria (M), few secretory granules (S), dispersed profiles of endoplasmic reticulum (E), clusters of microfilaments (arrowheads), and straight plasma membranes (arrows).

that medium aluminium concentrations, below that in plasma of patients with aluminium intoxication, resulted in an inhibition of PTH release. Subsequent studies utilizing medium aluminium concentrations from 20 to 500 ng/ml reported dose-dependent degenerative changes in chief cells ultrastructurally at the higher concentrations that were modulated by the extracellular calcium concentration. Degenerative changes produced in chief cells by high aluminium media were more extensive in a low calcium than a basal calcium environment. These findings were interpreted to suggest that sensitivity to aluminium occurs predominately in chief cells in the activated phase of the secretory cycle and that low extracellular calcium potentiates this effect (Bourdeau *et al.*, 1987).

The molecular mechanism by which aluminium inhibits PTH secretion appears to be similar to that of calcium ion by reducing diglyceride levels in chief cells (Morrissey & Slatopolsky, 1986). Aluminium appears to decrease diglyceride synthesis which is reflected in a corresponding decrease in synthesis of phosphatidylcholine and possible triglyceride; however, phosphatidylinositol synthesis was not affected by aluminium. The mechanism whereby aluminium decreases diglycerides and maintains phosphatidylinositol synthesis in parathyroid cells is not known.

## Parathyroid changes associated with metabolic disorders

### Renal hyperparathyroidism

Secondary hyperparathyroidism as a complication of chronic renal failure is a metabolic state characterized by an excessive, but not autonomous, rate of PTH secretion (Capen & Rosol, 1989). The secretion of hormone by the hyperplastic parathyroid glands usually remains responsive to fluctuations in blood calcium. The primary etiologic mechanism in this disorder is long-standing progressive renal disease resulting in severely impaired function. When the renal disease progresses to the point at which there is significant reduction in glomerular filtration rate, phosphorus is retained and progressive hyperphosphataemia develops. Although the concentration of blood phosphorus has no direct regulatory influence on the synthesis and secretion of PTH, when elevated it contributes to parathyroid stimulation by virtue of its ability to lower blood calcium levels.

Parathyroid stimulation associated with chronic renal disease can be attributed directly to the hypocalcaemia. An impaired intestinal absorption of calcium due to an acquired defect in vitamin D metabolism plays an important role in the development of hypocalcaemia associated with renal insufficiency. Chronic renal disease interferes with the production of $1,25\text{-}(OH)_2D_3$ by the kidney, thereby diminishing intestinal calcium transport. All parathyroids are considerably enlarged as a result initially of hypertrophy of chief cells and, subsequently, by hyperplasia as compensatory mechanisms to increase hormonal synthesis and secretion in response to the hypocalcaemic stimulus.

### Nutritional hyperparathyroidism

The increased secretion of PTH in this disorder is a compensatory mechanism directed against a disturbance in mineral homeostasis induced by nutritional imbalances (Capen, 1985a). The disease occurs in dogs, cats, monkeys, laboratory rodents, amongst other animals fed improper diets. Dietary mineral imbalances of etiologic importance in the pathogenesis are a low content of calcium, excessive phosphorus with normal or low calcium, and inadequate amounts of cholecalciferol (vitamin $D_3$) in New World non-human primates housed indoors without exposure to sunlight. The significant end result is hypocalcaemia, which results in parathyroid stimulation.

A diet low in calcium fails to supply the daily requirement, even though a greater proportion of ingested calcium is absorbed, and hypocalcaemia develops. Ingestion of excessive phosphorus results in increased intestinal absorption and elevation in blood phosphorus levels. Hyperphosphataemia does not stimulate the parathyroid gland directly but does so indirectly by virtue of its ability to lower blood calcium levels and suppress the synthesis of $1,25\text{-}(OH)_2$-cholecalciferol by the kidney. In response to the nutritionally-induced hypocalcaemia, all parathyroid glands undergo cellular hypertrophy and hyperplasia.

### Hypoparathyroidism

Hypoparathyroidism is a metabolic disorder in which either subnormal amounts of PTH are secreted by pathologic parathyroids or the hormone secreted is unable to interact normally with target cells (Capen, 1985b). Hypoparathyroidism often is associated with a diffuse lymphocytic parathyroiditis resulting in extensive degeneration of chief cells and replacement by fibrous connective tissue. In the early stages of lymphocytic parathyroiditis, there is infiltration of the gland with lymphocytes and plasma cells with nodular regenerative hyperplasia of the remaining chief cells. The lymphocytic parathyroiditis appears to develop by an immune-mediated mechanism, since a similar destruction of secretory parenchyma and lymphocytic infiltration has been produced experimentally by repeated injections of parathyroid tissue immulsions. The functional disturbances of hypoparathyroidism primarily are the result of increased neuromuscular excitability and tetany. Bone resorption is decreased because of a lack of PTH and blood calcium levels diminish progressively.

### Primary hyperparathyroidism

In primary hyperparathyroidism, PTH is produced in excess by a functional tumour in the gland. The normal control of PTH secretion by the concentration of blood calcium is lost in primary hyperparathyroidism. Hormone secretion is autonomous and the parathyroid produces excessive hormone in spite of the increased blood calcium. PTH acts initially on cells in the renal tubules to promote the excretion of phosphorus and retention of calcium. A prolonged increase secretion of PTH results in accelerated bone resorption and increased renal production of 1,25-$(OH)_2$-cholecalciferol. The lesion in the parathyroid gland responsible for the excessive secretion of PTH usually is an adenoma composed of active chief cells (Capen, 1990).

## Toxicity of parathyroid

### Agents influencing the development of proliferative lesions

#### Age

There are relatively few chemicals or experimental manipulations reported in the literature that significantly increase the incidence of parathyroid tumours. Long-standing renal failure with intense diffuse hyperplasia does not appear to increase the development of chief cell tumours in animals. The historical incidence of parathyroid adenomas in untreated control male F344 rats in studies conducted by the National Toxicology Program (NTP) (1986) was 4/1,315 (0.3%) and for female F344 rats was 2/1,330 (0.15%). Parathyroid adenomas in F344 rats are an example of a neoplasm whose incidence increases dramatically when comparing two-year studies to lifespan data. Solleveld, Haseman & McConnell (1984) reported that the incidence of parathyroid adenomas increased in males from 0.1% at 2 years to 3.1% in lifetime studies. Corresponding data for female F344 rats was 0.1% at 2 years and 0.6% in lifetime studies.

#### Irradiation and vitamin D

Wynford-Thomas, Wynford-Thomas & Williams (1982) reported that irradiation significantly increases the incidence of parathyroid adenomas in inbred Wistar albino rats and that the incidence could be modified by feeding diets with variable amounts of vitamin D. Neonatal Wistar rats were given either 5 or 10 μCi radioiodine ($^{131}$I) within 24 hours of birth. In rats 12 months of age and older, parathyroid adenomas were found in 33% of rats administered 5 μCi $^{131}$I and in 37% of rats given 10 μCi $^{131}$I compared to 0% in unirradiated controls. The incidence of parathyroid adenomas was highest (55%) in normocalcaemic rats fed a low vitamin D diet and lowest (20%) in irradiated rats fed a high vitamin D diet (40,000 IU/kg) that had a significant elevation in plasma calcium.

#### Gonadectomy

Oslapas *et al.* (1982) reported an increased incidence of parathyroid adenomas in female (34%) and male (27%) rats of the Long Evans strain administered 40 μCi sodium [131]I and saline at 8 weeks of age. There were no significant changes in serum calcium, phosphorus, and parathyroid hormone compared to controls. Gonadectomy performed at 7 weeks of age decreased the incidence of parathyroid adenomas in irradiated rats (7.4% in gonadectomy vs 27% in intact controls) but there was little change in incidence of parathyroid adenomas in irradiated females. X-irradiation of the thyroid-parathyroid region also increased the incidence of parathyroid adenomas. When female Sprague-Dawley rats received a single absorbed dose of X-rays at 4 weeks of age, they subsequently developed a 24% incidence of parathyroid adenomas after 14 months (Oslapas et al., 1981).

Xenobiotics

Parathyroid adenomas have been encountered infrequently following the administration of a variety of chemicals in 2-year bioassay studies in Fischer rats. In a study with F344 rats using the pesticide Rotenone, there appeared to be an increased incidence of parathyroid adenomas in high-dose (75 ppm) males compared to either low-dose (38 ppm) males, control males or NTP historical controls. It was uncertain whether the increased incidence of this uncommon tumour was a direct effect of Rotenone feeding or the increased survival in high dose males. Chief cell hyperplasia was not present in parathyroids that developed adenomas.

Fluoride

Drinking water containing large doses of fluoride (200 ppm) has been reported to cause parathyroid hyperplasia in sheep (Faccini & Care, 1965). Chief cells were primarily in the active stage of the secretory cycle after one month's exposure. The endoplasmic reticulum was aggregated into lamellar arrays and the Golgi apparatus was well developed in chief cells. Immunoreactive PTH levels in the blood were elevated five-fold after one week and remained elevated over the experimental period of a month. Faccini (1969) interpreted these changes suggesting stimulation of chief cells by fluoride as a response to an increased PTH demand resulting from decreased mobilization of calcium from fluoroapatite-containing bone. Apatite crystals in fluorotic bone are known to be of larger size than in normal bone and appear to be more stable and less reactive in surface exchange reactions.

Secondary hyperparathyroidism has been reported in patients with skeletal fluorosis (Teotia & Teotia, 1973). The parathyroid glands have morphologic evidence of hyperactivity and the patients have elevated circulating levels of immunoreactive PTH. Ream & Principato (1981) reported increased glycogen accumulation in hyperactive chief cells of rats following the ingestion of large doses (150 ppm) of fluoride in drinking water.

### Osteopetrosis virus (avian)

Osteopetrosis is a disease of several vertebrate species including mice, rabbits, chickens, and man (Simpson & Sanger, 1968). The skeletal lesions in avian osteopetrosis share certain similarities with Engleman's disease of progressive diaphysial dysplasia in children and Caffey's disease, and are characterized by excessive formation of periosteal new bone affecting mainly the diaphysis. Roentgenograms of involved bones reveal a marked increase in density, suggesting an underlying hypermineralization of the skeleton.

Hyperactive chief cells predominated in parathyroid glands of chickens with osteopetrosis (Youshak & Capen, 1970). The cytoplasmic area was more abundant and mitochondria were larger and more filamentous than in active chief cells of controls. The Golgi apparatus was large and associated with numerous prosecretory granules. Mature secretory granules were observed less frequently in chief cells from chickens with osteopetrosis. Viral particles, morphologically similar to the avian leukosis virus, were observed in the intercellular and extracellular spaces of parathyroid glands. Viral replication, as evidenced by viral budding from plasma membranes, was detected in chief cells. Invaginations of the plasma membrane as well as smooth membranous vesicles within the cytoplasm contain mature viral particles (Youshak & Capen, 1970).

The parathyroid hyperactivity reported in avian osteopetrosis appears to result from stimulation of chief cells by the serum calcium levels which are in the low normal range. The rapid growth rate and deposition of large amounts of mineral in both normal and abnormal fibrous bone most likely contribute to the lowered serum calcium (Youshak & Capen, 1970). The finding of large numbers of mature viral particles in the parathyroids was interpreted to be a reflection of the persistent viremic state in the osteopetrotic birds and the result of viral replication in parenchymal cells of the parathyroid and elsewhere.

### Diphosphonate-induced inhibition of bone resorption

Ethane-1-hydroxy-1, 1-diphosphonate (EHDP) is a synthetic analog of pyrophosphate and has a P-C-P bond instead of the P-O-P bond of the naturally occurring compound (Fleisch *et al.*, 1968; Francis, 1969). EHDP is a potent inhibitor of hydroxyapatite crystal precipitation and dissolution. These effects of EHDP are due to its ability to chemisorb to the surface of apatite crystals.

EHDP has a potent effect on resorption of bone. It can inhibit parathyroid extract-induced resorption of bone in mouse calvaria grown in tissue culture (Fleisch *et al.*, 1968) and in thyroparathyroidectomized rats *in vivo*. High doses of EHPD (40 mg/kg/day) given subcutaneously to rats caused a reduced rate of bone resorption, diminished efflux of $^{45}Ca$ from bone, and decreased urinary excretion of hydroxyproline (Gasser *et al.*, 1972).

The long term (70 days) effects of administering EHDP (4 mg/kg/day) on parathyroid function were investigated in pregnant animals fed a low calcium diet (Yarrington *et al.*, 1977b). Serum calcium and phosphorus were significantly lower at parturition and postpartum in EHDP-treated cows compared to pregnant controls fed the same diet. Plasma immunoreactive PTH levels were similar prepartum, at parturition, and postpartum in animals administered EHDP as in controls. Immediately available calcium reserves (at 10 days prepartum) were greater prepartum in controls than in animals receiving EHDP as indicated by a more rapid rate of return of serum calcium toward normal levels following EDTA-induced hypocalcaemia. EHDP-treated cows responded to the hypo-calcaemic challenge with similar changes in plasma immunoreactive PTH levels as in controls; however, urinary hydroxyproline excretion increased only in controls.

Chief cells in parathyroid glands of both groups of animals ultrastruc-turally were in an active stage of the secretory cycle with well developed secretory organelles (Yarrington *et al.*, 1977a,b). However, chief cells in animals administered EHDP were degranulated and contained fewer secretory granules in response to the hypocalcaemia than those in controls.

Dichloromethane diphosphonate ($Cl_2MDP$) is a synthetic analog of pyrophosphate which blocks the dissolution and growth of hydroxy-apatite crystals *in vitro* with activity similar to that of EHDP (Francis, 1969). However, $Cl_2MDP$ is 10 times more potent than EHDP as an inhibitor of bone resorption in bone tissue culture systems (Reynolds *et al.*, 1972). Similar differences in the potency of $Cl_2MDP$ and EHDP as inhibitors of bone resorption have been demonstrated by radiocalcium kinetic techniques in intact rats fed a low calcium diet (Gasser *et al.*, 1972).

The administration of dicholoromethane diphosphonate ($Cl_2MDP$) (4 mg/kg/day) subcutaneously to pregnant experimental cows fed a low calcium diet significantly reduced bone resorption as indicated by microradiographic evaluation of endosteal surfaces (Yarrington *et al.*, 1977a). Plasma PTH levels were similar between $Cl_2MDP$-treated and control cows prepartum, during EDTA infusions, and near parturition. Chief cells in the parathyroid glands of both groups of animals ultrastructurally were predominately in the active stage of the secretory cycle. The chronically stimulated chief cells from cows administered Cl$_2$MDP had an expanded cytoplasmic area containing many lipofuscin granules and lysosomal bodies but only a few secretory granules.

The administration of Cl$_2$MDP significantly reduced the rapidly mobilizable calcium reserves. Following an intravenous EDTA infusion and the spontaneous calcium drain associated with parturition and the beginning of lactation, Cl$_2$MDP-treated cows developed profound hypocalcaemia. The rapid mobilization of calcium reserves in animals administered Cl$_2$MDP prepartum was impaired mainly because of diminished resorption of bone despite an adequate PTH secretory response (Yarrington *et al.*, 1977a).

## Degenerative changes in parathyroid caused by:

### L-asparaginase

Tettenborn *et al.* (1970) and Chisari *et al.* (1972) reported that rabbits administered L-asparaginase develop severe hypocalcaemia and tetany characterized by muscle tremors, opisthotonos, carpopedal spasms, paralysis, and coma. This drug was of interest in cancer chemotherapy because of the beneficial effects of guinea pig serum against lymphosarcoma in mice.

Parathyroid chief cells appeared to be selectively destroyed by L-asparaginase (Young *et al.*, 1973). Chief cells were predominately in the inactive stage of the secretory cycle, degranulated, and large autophagic vacuoles were present in the cytoplasm of degenerating cells. Cytoplasmic organelles concerned with synthesis and packaging of secretory products were poorly developed in chief cells. The rabbits developed hyperphosphataemia, hypomagnesaemia, hyperkalaemia, and azotaemia in addition to the acute hypocalcaemia. Rabbits with clinical hypocalcaemic tetany did not recover spontaneously; however, administration of parathyroid extract prior to or during treatment with L-asparaginase decreased the incidence of hypocalcaemic tetany.

The development of hypocalcaemia and tetany have not been observed in other experimental animals administered L-asparaginase (Oettgen *et al.*, 1970). However, this response may not be limited to the rabbit since some human patients receiving the drug have also developed hypocalcaemia (Jaffe *et al.*, 1972). The L-asparaginase-induced hypoparathyroidism in rabbits is a valuable model to investigate drug-endocrine cell interactions, somewhat analogous to the selective destruction of pancreatic beta cells by alloxan with production of experimental diabetes mellitus.

Ozone

Inhalation of a single dose of ozone (0.75 ppm) for 4 to 8 hours has been reported to produce light and electron microscopic changes in parathyroid glands (Atwal & Wilson, 1974). Subsequent studies have utilized longer (48 hours) exposure to ozone in order to define the pathogenesis of the parathyroid lesions (Atwal, Samagh & Bhatnagar, 1975; Atwal, 1979). Initially (1 to 5 days post-ozone exposure), many chief cells undergo compensatory hypertrophy and hyperplasia with areas of capillary endothelial cell proliferation, interstitial oedema, degeneration of vascular endothelium, formation of platelet thrombi, leukocyte infiltration of the walls of larger vessels in the gland, and disruption of basement membranes. Chief cells had prominent Golgi complexes and endoplasmic reticulum, aggregations of free ribosomes, and swelling of mitochondria (Atwal & Pemsingh, 1981).

Inactive chief cells with few secretory granules predominate in the parathyroids in the later stages of exposure to ozone. There was evidence of parathyroid atrophy from 12 to 20 days post-ozone exposure, with mononuclear cell infiltration and necrosis of chief cells. The reduced cytoplasmic area contained vacuolated endoplasmic reticulum. A small Golgi apparatus, and numerous lysosomal bodies. Plasma membranes of adjacent chief cells were disrupted resulting in coalescence of the cytoplasmic area. Fibroblasts with associated collagen bundles were prominent in the interstitium and the basal lamina of the numerous capillaries often was duplicated. Atwal & Pemsingh (1984) reported unique Mallory body-like inclusions in ozone-treated dogs, especially after 10 to 13 days. There were numerous filaments accumulating in the perinuclear region with disruption of cytoplasmic organelles.

The parathyroid lesions in ozone-exposed animals are similar to isoimmune parathyroiditis in other species (Lupulescu et al., 1968a,b). Antibody against parathyroid tissue was localized near the periphery of chief cells by indirect immunofluorescence, especially 14 days following ozone injury in rabbits (Atwal et al., 1975). This suggests that ozone may react with residues of tyrosine and tryptophane in the PTH molecule, thereby altering its immunologic properties in such a way as to result in the formation of an auto-antigen that may initiate the isoimmune reaction in the parathyroid gland.

Immune-mediated injury

Lupulescu et al. (1968a,b) induced isoimmune hypoparathyroidism experimentally in dogs by repeated injections of parathyroid emulsions with Freund's adjuvant for four months. The parathyroids had lymphocytic infiltration, disorganization in the pattern of arrangement and atrophy of chief cells, and progressive fibrosis. Mitochondria in chief cells were irregularly swollen and cristae were disrupted giving a vacuolated appearance. The granular endoplasmic reticulum was poorly developed and secretory granules were reduced in number.

## Evaluation of toxicity

The parathyroid gland is infrequently injured directly by the acute or chronic administration of xenobiotics. However, parathyroid function may be altered by a wide variety of chemicals that either elevate or lower the blood concentration of calcium (particularly calcium ion). In response to hypocalcaemia, chief cells undergo hypertrophy and eventually hyperplasia. On formalin- or Bouin's-fixed sections the expanded cytoplasmic area is lightly eosinophilic and vacuolated compared with chief cells in normal animals. Perivascular spaces are narrow in hyperplastic parathyroids and there are few fat cells in the interstitium. In response to hypercalcaemia, the cytoplasmic area of chief cells is decreased and more densely eosinophilic often with a widening of intercellular and pericapillary spaces. If the hypercalcaemia is prolonged there is an overall reduction of glandular parenchyma with increased fibrous or adipose connective tissue in the interstitium. Subtle differences between treated and control groups can be best evaluated by morphometric evaluation of parenchyma:interstitium and cytoplasmic:nuclear area of chief cells.

Ultrastructural evaluation of chief cells is a sensitive means of morphologically assessing whether a particular drug or chemical affects the parathyroid gland (Roth & Capen, 1974). Perfusion of the thyroid-parathyroid area with glutaraldehyde-based fixatives followed by post-fixation in osmium tetroxide results in the best retention of structural detail in parathyroids of animals. Morphometric studies at the ultrastructural level can be used to quantitate total cytoplasmic area and area occupied by a particular organelle (e.g. secretory granules).

In response to an acute lowering of blood calcium a larger percentage of chief cells ultrastructurally will be in the active stage of synthesis and secretion than under steady-state conditions. This is indicated by a peripheral migration of secretory granules and alignment along the plasma membrane, aggregation of the endoplasmic reticulum into lamellar arrays, and enlargement of the Golgi apparatus associated with many small dense granules in the process of formation. Conversely, chief cells in response to hypercalcaemia are predominantly in the inactive stage of the secretory cycle as evaluated by electron microscopy with dispersed profiles of endoplasmic reticulum, small Golgi complexes with few granules, and often accumulations of either glycogen or lipid (depending upon species) in the cytoplasm. Secretory granules accumulate initially in response to an elevation in blood calcium but subsequently decrease due to degradation by lysosomal enzymes.

Atrophic chief cells develop in response to sustained and/or more severe hypercalcaemia. Their cytoplasm is more electron-dense and irregularly shrunken with widened intercellular spaces. Cytoplasmic organelles are poorly developed and may have early degenerative changes suggested by mitochondrial vacuolation with disruption of cristae and distension of endoplasmic reticulum with loss of ribosomes.

PTH in the circulation of animals can be measured by sensitive radio-immunoassays (RIA) or immunoradiometric assays (Potts *et al.*, 1983; Torrance & Nachriener, 1989). Although the hormone is secreted from chief cells primarily as a straight chain (1–84 amino acids) peptide, molecular fragments (amino and carboxy terminal) are formed in the periphery (primarily by Kupffer cells in the liver). The immunoheterogenicity created by the multiple circulating fragments of PTH has caused significant problems in the development of sensitive assays in both humans and animals. Since the amino (N-) terminal end of the molecule (that portion which interacts with the receptor in target cells) is highly conserved between man and other mammalian species, assays directed against this end of PTH are the most sensitive and accurate in assessing parathyroid function. The amino terminal assay is particularly useful in measuring ongoing or recent functional changes in the parathyroid following exposure to various xenobiotics or physiological perturbations.

The intact N-terminal PTH assay (kit available from Nichols Institute, P.O. Box 92797, Los Angeles, CA, USA) is useful for toxicity testing in a variety of animal species since the antibody is generated in chickens to the highly conserved end of the molecule (1–34 PTH synthetic human) (Potts, Segre & Endres, 1983). The assay can be run on either serum (preferred) or plasma that has been separated and frozen (−70 °C in either glass or plastic tubes) as soon as possible after collection. In contrast to some peptide hormones PTH as quantitated by RIA is relatively stable in serum at frozen or refrigerator temperatures so that it is possible to collect representative specimens from large numbers of experimental animals such as at the end of a chronic study. Circulating levels of PTH using N-terminal assays in most animals are near 20 pg/ml (e.g. dog $20\pm5$ pg/ml; mouse $19\pm3$ pg/ml; rat $29\pm7$ pg/ml; cat $17\pm2$ pg/ml) with levels in non-human primates being slightly lower.

Parathyroid hormone assays utilizing antibody generated against the carboxy (C-) terminal end of the human molecule usually give less consistent results in animals than in human patients. The amino acid sequence of the C-terminal portion of PTH is less well conserved between animal species and man than the N-terminal region, thereby, rendering the antibody less specific and the assay less sensitive. It is important to emphasize that the C-terminal fragment in the circulation is biologically inactive and has a longer plasma half-life than the N-terminal end of the PTH molecule. Therefore, C-terminal assays for PTH in species (e.g. humans) where a specific antibody is available, tend to give a more integrated evaluation of parathyroid function over time due to the slower turnover rate of this portion of the molecule in the circulation.

## References

Akatsu, T. *et al.* (1989). Parathyroid hormone (PTH)-related protein is a potent stimulator of osteoclast-like multinucleated cell formation to the same extent as PTH in mouse marrow cultures. *Endocrinology*, **125**, 20–7.

Atwal, O.S. (1979). Ultrastructural pathology of ozone-induced experimental parathyroiditis. IV. Biphasic activity in the chief cells of regenerating parathyroid glands. *Am. Journal of Pathology*, **95**, 611–22.

Atwal, O.S., Samagh, B.S. & Bhatnagar, M.K. (1975). A possible auto-immune parathyroiditis following ozone inhalation. II. A histopathologic, ultrastructural, and immunofluorescent study. *American Journal of Pathology*, **80**, 53–62.

Atwal, O.S. & Pemsingh, R.S. (1981). Morphology of microvascular changes and endothelial regeneration in experimental ozone-induced parathyroiditis. III. Some pathologic considerations. *The American Journal of Pathology*, **102**(3), 297–307.

Atwal, O.S. & Pemsingh, R.S. (1984). Occurrence of Mallory body-like inclusions in parathyroid chief cells of ozone-treated dogs. *Journal of Pathology*, **142**, 169–74.

Atwal, O.S. & Wilson, T. (1974). Parathyroid gland changes following oxone inhalation. A morphologic study. *Arch. Environmental Health*, **28**, 91–100.

Aurbach, G.D. & Potts, J.T., Jr (1964). The parathyroids. In *Advances in Metabolic Diseases*, vol. 1, ed. R. Levine & R. Luft, pp. 45–93. New York: Academic Press.

Ayer, L.M. *et al.* (1989). Analysis of parathyroid hormone in bovine parathyroid cysts. *Journal of Bone and Mineral Research*, **4**, 335–40.

Beck, N. *et al.* (1974). Direct inhibitory effect of hypercalcemia on renal actions of parathyroid hormone. *J. Clin. Invest.*, **53**, 717–25.

Black, H.E., Capen, C.C. & Arnaud, C.D. (1973). Ultrastructure of parathyroid glands and plasma immunoreactive parathyroid hormone in pregnant cows fed normal and high calcium diets. *Lab. Invest.*, **29**, 173–85.

Bourdeau, A.M. *et al.* (1986). Effects of aluminum addition on parathyroid tissue incubation medium composition. *Kidney Internat.*, **29**, 924–6.

Bourdeau, A.M. *et al.* (1987). Parathyroid responses to aluminum *in vitro*: Ultrastructural changes and PTH release. *Kidney International*, **31**, 15–24.

Broadus, A.E. (1988). Humoral hypercalcemia of malignancy. Identification of a novel parathyroid hormone-like peptide. *New England Journal of Medicine*, **319**, 556–63.

Brumbaugh, P.F., Hughes, M.R. & Haussler, M.R. (1975). Cytoplasmic and nuclear binding components for 1,25-dihydroxy-vitamin $D_3$ in chick parathyroid glands. *Proceedings of the National Academy of Science (USA)*, **72**, 4871–5.

Budayr, A.A. *et al.* (1989a). Increased serum levels of a parathyroid hormone-like protein in malignancy-associated hypercalcemia. *Annals of Internal Medicine*, **111**, 807–12.

Budayr, A.A. *et al.* (1989b). High levels of a parathyroid hormone-like protein in milk. *Proceedings of the National Academy of Science (USA)*, **86**, 7183–5.

Burtis, W.J. *et al.* (1987). Identification of a novel 17,000-dalton parathyroid hormone-like adenylate cyclase-stimulating protein from a tumor associated with humoral hypercalcemia of malignancy. *Journal of Biological Chemistry*, **262**, 7151–6.

Capen, C.C. (1983). Structural and biochemical aspects of parathyroid gland function in animals. In *Endocrine System*, ed. T.C. Jones, U. Mohr & R.D. Hunt, pp. 217–47. Berlin: Springer-Verlag.

Capen, C.C. (1985a). Calcium-regulating hormones and metabolic bone disease. In *Textbook of Small Animal Orthopaedics*, ed. C.D. Newton & D.M. Nunamaker, chapter 59, pp. 673–722. Philadelphia: Lippincott Co. Publishers.

Capen, C.C. (1985b). The endocrine glands. In *Pathology of Domestic Animals*, 3rd edn, ed. K.V.F. Jubb, P.C. Kennedy & N. Palmer, pp. 238–305. Orlando: Academic Press, Inc.

Capen, C.C. (1988). Endocrine system. In *Special Veterinary Pathology*, ed. R.G. Thomson, pp. 369–436. Philadelphia: B.C. Decker, Inc.

Capen, C.C. (1989a). Neoplasms of the parathyroid glands. In *Atlas of Tumor Pathology in the F344 Rat*, ed. S.F. Stinson & G. Reznik, pp. 367–78. Boca Raton: CRC Press, Inc.

Capen, C.C. (1989b). The calcium regulating hormones parathyroid hormone, calcitonin, and cholecalciferol. In *Veterinary Endocrinology and Reproduction*, 4th edn, ed. L.E. McDonald, chapter 4, pp. 92–185. Philadelphia: Lea & Febiger.

Capen, C.C. (1990). Tumors of the endocrine glands. In *Tumors in Domestic Animals*, 3rd edn, ed. J.E. Moulton, pp. 553–639. Berkeley and Los Angeles: University of California Press.

Capen, C.C., Cole, C.R. & Hibbs, J.W. (1968). The influence of vitamin D on calcium metabolism and the parathyroid glands of cattle. *Fed. Proc.*, **27**, 142–52.

Capen, C.C., Henry, H.L. & Norman, A.W. (1977). Ultrastructural alterations produced by vitamin D and its metabolites on the chick parathyroid gland. In *Vitamin D: Biochemical, Chemical and Clinical Aspects Related to Calcium Metabolism*, ed. A.W. Norman, K. Schaefer, J.W. Coburn, H.F. DeLuca, D. Fraser, H.G. Grigoleit & D.V. Herrath, pp. 101–4. New York: Walter de Gruyter.

Capen, C.C. & Rosol, T.J. (1989). Calcium regulating hormones and diseases of mineral (calcium, phosphorus, magnesium) metabolism. In *Clinical Biochemistry of Domestic Animals*, ed. J.J. Kaneko, chapter 15, pp. 682–766. New York: Academic Press Inc.

Capen, C.C., Koestner, A. & Cole, C.R. (1965). The ultrastructure, histopathology, and histochemistry of the parathyroid glands of pregnant and nonpregnant cows fed a high level of vitamin D. *Laboratory Investigation*, **14**, 1809–25.

Carillo, B.J. & Woker, N.A. (1967). Enteque seco: arteriosclerosis y calcificacion metastasica de origen toxico en animales a pastoreo. *Patologica Animales*, **4**, 9–11.

Chambers, T.J. (1980). The cellular basis of bone resorption. *Clinical Orthopaedic Related Research*, **151**, 283–93.

Chambers, T.J. *et al.* (1984). Resorption of bone by isolated rabbit osteoclasts. *Journal of Cell Science*, **66**, 383–99.

Chisari, F.V. *et al.* (1972). Parathyroid necrosis and hypocalcemic tetany induced in rabbits by L-asparaginase. *American Journal of Pathology*, **69**, 461–7.

Chu, L.L.H. *et al.* (1973). Studies on the biosynthesis of rat parathyroid hormone and proparathyroid hormone. Adaptation of the parathyroid gland to dietary restriction of calcium. *Endocrinology*, **93**, 915–24.

Civitelli, R. *et al.* (1988). PTH elevates inositol polyphosphates and diacylglycerol in a rat osteoblast-like cell line. *American Journal of Physiology*, **255**, E660–7.

Civitelli, R. *et al.* (1989). Parathyroid hormone-related peptide transiently increases cytosolic calcium in osteoblastic-like cells. Comparison with parathyroid hormone. *Endocrinology*, **125**, 1204–10.

Cohn, D.V. & MacGregor, R.R. (1981). The biosynthesis, intracellular processing, and secretion of parathormone. *Endocrine Reviews*, **2**, 1–26.

Cole, J.A. *et al.* (1987). A dual mechanism for regulation of kidney phosphate transport by parathyroid hormone. *Am. Journal of Physiology*, **253**, E221–7.

Collins, W.T. *et al.* (1977). Ultrastructural evaluation of parathyroid glands and thyroid C-cells of cattle fed *Solanum malacoxylon*. *American Journal of Pathology*, **87**, 603–14.

Corradino, R.A. & Wasserman, R.H. (1974). 1,25-dihydroxy-cholecalciferol-like activiity of *Solanum malacoxylon* extract on calcium transport. *Nature*, **252**, 716–18.

Danks, J. *et al.* (1989). Parathyroid hormone-related protein: Immunohistochemical localization in cancers and in normal skin. *Journal of Bone and Mineral Research*, **4**, 273–8.

de Vernejoul, M-C. *et al.* (1988). Bone resorption by isolated chick osteoclasts in culture is stimulated by murine spleen cell supernatant fluids (osteoclast-activating factor) and inhibited by calcitonin and prostaglandin E2. *Journal of Bone and Mineral Research*, **3**, 69–80.

Delaisse, J-M. *et al.* (1985). A new synthetic inhibitor of mammalian tissue collagenase inhibits bone resorption in culture. *Biochemical and Biophysical Research Communications*, **133**, 483–90.

Dirksen, G. *et al.* (1975). Experimental investigations on the etiology of an enzootic calcinosis in cattle. In *Vitamin D and Problems Related to Uremic Bone Disease*, ed. A.W. Norman, K. Schaffer, H.G. Grigoleit, D.V. Herrath & E. Ritz, pp. 697–702. New York: Walter de Gruyter.

Döbereiner, J. *et al.* (1971). 'Espichamento', intoxicacao de bovinos por *Solanum malacoxylon*, no pantanal de Mato Gross. *Pesq Agropee Bras (Ser Vet)*, **6**, 91–117.

Döbereiner, J., Done, S.H. & Beltran, L.E. (1975). Experimental *Solanum malacoxylon* poisoning in calves. *British Veterinary Journal*, **131**, 175–85.

Donahue, H.J. *et al.* (1988). Differential effects of parathyroid hormone and its analogues on cytosolic calcium ion and cAMP levels in cultured rat osteoblast-like cells. *Journal of Biological Chemistry*, **263**, 13522–7.

Ebeling, P.R. *et al.* (1989). Actions of synthetic parathyroid hormone-related protein (1–34) on the isolated rat kidney. *Journal of Endocrinology*, **120**, 45–50.

Eeckhout, Y. *et al.* (1988). The proteinases of bone resorption. In *The Control of Tissue Damage*, ed. A.M. Glauert, pp. 297–313. Amsterdam: Elsevier Science Publishers.

Faccini, J.M. (1969). Fluoride-induced hyperplasia of the parathyroid glands. *Proceedings of the Royal Society of Medicine*, **62**, 241.

Faccini, J.M. & Care, A.D. (1965). Effect of sodium fluoride on the ultrastructure of the parathyroid glands of the sheep. *Nature*, **207**, 1399–401.

Farndale, R.W. *et al.* (1988). Parathyroid hormone and prostaglandin E2 stimulate both inositol phosphates and cyclic AMP accumulation in mouse osteoblast cultures. *Biochemistry Journal*, **252**, 263–8.

Fleisch, H. *et al.* (1968). The influence of pyrophosphate analogues (diphosphonates) on the precipitation and dissolution of calcium phosphate *in vitro* and *in vivo*. *Classified Tissue Research*, **2**(Suppl), 10–10a.

Francis, M.D. (1969). The inhibition of calcium hydroxyapatite crystal growth by polyphosphonates. *Calcified Tissue Res.*, **3**, 151–62.

Fukumoto, S. *et al.* (1989). Secretion of parathyroid hormone-like activity from human T-cell lymphotropic virus type I-infected lymphocytes. *Cancer Research*, **49**, 3849–52.

Gasser, A.B. *et al.* (1972). The influence of two diphosphonates on calcium metabolism in the rat. *Clinical Science*, **43**, 31–45.

Goltzman, D. *et al.* (1986). Studies of the multiple molecular forms of bioactive parathyroid hormone and parathyroid hormone-like substances. *Recent Progress in Hormone Research*, **42**, 665–703.

Goltzman, D., Hendy, G.N. & Banville, D. (1989). Parathyroid hormone-like peptide: molecular characterization and biological properties. *Trends in Endocrinology Metabolism*, **1**, 39–44.

Habener, J.F. (1981). Recent advances in parathyroid hormone research. *Clinical Biochemistry*, **14**, 223–9.

Habener, J.F. & Potts, J.T. Jr (1978). Biosynthesis of parathyroid hormone. *New England Journal of Medicine*, **299**, 580–5; 635–44.

Habener, J.F. and Potts, J.T. Jr (1979). Subcellular distribution of parathyroid hormone hormonal precursors and parathyroid secretory protein. *Endocrinology*, **104**, 265–75.

Hanai, H. *et al.* (1986). Parathyroid hormone increases sodium/calcium exchange activity in renal cells and the blunting of the response in aging. *Journal of Biological Chemistry*, **261**, 5419–25.

Haussler, M.R. *et al.* (1976). 1,25-dihydroxyvitamin $D_3$-glycoside. Identification of a calcinogenic principle of *Solanum malacoxylon*. *Life Science*, **18**, 1049–56.

Hayman, J.A. *et al.* (1989). Expression of parathyroid hormone related protein in normal skin and in tumors of skin and skin appendages. *Journal of Pathology*, **158**, 293–6.

Henry, H.L. (1985). Parathyroid hormone modulation of 25-hydroxyvitamin D3 metabolism by cultured chick kidney cells is mimicked and enhanced by Forskolin. *Endocrinology*, **116**, 503–10.

Henry, H.L. & Norman, A.W. (1975). Studies on the mechanism of action of calciferol VII. Localization of 1,25-dihydroxyvitamin $D_3$ in chick parathyroid glands. *Biochemical & Biophysical Research Communications*, **62**, 781–8.

Henry, H.L., Taylor, A.N. & Norman, A.W. (1977). Response of chick parathyroid glands to the vitamin D metabolites, 1,25-dihydroxycholecalciferol and 24,25-dihydroxycholecalciferol. *Journal of Nutrition*, **107**, 1918–26.

Herrmann-Erlee, M.P.M. *et al.* (1988). Different roles for calcium and cyclic AMP in the action of PTH: studies in bone explants and isolated bone cells. *Bone*, **9**, 93–100.

High, W.B., Black, H.E. & Capen, C.C. (1981). Histomorphometric evaluation of the effects of low dose parathyroid hormone administration on cortical bone remodeling in adult dogs. *Laboratory Investigation*, **44**, 449–54.

Holick, M.F., Nussbaum, S. & Persons, K.S. (1988). PTH-like humoral hypercalcemia factor (HHF) of malignancy may be an epidermal differentiation factor: synthetic hHHF(1–34)amide inhibits terminal differentiation of cultured human keratinocytes. *Journal of Bone and Mineral Research*, **3**, S214. (Abstract No. 582.)

Hruska, K.A. *et al.* (1977). Degradation of parathyroid hormone and fragment production by the isolated perfused dog kidney. The effect of glomerular filtration rate and perfusate $Ca^{++}$ concentrations. *Journal of Clinical Investigations*, **60**, 501–10.

Hruska, K.A. *et al.* (1987). Stimulation of inositol trisphosphate and diacylglycerol production in renal tubular cells by parathyroid hormone. *Journal of Clinical Investigation*, **79**, 230–39.

Ikeda, K. *et al.* (1988a). Identification of transcripts encoding a parathyroid hormone-like peptide in messenger RNAs from a variety of human and animal tumors associated with humoral hypercalcemia of malignancy. *Journal of Clinical Investigation*, **81**, 2010–14.

Ikeda, K. *et al.* (1988b). Expression of messenger ribonucleic acids encoding a parathyroid hormone-like peptide in normal human and animal tissues with abnormal expression in human parathyroid adenomas. *Molecular Endocrinology*, **2**, 1230–6.

Jaffe, N. *et al.* (1972). Comparison of daily and twice-weekly schedule of L-asparaginase in childhood leukemia. *Pediatrics*, **49**, 590–5.

Klausner, J.S. *et al.* (1990). Hypercalcemia in two cats with squamous cell carcinomas. *Journal of the American Veterinary Medical Association*, **196**, 103–5.

Knox, F.G. & Haramati, A. (1985). Renal regulation of phosphate excretion. In *The Kidney: Physiology and Pathophysiology*, ed. D.W. Seldin & G. Giebisch, pp. 1381–96. New York: Raven Press.

Kronenberg, H.M. *et al.* (1986). Structure and expression of the human parathyroid hormone gene. *Rec. Prog. Horm. Res.*, **42**, 641–63.

Krook, L. *et al.* (1975). Hypercalcemia and calcinosis in Florida horses. Implication of the shrub, *Cestrum diurnum*, as the causative agent. *Cornell Veterinarian*, **65**, 26–56.

Kukreja, S.C. *et al.* (1988). Antibodies to parathyroid hormone-related protein lower serum calcium in athymic mouse models of malignancy-associated hypercalcemia due to human tumors. *Journal of Clinical Investigation*, **82**, 1798–1802.

Loveridge, N. *et al.* (1988). Further evidence for a parathyroid hormone-related protein in fetal parathyroid glands of sheep. *Quarterly Journal of Experimental Physiology*, **73**, 781–4.

Lupulescu, A. *et al.* (1968a). Experimental investigation on immunology of the parathyroid gland. *Immunology*, **14**, 475–82.

Lupulescu, A. *et al.* (1968b). Electron microscopic observations on the parathyroid gland in experimental hypoparathyroidism. *Experientia*, **24**, 62–3.

Mangin, M. *et al.* (1988). Identification of a cDNA encoding a parathyroid hormone-like peptide from a human tumor associated with humoral hypercalcemia of malignancy. *Proceedings of the National Academy Science (USA)*, **85**, 597–601.

Mangin, M. *et al.* (1989). Isolation and characterization of the human parathyroid hormone-like peptide gene. *Proceedings of the National Academy Science (USA)*, **86**, 2408–12.

Mayer, G.P. & Hurst, J.G. (1978). Comparison of the effects of calcium and magnesium on parathyroid hormone secretion rate in calves. *Endocrinology*, **102**, 1803–7.

McSheehy, P.M.J. & Chambers, T.J. (1986). Osteoblastic cells mediate osteoclastic responsiveness to parathyroid hormone. *Endocrinology*, **118**, 824–8.

Merendino, J.J. *et al.* (1986). Cultured human keratinocytes produce a parathyroid hormone-like protein. *Science*, **231**, 388–90.

Merryman, J.I., Rosol, T.J., Brooks, C.L. & Capen, C.C. (1989). Separation of parathyroid hormone-like activity from transforming growth factor alpha and beta in the canine adenocarcinoma (CAC-8) model of humoral hypercalcemia of malignancy. *Endocrinology*, **124**, 2456–63.

Meuten, D.J. *et al.* (1978). Gastric carcinoma with pseudohyper-parathyroidism in a horse. *Cornell Veterinarian*, **68**, 179–95.

Meuten, D.J. *et al.* (1983a). Hypercalcemia in dogs with adeno-carcinoma derived from apocrine glands of the anal sac: biochemical and histomorphometric investigations. *Laboratory Investigation*, **48**, 428–35.

Meuten, D.J. *et al.* (1983b). Hypercalcemia in dogs with lympho-sarcoma: biochemical, ultrastructural, and histomorphometric investigations. *Laboratory Investigation*, **49**, 553–62.

Meuten, D.J., Capen, C.C., Thompson, K.G. & Segre, G.V. (1984). Syncytial chief cells in canine parathyroid glands. *Veterinary Pathology*, **21**, 463–8.

Morrissey, J. *et al.* (1983). Suppression of parathyroid hormone secretion by aluminum. *Kidney International*, **23**, 699–704.

Morrissey, J. & Slatopolsky, E. (1986). Effect of aluminum on parathyroid hormone secretion. *Kidney International*, **29**, S41–4.

Moseley, J.M. *et al.* (1987). Parathyroid hormone-related protein purified from a human lung cancer cell line. *Proceedings of the National Academy of Science (USA)*, **84**, 5048–52.

Motokura, T. *et al.* (1988). Expression of parathyroid hormone-related protein in a human T cell lymphotrophic virus type I-infected T cell line. *Biochemical and Biophysical Research Communications*, **154**, 1182–8.

Motokura, T. *et al.* (1989). Parathyroid hormone-related protein in adult T-cell leukemia-lymphoma. *Annals of Internal Medicine*, **111**, 484–8.

Mundy, G.R. (1988). Hypercalcemia of malignancy revisited. *Journal of Clinical Investigation*, **82**, 1–6.

Mundy, G.R. (1989). Hypercalcemic factors other than parathyroid hormone-related protein. *Clinics of Endocrinology and Metabolism in North America*, **18**, 795–806.

National Toxicology Program (1986). *Toxicology and Carcinogenesis Studies of Rotenone in F344/N Rats and B6C3F1 Mice* (CAS No. 83-79-4). NIH Publication No. 86-2576. Washington D.C.: U.S. Department of Health and Human Services, Public Health Services, National Institute of Health.

Nemere, I. & Norman, A.W. (1986). Parathyroid hormone stimulates calcium transport in perfused duodena from normal chicks. Comparison with the rapid (transcaltachic) effect of 1,25-dihydroxyvitamin D3. *Endocrinology*, **119**, 1406–8.

Nickols, G.A. *et al.* (1989). Hypotension and cardiac stimulation due to the parathyroid hormone-related protein, humoral hypercalcemia of malignancy factor. *Endocrinology*, **125**, 834–41.

Nissenson, R.A., Diep, D. & Strewler, G.J. (1988). Synthetic peptides comprising the amino-terminal sequence of a parathyroid hormone-like protein from human malignancies. Binding to parathyroid hormone receptors and activation of adenylate cyclase in bone cells and kidney. *Journal of Biological Chemistry*, **263**, 12866–71.

Oettgen, H.F. *et al.* (1970). Toxicity of *E. coli* L-asparaginase in man. *Cancer*, **25**, 253–78.

Orloff, J.J. *et al.* (1989a). Characterization of canine renal receptors for the parathyroid hormone-like protein associated with humoral hypercalcemia of malignancy. *Journal of Biological Chemistry*, **264**, 6097–103.

Orloff, J.J., Wu, T.L. & Stewart, A.F. (1989b). Parathyroid hormone-like proteins. Biochemical responses and receptor interactions. *Endocrine Review*, **10**, 476–94.

Oslapas, R. *et al.* (1981). Incidence of radiation-induced parathyroid tumours in male and female rats. *Clinical Research*, **29**, 734A.

Oslapas, R., Shah, K.H., Hoffman, C., Ernst, K., Ku, W., Lawrence, A.M. & Paloyan, E. (1982). Effect of gonadectomy on the incidence of radiation-induced parathyroid tumors in male and female rats. *Clinical Research*, **30**, 401A.

Parsons, J.A. & Robinson, C.J. (1971). Calcium shift into bone causing transient hypocalcemia after injection of parathyroid hormone. *Nature*, **230**, 581–2.

Pliam, N.B., Nviredy, K.O. & Arnaud, C.D. (1982). Parathyroid hormone receptors in avian bone cells. *Proc. National Academy of Science (USA)*, **79**, 2061–3.

Potts, J.T., Segre, G.V. & Endres, D.B. (1983). Current clinical concepts. Assessment of parathyroid gland function with an N-terminal specific radioimmunoassay for intact parathyroid hormone. San Juan Capistrano: *Nichols Institute Note*, pp. 1–6.

Proscal, D.A. *et al.* (1976). 1,25-dihydroxyvitamin D₃-like component present in the plant *Solanum glaucophyllum*. *Endocrinology*, **99**, 437–44.

Pun, K.K., Arnaud, C.D. & Nissenson, R.A. (1988). Parathyroid hormone receptors in human dermal fibroblasts. Structural and functional characterization. *Journal of Bone and Mineral Research*, **3**, 453–60.

Rabbani, S.A. *et al.* (1988). Influence of the amino-terminus on in vitro and in vivo biological activity of synthetic parathyroid hormone-like peptides of malignancy. *Endocrinology*, **123**, 2709–16.

Raisz, L.G. & Kream, B.E. (1983). Regulation of bone formation. *New England Journal of Medicine*, **309**, 83–9.

Ream, L.J. & Principato, R. (1981). Glycogen accumulation in the parathyroid gland of the rat after fluoride ingestion. *Cell and Tissue Research*, **220**, 125–30.

Reynolds, J.J. *et al* (1972). The effect of two diphosphonates on the resorption of mouse calvaria *in vitro*. *Calcified Tissue Res.*, **10**, 302.

Rodan, G.A. & Martin, T.J. (1981). The role of osteoblasts in hormonal control of bone resorption – a hypothesis. *Calcified Tissue International*, **33**, 349–51.

Rodda, C.P. *et al.* (1988). Evidence for a novel parathyroid hormone-related protein in fetal lamb parathyroid glands and sheep placenta. Comparisons with a similar protein implicated in humoral hypercalcemia of malignancy. *Journal of Endocrinology*, **117**, 261–71.

Rosol, T.J. *et al.* (1990). Identification of parathyroid hormone-related protein in canine apocrine adenocarcinoma of the anal sac. *Veterinary Pathology*, **27**, 89–95.

Rosol, T.J. & Capen, C.C. (1988). Pathogenesis of humoral hypercalcemia of malignancy. *Dom. Anim. Endocrinol.*, **5**, 1–21.

Rosol, T.J., Capen, C.C. & Brooks, C.L. (1987). Bone and kidney adenylate cyclase-stimulating activity produced by a hypercalcemic canine adenocarcinoma line (CAC-8) maintained in nude mice. *Cancer Research*, **47**, 690–5.

Rosol, T.J., Capen, C.C. & Horst, R.L. (1988). Effects of infusion of human parathyroid hormone-related protein (1–40) in nude mice. Histomorphometric and biochemical investigations. *Journal of Bone and Mineral Research*, **3**, 699–706.

Rosol, T.J., Capen, C.C. & Minkin, C. (1986). *In vitro* bone resorption activity produced by a hypercalcemic adenocarcinoma tumor line (CAC-8) in nude mice. *Calcified Tissue International*, **39**, 334–41.

Rosol, T.J., Capen, C.C., Weisbrode, S.E. & Horst, R.L. (1986). Humoral hypercalcemia of malignancy in nude mouse model of a canine adenocarcinoma derived from apocrine glands of the anal sac. *Laboratory Investigation*, **54**, 679–88.

Roth, S.I. & Capen, C.C. (1974). Ultrastructural and functional correlations of the parathyroid glands. In *International Review of Experimental Pathology*, vol. 13, ed. G.W. Richter & M.A. Epstein, pp. 162–221. New York: Academic Press.

Roth, S.I. & Raisz, L.G. (1964). Effect of calcium concentration on the ultrastructure of rat parathyroid in organ culture. *Laboratory Investigation*, **13**, 331–45.

Silve, C.M. *et al.* (1982). Parathyroid hormone receptor in intact embryonic chicken bone: characterization and cellular localization. *Journal of Cell Biology*, **94**, 379–86.

Simpson, E.L. *et al.* (1983). Absence of parathyroid hormone messenger RNA in nonparathyroid tumors associated with hypercalcemia. *New England Journal of Medicine*, **309**, 325–30.

Simpson, C.F. & Sanger, V.L. (1968). A review of avian osteoporosis. Comparisons with other bone diseases. *Clinical Orthopedics and Related Research*, **58**, 271–81.

Solleveld, H.A., Haseman, J.K. & McConnell, E.E. (1984). National history of body weight gain, survival and neoplasia in the F344 rat. *Journal of the National Cancer Institute*, **72**, 929–40.

Stewart, A.F. *et al.* (1986). Frequency and partial characterization of adenylate cyclase-stimulating activity in tumors associated with humoral hypercalcemia of malignancy. *Journal of Bone and Mineral Research*, **1**, 267–76.

Stewart, A.F. *et al.* (1988). Synthetic human parathyroid hormone-like protein stimulates bone resorption and causes hypercalcemia in rats. *Journal of Clinical Investigation*, **81**, 596–600.

Sutton, R.A.L. & Dirks, J.H. (1978). Renal handling of calcium. *Federation Proceedings*, **37**, 2112–19.

Strewler, G.J. *et al.* (1987). Parathyroid hormone-like protein from human renal carcinoma cells. Structural and functional homology with parathyroid hormone. *Journal of Clinical Investigation*, **80**, 1803–7.

Suva, L.J. *et al.* (1987). A parathyroid hormone-related protein implicated in malignant hypercalcemia. Cloning and expression. *Science*, **237**, 893–6.

Suva, L.J. *et al.* (1989). Structure of the 5' flanking region of the gene encoding human parathyroid-hormone-related protein (PTHrP). *Gene*, **77**, 95–105.

Teotia, S.P.S. & Teotia, M. (1973). Secondary hyperparathyroidism in patients with endemic fluorosis. *British Medical Journal*, **1**, 637–40.

Tettenborn, D., Hobik, H.P. & Luckhaus, G. (1970). Hypoparathyroidismus beim Kaninchen nach Verabreichung von L-asparaginase. *Arzneimit Forsch*, **20**, 1753–5.

Thiede, M.A. (1989). The mRNA encoding a parathyroid hormone-like peptide is produced in mammary tissue in response to elevations in serum prolactin. *Molecular Endocrinology*, **3**, 1443–7.

Thiede, M.A. & Rodan, G. (1988). Expression of a calcium-mobilizing parathyroid hormone-like peptide in lactating mammary tissue. *Science*, **242**, 278–80.

Torrance, A.G. & Nachreiner, R. (1989). Human-parathormone assay for use in dogs. Validation, sample handling studies, and parathyroid function testing. *American Journal of Veterinary Research*, **50**, 1123–7.

Vaes, G. (1988). Cellular biology and biochemical mechanism of bone resorption. A review of recent developments on the formation, activation, and mode of action of osteoclasts. *Clinical Orthopaedic Related Research*, **231**, 239–71.

van Leeuwen, J.P.T.M. *et al.* (1988). Effect of parathyroid hormone and parathyroid hormone fragments on the intracellular ionized calcium concentration in an osteoblast cell line. *Bone and Mineral*, **4**, 177–88.

Wasserman, R.H. (1975). Active vitamin D-like substances in *Solanum malacoxylon* and other calcinogenic plants. *Nutrition Review*, **33**, 1–5.

Wasserman, M.R. *et al.* (1976). Calcinogenic factor in *Solanum malacoxylon*. Evidence that it is a 1,25-dihydroxyvitamin $D_3$-glycoside. *Science*, **194**, 853–5.

Wasserman, R.H., Corradino, R.A. & Krook, L. (1975). *Cestrum diurnum*. A domestic plant with 1,25-dihydroxycholecalciferol-like activity. *Biochemical & Biophysical Research Communications*, **62**, 85–91.

Weir, E.C. *et al.* (1988a). Humoral hypercalcemia of malignancy in canine lymphosarcoma. *Endocrinology*, **122**, 602–8.

Weir, E.C. *et al.* (1988b). Isolation of 16,000-dalton parathyroid hormone-like proteins from two animal tumors causing humoral hypercalcemia of malignancy. *Endocrinology*, **123**, 1744–51.

Weir, E.C. *et al.* (1988c). Hypercalcemia in canine lymphosarcoma is associated with the T-cell sub-type and with secretion of a PTH-like factor. *Journal of Bone and Mineral Research*, **3**, S106 (Abst.).

Wong, G.L. (1986). Skeletal effects of parathyroid hormone. In *Bone and Mineral Research*, 4th edn, ed. W.A. Peck, pp. 103–29. Amsterdam: Elsevier Science Publishers.

Wynford-Thomas, V., Wynford-Thomas, D. & Williams, E.D. (1982). Experimental induction of parathyroid adenomas in the rat. *Journal of the National Cancer Institute*, **70**, 127–34.

Yamaguchi, D.T., Kleeman, C.R. & Muallem, S. (1987). Protein kinase C-activated calcium channel in the osteoblast-like clonal osteosarcoma cell line UMR-106. *Journal of Biological Chemistry*, **262**, 14967–73.

Yamamoto, I. *et al.* (1988). Properties of parathyroid hormone receptors on circulating bovine lymphocytes. *Journal of Bone and Mineral Research*, **3**, 289.

Yarrington, J.T. *et al.* (1977a). Effect of dichloromethane diphos-phonate on calcium homeostatic mechanisms in pregnant cows. *American Journal of Pathology*, **87**, 615–30.

Yarrington, J.T. *et al.* (1977b). Effect of ethane-1-hydroxy-1, 1-diphos-phonate (EHDP) on the ultrastructure of parathyroid glands and plasma immunoreactive parathyroid hormone in pregnant cows fed a low-calcium diet. *Laboratory Investigation*, **36**, 402–12.

Yasuda, T. *et al.* (1989). Rat parathyroid hormone-like peptide. Com-parison with the human homologue and expression in malignant and normal tissue. *Molecular Endocrinology*, **3**, 518–25.

Yates, A.J.P. *et al.* (1988). Effects of a synthetic peptide of a parathyroid hormone-related protein on calcium homeostasis, renal tubular calcium reabsorption, and bone metabolism *in vivo* and *in vitro* in rodents. *Journal of Clinical Investigation*, **81**, 932–8.

Young, D.M. *et al.* (1973). Clinicopathologic and ultrastructural studies of L-asparaginase-induced hypocalcemia in rabbits. An experimental animal model of acute hypoparathyroidism. *Laboratory Investigation*, **29**, 374–86.

Youshak, M.S. & Capen, C.C. (1970). Fine structural alterations in parathyroid glands of chickens with osteopetrosis. *American Journal of Pathology*, **60**, 257–73.

# IV    Adrenal toxicology

HOWARD D. COLBY AND PENELOPE A.
LONGHURST

# 8    Toxicology of the adrenal gland

## Introduction

The adrenal gland is a compound endocrine organ consisting of the inner medulla and the outer cortex (see Colby, 1987a,b). Although the cortex and medulla are anatomically juxtaposed, the functions and regulation of each are independent of one another. The medulla is comprised of chromaffin cells which synthesize catecholamines, principally epinephrine, and hormone secretion is controlled by the sympathetic innervation of the gland. The cortex, by contrast, produces a variety of steroid hormones as its secretory products, and regulation involves a hypothalamic-anterior pituitary negative feedback loop, the renin-angiotensin system, and other humoral factors. Probably because of the vast structural and functional differences between the cortex and medulla, adrenal toxins tend to be specific for one or the other. Thus, the cortex and medulla are distinct with respect to both physiology and toxicology, and each is most readily studied independently of the other.

In this chapter, an overview of adrenal medullary and cortical physiology will be presented before any consideration of toxicology. A full understanding of the functional changes effected by toxic chemicals requires some knowledge of the underlying physiological processes characteristic of the target organs. In the discussion of adrenal toxicology, the focus will be on the functional lesions induced by adrenal toxins; morphologic alterations have been described by others (Ribelin, 1984; Szabo & Lippe, 1989). Since the functional consequences of adrenal cortical toxins have been more thoroughly characterized and seem to be far more common than those of the medulla, this chapter will emphasize the toxicology of the cortex. Some general characteristics will be discussed followed by specific examples taken from our own investigations with the drug, spironolactone, and the solvent, carbon tetrachloride.

## Adrenal medulla

## Physiology (see Colby, 1987a)

The adrenal medulla comprises the inner 20% of the adrenal gland. Histologically, the medulla consists of chromaffin cells, which characteristically synthesize and store catecholamines, surrounded by large venous sinusoids. The gland is structurally and functionally analogous to a post-ganglionic sympathetic neuron. Like sympathetic neurons, the adrenal medulla receives central nervous system input from the medulla, pons, and hypothalamus via the thoracolumbar spinal cord. However, in contrast to most preganglionic sympathetic nerve fibers which synapse in the ganglia of the sympathetic chain, the preganglionic nerve fibers to the adrenal medulla exit the spinal cord without passing through the sympathetic chain and synapse directly on the chromaffin cells of the gland. It is this sympathetic innervation which controls catecholamine secretion by the chromaffin cells.

The major physiological functions of adrenal medullary cells are the synthesis and secretion of catecholamines. The normal substrates for catecholamine synthesis are phenylalanine and tyrosine. Phenylalanine may be converted to tyrosine by the enzyme, phenylalanine hydroxylase, but most of the catecholamine synthesis in the adrenal medulla utilizes tyrosine as the initial substrate (Fig. 8.1). Tyrosine is oxidized to dihydroxyphenylalanine (DOPA) by the cytosolic enzyme tyrosine hydroxylase. This reaction is the rate limiting step in catecholamine synthesis, and requires molecular oxygen, tetrahydropteridine, and NADPH as co-factors. Catecholamines exert a negative feedback effect on tyrosine hydroxylase by competing for the pteridine co-factor binding site on the enzyme. DOPA is converted to dopamine by another cytosolic enzyme, dopa decarboxylase (aromatic-L-amino acid decarboxylase) which requires pyridoxal phosphate as a co-factor. Dopamine is then actively transported into vesicles known as chromaffin granules which are found in all chromaffin cells. Within the vesicles, dopamine is converted to norepinephrine by the enzyme dopamine-β-hydroxylase (DBH). Molecular oxygen and ascorbic acid are co-factors for the reaction. Norepinephrine is then released into the cytoplasm for conversion to epinephrine by phenylethanolamine-N-methyltransferase (PNMT). The reaction involves the donation of a methyl group by S-adenosyl-methionine to the primary nitrogen group of norepinephrine. Once formed, epinephrine is actively transported into medullary chromaffin granules which are distinct from those containing norepinephrine, and stored.

It is generally believed that there are two different populations of

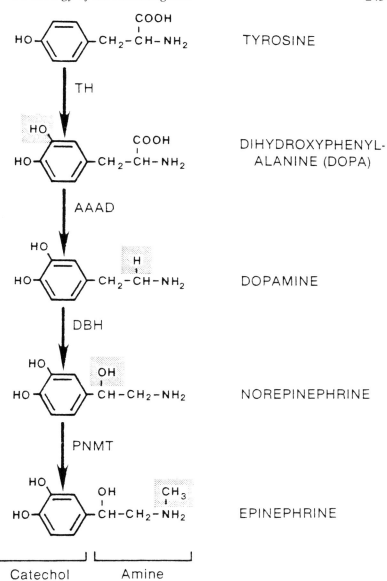

Fig. 8.1. Pathway of catecholamine synthesis in the adrenal medulla. (TH, tyrosine hydroxylase; AAAD, aromatic L-amino acid decarboxylase; DBH, dopamine β-hydroxylase; PNMT, phenylethanolamine N-methyl transferase). (From Hedge, Colby & Goodman, *Clinical Endocrine Physiology*, Saunders, 1987.)

chromaffin cells within the medulla, one that stores and secretes epinephrine, and the other norepinephrine. PNMT is localized exclusively in
the cytosol of the epinephrine-containing cells of the adrenal medulla and
of a few central nervous system neurons. The formation of epinephrine,
therefore, is restricted to these same cells. Synthesis of PNMT is induced
by glucocorticoids, and the portal venous sinusoids which drain from the
adrenal cortex to the medulla contain high concentrations of the cortical
hormone, cortisol, a potent glucocorticoid. Thus, the anatomic relationship of the cortex and medulla contributes to maintaining adequate
PNMT levels and epinephrine synthesis.

Epinephrine is the major catecholamine that is synthesized and stored
in the adrenal medulla, comprising approximately 80% of the total hormonal output of the gland. Secretion of catecholamines by the adrenal
medulla is influenced by a number of factors, some of which are included
in Table 8.1. Neural pathways mediate the stimulation of catecholamine
secretion by the adrenal medulla in response to hypoglycaemia, exercise,
hypothermia, hypoxia, hypercapnia, and stress. These pathways originate
in the same regions of the central nervous system as those that control
sympathetic nerve activity, reaching the adrenal gland via splanchnic
nerve fibers. The overall sequence of events leading to catecholamine
secretion by adrenal medullary cells is known as stimulus-secretion coupling (Fig. 8.2). Release of acetylcholine from the preganglionic nerve
synapses at the chromaffin cells causes depolarization of the cell membrane and a concomitant increase in calcium permeability. The resulting
increases in intracellular calcium levels stimulate release of epinephrine
or norepinephrine from the chromaffin cells by the process of exocytosis.
The chromaffin granules migrate to the cell membrane, the granule and
cell membranes fuse, and catecholamines, as well as the other contents of
the granules, are released into the extracellular space. The fused membrane is pinched off to form a new vesicle which returns to the cytosol and
is re-used. Approximately 50% of the catecholamines secreted by the
adrenal medulla circulate in the blood as free hormones, the rest is bound
to albumin.

Catecholamines exert effects on most of the tissues of the body. Cannon described the actions of catecholamines as producing a 'fight or
flight' response, meaning that the body is mobilized to meet an
emergency. That description is indeed appropriate for many of the effects
of catecholamines (Table 8.2). There are two major types of receptors,
known as $\alpha$- and $\beta$-adrenergic receptors, which are involved in mediating
the actions of epinephrine and norepinephrine. The $\alpha$- and $\beta$-receptors
are further divided into at least two subtypes of each, $\alpha_1$ and $\alpha_2$, and $\beta_1$
and $\beta_2$. Each receptor type is differentially distributed throughout the

Table 8.1. *Stimuli for catecholamine secretion by the adrenal medulla*

| | |
|---|---|
| Hypoglycaemia | Exercise |
| Physical or psychological trauma | Illness |
| Circulatory failure (Haemorrhage) | Hypoxia |
| Stress | Cold Exposure |

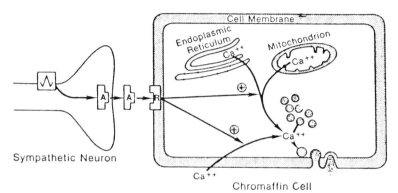

Fig. 8.2. Stimulus-secretion coupling in the adrenal chromaffin cell. (A, acetylcholine; R, receptor.) (From Hedge, Colby & Goodman, *Clinical Endocrine Physiology*, Saunders, 1987.)

body, and it is the relative distribution of these receptors, in part, that determines the type of response of a tissue to catecholamines. $\alpha_1$-Receptors predominate at postsynaptic nerve endings, while $\alpha_2$-receptors are presynaptic where they control the release of catecholamines from sympathetic nerve endings. $\beta_1$-Receptors are of greatest importance in the heart and $\beta_2$-receptors participate in catecholamine effects on smooth muscle function and on intermediary metabolism. Epinephrine and norepinephrine have different relative affinities for $\alpha$- and $\beta$-receptors. However, neither is totally specific for either receptor type, and both stimulate $\alpha$- and $\beta$-receptors to some degree. The relative affinity of epinephrine for $\alpha_1$-receptors is equal to, or greater than that of norepinephrine and the opposite is true for $\alpha_2$-receptors. Epinephrine and norepinephrine are equipotent at $\beta_1$-receptors, but at $\beta_2$-receptors, epinephrine is at least 10 times more potent than norepinephrine.

In general, the responses to $\alpha$-stimulation are excitatory (Table 8.2). Stimulation of $\alpha$-receptors causes vasoconstriction, contraction of the radial muscle of the eye resulting in mydriasis, constriction of the sphincters of the stomach, intestine, and bladder, contraction of the pregnant

Table 8.2. *Responses of target tissues to catecholamines*

| Target tissue | Receptor type | Response |
|---|---|---|
| Adipose tissue | $\beta_2$ | Lipolysis |
| Bronchial muscle | $\beta_2$ | Relaxation |
| CNS | $\alpha$ | Stimulation |
| Cardiovascular system | $\alpha$ | Vasoconstriction |
| | $\beta_1$ | Tachycardia, increased contractility, increased conduction velocity |
| | $\beta_2$ | Vasodilation of skeletal muscle anterioles, coronary arteries, and veins |
| Eye | $\alpha_1$ | Radial muscle contraction |
| | $\beta_2$ | Ciliary muscle relaxation |
| Gastrointestinal tract | $\beta_2$ | Decreased contractility |
| | $\alpha$ | Sphincter contraction |
| Liver | $\beta_2$ | Glycogenolysis, lipolysis, gluconeogenesis |
| Male sex organs | $\alpha$ | Ejaculation, detumescence |
| | $\beta_2$ | Erection? |
| Pancreas | $\alpha_2$ | Decreased insulin secretion |
| | $\beta_2$ | Increased insulin secretion |
| Renin secretion | $\beta_1$ | Stimulation |
| Skeletal muscle | $\beta_2$ | Glycogenolysis |
| Skin | $\alpha$ | Piloerection, sweat production |
| Urinary bladder | $\alpha$ | Sphincter contraction |
| | $\beta_2$ | Detrusor relaxation |
| Uterus | $\alpha$ | Contraction |
| | $\beta_2$ | Relaxation |

CNS = central nervous system

uterus, ejaculation, piloerection, and sweating. Activation of $\beta_1$-receptors in the heart produces excitatory effects, including increases in contractility, heart rate, and conduction velocity. $\beta_2$-Receptors mediate the metabolic effects of catecholamines including stimulation of glycogenolysis, lipolysis, and gluconeogenesis. Other actions resulting from $\beta_2$-receptor activation are arteriolar dilatation, relaxation of the bronchi, decreased stomach and intestinal motility, stimulation of renin secretion, urinary bladder body relaxation, and relaxation of the non-pregnant uterus (Table 8.2). In addition, a $\beta_3$-receptor has recently been cloned (Emorine *et al.*, 1989). This may be the same receptor responsible for atypical $\beta$-receptor-mediated effects in adipocytes, stomach fundus, ileum, and colon smooth muscle, cardiac muscle, and skeletal muscle (Zaagsma & Nahorski, 1990). The functional significance of these $\beta_3$-receptors is, at present, unknown.

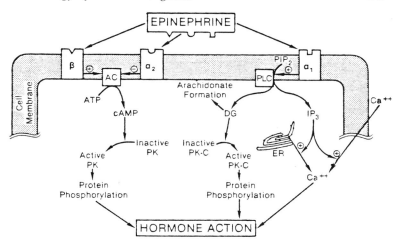

Fig. 8.3. Mechanisms of action of epinephrine in target cells mediated by β-, α$_2$- and α$_1$-adrenergic receptors. (PIP$_2$, phosphatidylinositol-4,5-biphosphate; PLC, phospholipase C; DG, diacylglycerol; IP$_3$, inositol-1,4,5-triphosphate; AC, adenylate cyclase; PK, protein kinase; PK-C, protein kinase C; ER, endoplasmic reticulum.) (From Hedge, Colby & Goodman, *Clinical Endocrine Physiology*, Saunders, 1987.)

The cellular mechanism of action of the catecholamines depends on which receptor subtype is activated. Activation of β-receptors involves binding of the catecholamine to the three-compartment adenylate cyclase system and subsequent stimulation of cyclic AMP (cAMP) formation (Fig. 8.3). By contrast, catecholamine binding to α$_2$-receptors inhibits adenylate cyclase, thereby decreasing AMP production. The activation of α$_1$-receptors involves a different pathway, one that is associated with a rapid breakdown of membrane polyphosphoinositides and an increase in intracellular calcium levels (Fig. 8.3).

Catecholamines have very short biological half-lives and are cleared from plasma or synaptic pools by three methods, enzymatic conversion to inactive products, neuronal and extraneuronal uptake, and excretion. Neuronally-released catecholamines are rapidly transported into the nerves and stored for re-use. In contrast, catecholamines secreted by the adrenal medulla into the blood are generally inactivated by enzymatic degradation in the liver and kidneys. The degradative metabolism of catecholamines involves two major pathways—deamination by the enzyme monoamine oxidase (MAO) and methylation by the enzyme catechol-O-methyltransferase (COMT). MAO is most abundantly found in liver, kidney, stomach, and intestine and the highest activities of

COMT are found in liver and kidney. The catecholamine metabolites produced by these enzymes as well as unaltered parent compounds are normally excreted in the urine.

## Toxicology

Diseases of the adrenal medulla are limited to the development of tumours some of which are functional, that is they secrete catecholamines. Pheochromocytomas are chromaffin cell tumours that secrete large quantities of epinephrine or norepinephrine. Although pheochromocytomas are usually benign, they are potentially dangerous because the excessive secretion of catecholamines can cause severe hypertension and arrhythmias. Pheochromocytomas may occur in the adrenal medulla or in extra-medullary chromaffin tissues such as the sympathetic chain or the organ of Zuckerkandl (Landsberg & Young, 1980).

Relatively little is known about the toxic effects of chemicals on adrenal medullary structure or function. This may be related at least in part, to the difficulty of defining a toxic effect on the gland. Many chemicals can non-specifically elicit activation of the sympathetic nervous system, resulting in stimulation of catecholamine secretion and depletion of catecholamine stores in the adrenal medulla. Such changes are rapidly reversed by removal of the noxious stimulus. Most investigators use histological evidence of hypertrophy or hyperplasia accompanied by changes in epinephrine or norepinephrine content as an indication of medullary toxicity. However, some of the laboratory animals commonly used for toxicity testing have a high incidence of spontaneous adrenal medullary hypertrophy or hyperplasia, which often makes interpretation of toxicity data difficult (Thompson *et al.*, 1981; Tischler & DeLellis, 1988; Tischler, 1989). In addition, the composition of animal diets can influence the development of adrenal medullary tumours, further complicating analysis of toxicity studies (Roe & Bär, 1985). Interestingly, several of the substances which have been shown to be toxic to the adrenal medulla affect medullary content of epinephrine or norepinephrine, but not necessarily both. Apparently, such compounds have selective effects on the epinephrine- or norepinephrine-producing cells of the medulla.

A number of reports indicate that the morphology and/or function of the adrenal medulla may be adversely affected by several hormonal factors. However, many of the observations on hormonal effects in the literature are conflicting, which may be the result of differences in species studied, dose and purity of hormone preparations used, and duration of hormone treatment. The endocrine effects on the adrenal medulla that have been most thoroughly investigated are those of the thyroid hormones and of growth hormone. The thyroid hormones have been found to cause hypertrophy of the entire adrenal gland, but particularly the medulla (Hopsu, 1960). The effects of thyroid hormones on adrenal weight are prevented by hypophysectomy indicating that they are mediated by the pituitary gland. In general, the norepinephrine-containing cells of the adrenal medulla seem to be more sensitive to thyroid hormones than are the epinephrine-containing cells. Increases in thyroid hormone levels decrease the volumes and catecholamine content of the norepinephrine-containing but not the epinephrine-containing cells. Decreases in thyroid hormone levels tend to produce the opposite effects and also cause increases in medullary epinephrine content (Marine & Baumann, 1945; Hopsu, 1960).

The results of several studies indicate that growth hormone (GH) also has effects on the adrenal medulla. Chronic GH administration to rats is associated with hypertrophy and hyperplasia of the medulla. The morphologic characteristics of medullary cells resulting from GH treatment include pale cytoplasm and large vesicular nuclei, often with prominent nucleoli. There were no apparent effects of GH in rats on norepinephrine or epinephrine content of the medulla (Evans *et al.*, 1948; Simpson, Evans & Li, 1949; Moon *et al.*, 1950). By contrast, treatment of mice with GH had no effects on adrenal weights, but increased the volume and catecholamine content of both epinephrine- and norepinephrine-containing chromaffin cells (Hopsu, 1960). The reasons for the species differences in the effects of GH on the adrenal medulla are not known.

Relatively few reports of xenobiotic effects on the adrenal medulla have appeared in the literature (Table 8.3). From the limited data available it is difficult to draw any general conclusions about the chemical characteristics of medullary toxins. In addition, the mechanisms responsible for the toxic effects are largely unknown. Some drugs, such as reserpine and nicotine may produce their toxicity as a result of effects on catecholamine release from the adrenal. Somewhat conflicting results have been obtained with nicotine, but this may be related to differences in experimental protocols and/or species studied. Eränkö (1955) found that chronic administration of nicotine to rats had no effects on body weight, whole adrenal gland weight, or adrenal cortex volume. However, there was a two-fold increase in adrenal medullary volume and histologic changes in the medulla. Small nodules were present, the medullae appeared less vascularized, and there were increases in the number of nuclei per unit area. There were significant increases in medullary norepinephrine stores and decreases in epinephrine content. Similarly, Boelsterli, Cruz-Orive & Zbinden (1984) found that nicotine administra-

Table 8.3. *Compounds producing lesions in the adrenal medulla*

| | |
|---|---|
| Acrylonitrile | (Szabo *et al.*, 1980) |
| ACTH | (Szabo *et al.*, 1980) |
| Alloxan | (Grasso, 1963) |
| Blocadren | (Ribelin, 1984) |
| Chlordecone | (Baggett *et al.*, 1980) |
| o-Chlorobenzylidine malononitrile | (Chowdhury *et al.*, 1978) |
| Cysteamine | (McComb *et al.*, 1981) |
| Dichloromethane | (Marzotko & Pankow, 1987) |
| 7, 12-Dimethylbenzanthracene | (Harris, 1968) |
| Oestrogens | (Tischler & De Lellis, 1988) |
| Growth hormone | (Moon *et al.*, 1950) |
| Interleukin-2 | (Anderson & Hayes, 1989) |
| Lactitol | (Roe & Bär, 1985) |
| Lactose | (Roe & Bär, 1985) |
| Malathion | (Gowda *et al.*, 1975) |
| Mannitol | (Roe & Bär, 1985) |
| 1-Methyl-4-phenyl-1, 2, 3, 6-tetrahydropyridine, MPTP | (Barbeau *et al.*, 1985) |
| Neuroleptics | (Roe & Bär, 1985) |
| Nicotine | (Boelsterli *et al.*, 1984) |
| Pyrazole | (Szabo *et al.*, 1981) |
| Reserpine | (USDHHR, 1982) |
| Retinol acetate | (Kurokawa, *et al.*, 1985) |
| Sorbitol | (Salsburg, 1980) |
| Thiouracil | (Hopsu, 1960) |
| TSH | (Hopsu, 1960) |
| Thyroid Hormones | (Hopsu, 1960) |
| 1, 1, 2-Trichloroethane | (USDHEW, 1978) |
| Xylitol | (Boelsterli & Zbinden, 1985) |

tion to rats caused medullary hypertrophy and hyperplasia which was accompanied by increases in adrenal catecholamine levels. In contrast the short-term treatment of guinea-pigs with the nicotine equivalent of two-packs of cigarettes per day had no effects on adrenal norepinephrine or epinephrine stores but increased serum epinephrine levels (Hexum & Russett, 1987). Reserpine, which depletes adrenal catecholamine stores, has been found to increase the incidence of tumours resembling pheo-chromocytomas in male Fischer 344 rats (USDHHR, 1982).

Insecticides can have toxic effects on several endocrine organs including the adrenal medulla. Dietary administration of the chlorocarbon insecticide, Chlordecone, to rats significantly reduced medullary epinephrine but increased norepinephrine content (Baggett, Thureson-Klein

& Klein, 1980). By contrast, Mirex, another chlorocarbon insecticide, had no effect on adrenal catecholamine content. The differences between the actions of Chlordecone and Mirex were attributed to possible effects of Chlordecone to decrease PNMT activity and thereby decrease epinephrine synthesis, and/or to inhibit mitochondrial $Mg^{++}$-ATPase activity, resulting in decreased uptake of epinephrine into the medullary storage granules (Baggett *et al.*, 1980). Several studies have been done to evaluate the effects of 1-methyl-4-phenyl-1,2,3,6-tetrahydropyridine (MPTP), an insecticide structurally similar to paraquat, and of 1-methyl-4-phenylpyridinium ($MPP^+$), its major metabolite (Langston *et al.*, 1987), on adrenal medullary function. Following injection of MPTP, the concentration of $MPP^+$ is greater in the adrenal than in any other organ in the body (Johannessen *et al.*, 1986). Administration of MPTP to frogs decreased adrenal medullary dopamine and norepinephrine content (Barbeau *et al.*, 1985; Neafsey *et al.*, 1986). $MPP^+$ almost totally depleted the medulla of dopamine and decreased epinephrine and norepinephrine content by approximately 50%. Paraquat, by contrast, had no effect on medullary content of any of the three catecholamines measured (Barbeau *et al.*, 1985). In rats, MPTP and $MPP^+$ decreased adrenal epinephrine content and tyrosine hydroxylase activity (Ambrosio & Mahy, 1989). Bovine adrenal chromaffin cells were found to accumulate $MPP^+$, an effect which was blocked by the catecholamine uptake inhibitor, desmethylimipramine. The $MPP^+$ was found to be co-localized with catecholamines in chromaffin granules and co-secreted with the catecholamines. Blockade of the uptake of $MPP^+$ by tetrabenazine resulted in $MPP^+$-induced toxicity, manifested by decreases in catecholamine content, protein content, and tyrosine hydroxylase activity (Reinhard *et al.*, 1987). These observations suggest that the storage of $MPP^+$ in the chromaffin vesicles may in some way protect the cells from its toxic effects.

A number of reports indicate that dietary administration of xylitol and other sugar alcohols (polyols) to rodents causes hypertrophy of the adrenal medulla (Salsburg, 1980; Boelsterli & Zbinden, 1985). The mechanism of action of these chemicals is thought to be related to effects on calcium homeostasis, since they also increase calcium absorption from the intestinal tract (Roe & Bär, 1985). However, in man, there is no evidence of any link between calcium absorption and adrenal medullary proliferative disease. A variety of other compounds which have been reported to have effects on adrenal medullary structure or function are listed in Table 8.3. For most, relatively few studies on their medullary toxicity have appeared in the literature and very little is known about their mechanisms of action on the adrenal medulla.

## Adrenal cortex

## Physiology (See Colby, 1987b)

The adrenal cortex secretes a variety of steroid hormones which impact upon numerous metabolic processes throughout the body (Table 8.4). The relative amounts of the different hormones produced varies among the three anatomical zones of the cortex, effecting what is known as a functional zonation which coincides with the gland's anatomical zonation (Table 8.5). The outermost zone of the cortex, the zona glomerulosa, is the only region that can synthesize aldosterone, the major mineralocorticoid secreted by the adrenal cortex. The actions of mineralocorticoids are concerned principally with electrolyte balance and blood pressure homeostasis. The middle and inner zones of the cortex, the zona fasciculata and zona reticularis, respectively, are the major sites of glucocorticoid and androgen production. There are many species differences in the profiles of adrenal glucocorticoids and androgens as a result of differences in the relative activities of various steroidogenic enzymes in these zones. Cortisol, the physiologically most important glucocorticoid secreted by the human adrenal, exerts a variety of effects on intermediary metabolism, particularly on protein and carbohydrate metabolism. Adrenal androgens are far less potent than the testicular androgen, testosterone, but otherwise have similar actions. The quantitatively most significant adrenal androgen in humans is dehydroepiandrosterone (DHEA) which is also secreted by the gland as a sulphated conjugate (DHEA-sulphate).

All of the steroid hormones are synthesized from the common precursor, cholesterol. Large amounts of cholesterol in the form of cholesterol esters are stored within lipid droplets in adrenocortical cells. Adrenal cholesterol is derived from circulating lipoproteins by a receptor-mediated uptake process and by *de novo* synthesis from acetate in adrenal cells. Stored cholesterol esters can be hydrolyzed enzymatically as needed, to provide free cholesterol as substrate for steroidogenesis.

Synthesis of steroid hormones involves the step-by-step enzymatic modification of the cholesterol molecule (Fig. 8.4). Hydroxylations at several sites on the steroid nucleus are key reactions for hormone production and the enzymes involved are targets for a number of adrenal toxins. One of the components of these steroid hydroxylases, the haemprotein, cytochrome P-450, seems particularly vulnerable to the actions of exogenous chemicals. Different cytochrome P-450 isozymes serve as the substrate-binding sites for the different steroid hydroxylases and thereby confer the substrate specificity characteristic of each enzyme (Hall, 1986).

It is the first step in the steroidogenic pathway, the conversion of

Table 8.4. *Major steroids secreted by the human adrenal cortex*

| Steroid | Type of hormone | Secretion rate (mg/day) |
|---|---|---|
| Cortisol | Glucocorticoid | 10–30 |
| Aldosterone | Mineralocorticoid | 0.05–0.15 |
| DHEA + DHEA-sulphate | Androgen | 15–40 |

DHEA = dehydroepiandrosterone

Table 8.5. *Functional zonation of the adrenal cortex*

| Zone | Hormone(s) produced |
|---|---|
| Zona glomerulosa | Aldosterone |
| Zona fasciculata | Cortisol, DHEA |
| Zona reticularis | Cortisol, DHEA |

DHEA = dehydroepiandrosterone

cholesterol to pregnenolone, that is rate-limiting for steroid hormone production. Accordingly, the regulation of steroidogenesis occurs principally by hormonal modulation of the rate of this reaction. Unlike other types of hormones, steroids are not stored to any significant degree within their cells of origin. Since steroids are highly lipid-soluble, once synthesized, they can freely diffuse across cell membranes and into the blood. Thus, synthesis and secretion of steroid hormones tend to be tightly coupled processes, with regulation of secretion occurring by control of biosynthesis.

The profile of secretory products for any steroid-producing cell is determined by the relative amounts and activities of the various steroidogenic enzymes characteristic of each cell. Thus, the functional zonation within the adrenal cortex is explained by enzymatic differences between the zona glomerulosa and the inner zones of the gland, the zona fasciculata and the zona reticularis. The cells of the zona glomerulosa lack the steroid 17α-hydroxylase, an enzyme required for cortisol and androgen synthesis, but have all of the enzymatic machinery required for aldosterone production. By contrast, the cells of the zona fasciculata and zona reticularis can effect 17α-hydroxylation but are unable to catalyze the final step in aldosterone formation. Consequently, aldosterone production is limited to the zona glomerulosa and glucocorticoid and androgen production to the zona fasciculata and zona reticularis.

After secretion by adrenocortical cells, steroid hormones, because of

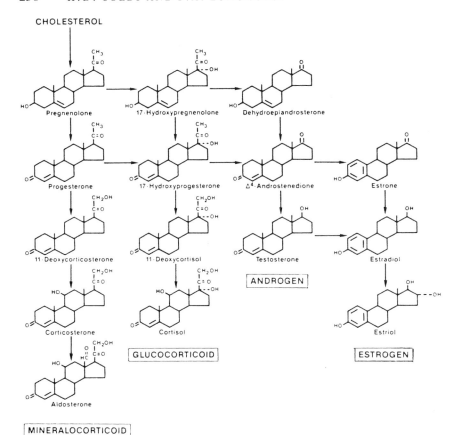

Fig. 8.4. Pathways involved in the production of the major steroid hormones. (From Hedge, Colby & Goodman, *Clinical Endocrine Physiology*, Saunders, 1987.)

their lipophilicity, are largely protein bound as they circulate in the blood. The unbound or 'free' hormone is in reversible equilibrium with the protein-bound pool, the relative amounts of each depending upon the affinity of the steroid for its binding protein(s) and the concentrations of the binding proteins. It is important to recognize that only the free hormone has access to receptors in target tissues and, therefore, is able to initiate the actions characteristic of the hormone. However, because of the equilibrium between the free and protein-bound hormone pools, the latter can serve as a source of additional free hormone when needed. In addition, the protein-bound fraction is relatively resistant to metabolism, which increases the plasma half-life of steroid hormones.

The mechanism of action of all adrenocortical hormones follows the general model for lipophilic hormone actions. According to this model, steroid hormones diffuse across cell membranes in their target cells and interact with highly specific cystolic receptors. The hormone-receptor complexes are then translocated to the nucleus of the target cells, effecting the transcription of specific genes and ultimately the synthesis of certain proteins. The proteins synthesized, which are characteristic of both the target cell and effector hormone, mediate the biological actions of the hormone.

## Glucocorticoids

The major physiological effects of glucocorticoids are associated with carbohydrate, protein, and lipid metabolism. These effects are summarized in Table 8.6.

One of the most prominent actions of glucocorticoids is stimulation of hepatic gluconeogenesis, resulting from induction of several of the enzymes in the gluconeogenic pathway. Glucocorticoids also increase the amounts of amino acid substrates available for gluconeogenesis by promoting the degradation of muscle protein. The net effects of augmenting the conversion of amino acids to carbohydrate include increases in hepatic glycogen content and in blood glucose levels. In addition, the catabolic effects on protein metabolism increase urinary excretion, causing a negative nitrogen balance.

The effects of glucocorticoids on fat metabolism are not as well understood as those on carbohydrate and protein metabolism. Cortisol seems to enhance the actions of lipolytic hormones such as epinephrine. Thus glucocorticoids are sometimes described as having 'permissive' effects on lipolysis, increasing plasma free fatty acid levels.

Other effects of glucocorticoids which are poorly understood include their roles in adaptation to stress and in the modulation of behaviour. Stress is one of the most potent stimuli for cortisol secretion and is poorly tolerated by individuals with adrenal insufficiency. However, the nature of glucocorticoid actions in the response to stress has not been resolved. Adrenocortical dysfunction is also associated with a variety of behavioural disorders. The mechanism(s) responsible for glucocorticoid effects on behaviour, like those involved in the response to stress, have not been clearly defined.

The secretion of cortisol is controlled principally by a negative feed-

Table 8.6. *Major physiological effects of glucocorticoids*

Stimulate hepatic gluconeogenesis
Increase hepatic glycogen content
Increase blood glucose concentrations
Promote lipolysis
Catabolic (cause negative nitrogen balance)
Response to stress
Behavioral effects
Inhibit ACTH secretion

back loop involving the hypothalamus and anterior pituitary gland (Fig. 8.5). Corticotrophin releasing hormone (CRH) is secreted by the hypothalamus into the hypophyseal portal vessels which transport it to the anterior pituitary gland. In response to CRH stimulation, the pituitary corticotrophin (ACTH)-producing cells secrete ACTH into the blood. ACTH interacts with membrane bound receptors on adrenocortical cells, principally those of the zona fasciculata and zona reticularis, activating adenylate cyclase and stimulating cAMP production. Both the chronic and acute effects of ACTH on the adrenal cortex appear to be mediated by cAMP. The chronic actions include an overall stimulation of adrenal protein synthesis and growth of the gland. Thus, conditions associated with chronic hyper- or hyposecretion of ACTH result in adrenal hypertrophy or atrophy, respectively.

The acute actions of ACTH relate primarily to its stimulation of cortisol secretion. Acting via cAMP, ACTH exerts several effects which rapidly increase the rate of conversion of cholesterol to pregnenolone, the rate-limiting step in cortisol production. ACTH increases the amount of free cholesterol available for steroidogenesis and also promotes the binding of cholesterol to the cholesterol side-chain cleavage enzyme, a critical step in the initiation of enzyme activity. As a result, cholesterol metabolism is accelerated, increasing the synthesis and secretion of cortisol by the cells of the zona fasciculata and zona reticularis.

It is the cortisol circulating in the blood that is the final component of the regulatory system for adrenal cortisol secretion. Plasma free cortisol exerts inhibitory effects on the secretion of CRH and ACTH by the hypothalamus and anterior pituitary gland respectively. The net effect is that increases or decreases in plasma cortisol levels cause the opposite changes in ACTH and cortisol secretion, tending to preserve blood hormone concentrations in the normal range. Thus, the regulatory system serves to monitor free cortisol levels in blood and adjust adrenal secretion in accordance with need.

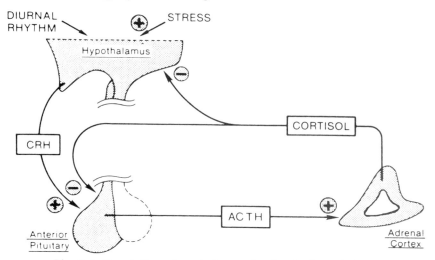

Fig. 8.5. Regulation of cortisol secretion by the hypothalamo-pituitary axis (+, stimulation; −, inhibition). (From Hedge, Colby & Goodman, *Clinical Endocrine Physiology*, Saunders, 1987.)

Superimposed upon the primary regulatory system for cortisol secretion described above are two additional factors, diurnal rhythm and stress (Fig. 8.5). In humans, cortisol secretion is maximal in the early morning and at a minimum late at night. The reverse pattern occurs in nocturnal species such as rats. This diurnal variation in adrenal secretion is the result of hypothalamic rhythms in CRH release and therefore, is intrinsic to the regulatory system for cortisol secretion and not to the adrenal gland itself.

It has long been recognized that all types of stress non-specifically stimulate ACTH and consequently cortisol secretion. The effects of stress are mediated through the central nervous system and override the inhibitory effects of cortisol on CRH and ACTH secretion. Thus, during periods of stress plasma cortisol levels may increase dramatically. As noted earlier, there is evidence to indicate that cortisol has a role in the body's adaptation to stress. However, the precise nature of that role has not yet been determined.

## Mineralocorticoids

The most important physiological effects of mineralocorticoids are related to blood pressure homeostasis and electrolyte balance, and are the results of hormone actions on the distal tubules in the nephrons of the

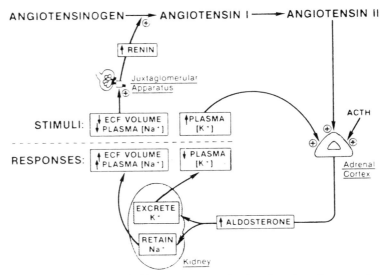

Fig. 8.6. Regulation of aldosterone secretion by the adrenal cortex. (+, stimulation; −, inhibition; ECF, extracellular fluid.) (From Hedge, Colby & Goodman, *Clinical Endocrine Physiology*, Saunders, 1987.)

kidney. Mineralocorticoids interact with cytosolic receptors in renal tubular cells and stimulate RNA transcription and protein synthesis. The net effect of these newly synthesized proteins is to increase the renal reabsorption of sodium ions, thereby increasing plasma sodium concentrations. The osmotic effect of sodium tends to promote expansion of the extracellular fluid volume. The reabsorption of sodium in response to mineralocorticoids is accompanied by an increase in the excretion of potassium and hydrogen ions. As a consequence of these hormonal effects, mineralocorticoid excess is usually characterized by hypertension (volume expansion), hypernatraemia, hypokalaemia, and metabolic alkalosis. Mineralocorticoid insufficiency causes the opposite changes.

The mineralocorticoid of greatest physiological significance is aldosterone, the principal secretory product of the zona glomerulosa. One of the major regulators of aldosterone production is the renin-angiotensin system (Fig. 8.6). Renin is an enzyme produced by the juxtaglomerular apparatus of the kidney and catalyzes the conversion of a circulating globulin, angiotensinogen, to angiotensin I. Angiotensin converting enzyme, which is found in high concentrations in the pulmonary vasculature, then catalyzes the conversion of angiotensin I to angiotensin II. Angiotensin II interacts with cell membrane receptors in the zona glomerulosa of the adrenal cortex, initiating a series of changes which results in a stimulation of aldosterone secretion.

Blood pressure and plasma sodium concentrations are the major factors involved in the regulation of the renin-angiotensin system (Fig. 8.6). A decrease in pressure in the afferent arteriole of the kidney elicits an increase in renin release and ultimately in aldosterone secretion. The effects of aldosterone promote plasma volume expansion, thereby restoring blood pressure to normal. An increase in blood pressure, on the other hand, decreases renin and aldosterone secretion, resulting in a decline in blood pressure. Thus, the components of the renin-angiotensin system form a type of feedback loop which serves to prevent any large deviations from normal blood pressure.

The effects of sodium concentrations on the renin-angiotensin system are apparently mediated by the macula densa, a group of cells located at the distal tubule of the nephron. A decrease in tubular fluid sodium concentration elicits an increase in renin secretion whereas an increase in sodium levels inhibits renin secretion. In both cases, the resulting changes in aldosterone secretion return sodium concentrations to normal levels.

Plasma potassium concentrations also have a regulatory influence on adrenal secretion of aldosterone, but act independently of the renin-angiotensin system (Fig. 8.6). Changes in plasma potassium levels seem to have direct effects on the cells of the zona glomerulosa. An increase in plasma potassium stimulates aldosterone secretion, and a decrease inhibits aldosterone output. In each situation, the effect of aldosterone on renal potassium excretion results in restoration of plasma potassium levels to normal.

Receptors for ACTH have been demonstrated on zona glomerulosa cells and under certain circumstances, ACTH stimulates aldosterone secretion. However, the overall physiological role of ACTH in the regulation of aldosterone production is minor in comparison with the renin-angiotensin system and plasma potassium concentrations.

## Adrenal androgens

Large amounts of androgenic steroids are produced by the adrenal cortex, but because they are far less potent than the testicular hormone, testosterone, adrenal androgens are of little physiological significance in males. In females, by contrast, adrenal androgens such as DHEA and androstenedione represent a major source of androgenic steroids. Thus, adrenal androgens are needed for androgen-dependent processes in females, including the development of libido and growth of pubertal hair.

The secretion of adrenal androgens and cortisol generally parallel one another, suggesting that ACTH is the major regulator of adrenal androgen output. However, there are times when adrenal androgen secretion changes without concurrent changes in cortisol production. This occasional divergence had led some to postulate the existence of factors other than ACTH which are involved in the regulation of adrenal androgen secretion. However, at present, the existence and physiological significance of such factors remains unresolved.

## Toxicology

A survey of the literature done several years ago by Ribelin (1984) revealed that chemical induced lesions in endocrine organs most frequently involved the adrenal gland (Table 8.7). In fact, the adrenal gland and testes collectively accounted for 90% of the total number of publications identified. The preponderance of reports citing the adrenals involved lesions in the cortex of the gland. Although the relative organ frequencies of endocrine toxicities reported in the literature may have changed somewhat over the past few years, these data clearly identify the adrenal cortex as a major endocrine target for exogenous chemicals.

The review by Ribelin (1984) included a list of 50–60 compounds which had been reported to cause adrenocortical lesions. The substances indicated in Table 8.8 include a few of the more widely recognized adrenal toxins previously noted by Ribelin, but most represent additional compounds that have been found to alter adrenocortical structure and/or function. Only a single citation is provided for each, but for most, multiple reports have appeared in the literature. Still other adrenal toxins are identified in a recent review by Szabo & Lippe (1989). Collectively, these reports indicate that a wide range of substances can adversely affect the adrenal cortex. There is obviously great diversity in the chemical characteristics of the compounds delineated. Some cause both structural and functional lesions in the cortex; others cause morphological or functional changes, but not both. The latter may in some cases simply indicate that appropriate investigations have not been done. Certain adrenal toxins are species-specific in their actions, others seem to have similar effects in most species studied. For some compounds, information on species-specificity is not available because investigations have been limited to a single species. Factors affecting adrenal toxicity such as age, sex, nutritional, or endocrine status have been determined for relatively few substances, and as one might predict, the effects of such factors are highly variable.

Table 8.7. *Chemical induced endocrine lesions*
(by organ frequency)

1. Adrenal gland
2. Testis
3. Thyroid gland
4. Ovary
5. Pancreas
6. Pituitary gland
7. Parathyroid gland

(Based upon Ribelin, 1984.)

Table 8.8. *Compounds producing lesions in the adrenal cortex*

| | |
|---|---|
| Adriamycin | (Cuellar *et al.*, 1984) |
| Aminoglutethimide | (Dexter *et al.*, 1967) |
| 4-aminopyrazolo(3, 4-d)pyrimidine | (Almeida *et al.*, 1987) |
| Cadmium | (Nishiyama & Nakamura, 1984) |
| Carbon tetrachloride | (Brogan *et al.*, 1984) |
| Chloramphenicol | (Mazzocchi & Nussdorfer, 1985) |
| Chlordane | (Cranmer *et al.*, 1984) |
| Chloroform | (Hoerr, 1931) |
| Chlorphentermine | (Hartmann & Jentzen, 1979) |
| Chlorpromazine | (Chan & Hung, 1983) |
| Copper | (Veltman & Maines, 1986) |
| Cyclosporin | (Rebuffat *et al.*, 1989) |
| Cyproterone | (Panesar *et al.*, 1979) |
| *o,p'*-DDD | (Hart *et al.*, 1973) |
| Danazol | (Barbieri *et al.*, 1980) |
| Dichlorvos | (Civen *et al.*, 1980) |
| 7, 12-Dimethylbenzanthracene | (Huggins & Morii, 1961) |
| Etomidate | (Preziosi & Vacca, 1988) |
| 5-Fluorouracil | (Morgan & O'Hare, 1979) |
| Kepone | (Eroschenko & Wilson, 1975) |
| Ketoconazole | (Feldman, 1986) |
| Nicotine | (Barbieri *et al.*, 1987) |
| Phenobarbital | (Rivera-Calimlim *et al.*, 1978) |
| Polychlorinated biphenyls | (Inao, 1970) |
| Spironolactone | (Sherry *et al.*, 1986) |
| Tamoxifen | (Lullman & Lullman-Rauch, 1981) |
| TCDD | (DiBartolomeis *et al.*, 1987) |
| Tetrahydrocannabinol | (Warner *et al.*, 1977) |
| Toxaphene | (Mohammed *et al.*, 1985) |

For most of the adrenal toxins identified, mechanisms of action have not been clearly defined. Those that have been determined include some of the general mechanisms applicable to most toxic substances. Thus, for some compounds, covalent interactions with adrenal cellular macromolecules such as proteins have been identified as the basis for toxicity. For others, oxygen activation resulting in the formation of highly reactive oxygen species has been implicated. The latter may initiate peroxidation of adrenal membrane lipids, ultimately compromising membrane integrity and a host of membrane functions. Some compounds interfere with adrenocortical function by reversible interactions with steroidogenic enzymes, thereby decreasing hormone production. Several of the latter inhibitors of steroidogenesis had, in fact, been developed for clinical use in the differential diagnosis of adrenocortical dysfunction and/or treatment of hypersecretory conditions.

Adrenal toxins include both direct-acting compounds and those whose effects are mediated by metabolites. It is now widely recognized that the metabolism of drugs and other xenobiotics may result in the formation of products with greater biological activity than the parent compounds (Fig. 8.7). The production of active metabolites from inactive precursors, known as bioactivation, is involved in the beneficial (therapeutic) as well as the adverse effects of many chemicals. Highly reactive metabolites have been implicated in the adrenal toxicity of several compounds including carbon tetrachloride, the DDT derivative, o, p'-DDD, and the diuretic drug, spironolactone. For most adrenal toxins, the role of metabolites in mediating the adverse effects has not been determined. When toxic metabolites are involved, they are usually produced within their target tissues. Formation at peripheral sites and subsequent transport to the target tissues rarely occur because of the high reactivity and short half-lives characteristic of most toxic metabolites. Thus, local metabolism in target tissues plays a major role in the mechanisms of action of those toxins requiring bioactivation, and the presence of unique metabolic pathways within certain organs probably contributes to the organ-specific effects of many toxic chemicals.

There probably are numerous factors which contribute to the high vulnerability of the adrenal cortex to exogenous chemicals. As a result of the multiple levels of regulation of adrenocortical function, there are many potential sites of action at which chemicals can interfere with adrenal homeostasis. Effects of chemicals on the brain or pituitary gland to alter ACTH secretion will, of course, change the rate of adrenal glucocorticoid and androgen secretion. Similarly, substances affecting the renin-angiotensin system may have selective effects on mineralocorticoid production. Chemicals may also interfere with adrenocortical function by

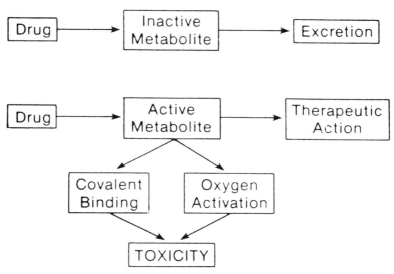

Fig. 8.7. Metabolic fate of drugs and other foreign compounds in the body.

acting directly at the level of the adrenal gland. The response of the adrenal to ACTH, for example, may be compromised by chemical effects on membrane receptors, cyclic nucleotide levels, protein synthesis, and other processes required for the stimulation of steroidogenesis. Foreign compounds may also influence plasma levels of adrenal hormones via effects on hepatic steroid metabolism or on the synthesis of plasma-binding proteins. Finally, chemicals may have direct effects on target tissues, interfering with or enhancing the actions of adrenal steroids.

Other characteristics of the adrenal cortex may further contribute to its vulnerability (Table 8.9). The excellent blood supply to the gland assures delivery of potentially toxic foreign compounds that enter the circulation. Most xenobiotics that enter the body are relatively insoluble in water and the hydrophobic nature of the adrenal cortex, resulting from its high lipid content, promotes the deposition and accumulation of various lipophilic substances including toxins. In addition, the potential for bioactivation of foreign compounds, effecting the formation of toxic metabolites, appears to be greater for the adrenal cortex than for other endocrine organs (Colby & Rumbaugh, 1980; Hallberg, 1990). The enzyme systems most commonly involved in bioactivation reactions are the cytochrome P-450-containing monooxygenases, the same types of enzymes that catalyze steroid hydroxylation reactions in the adrenal. Until recent years, adrenal cytochrome P-450 isozymes were thought to participate in steroid metab-

Table 8.9. *Factors affecting adrenocortical vulnerability to chemicals*

1. Blood supply
2. Lipophilic nature of gland
3. Bioactivation processes
4. Steroidogenesis-related production of reactive oxygen species
5. Potential for lipid peroxidation

olism only, and not to catalyze the metabolism of xenobiotics. However, it is now apparent that adrenal monooxygenases can effect the metabolism of a wide variety of foreign compounds, in some cases producing toxic products.

The mechanism of action of the adrenal steroid hydroxylases may also enhance the potential for local toxicity (Hall, 1986; Hornsby, 1989). The catalytic cycle for these cytochrome P-450-dependent enzymes involves oxygen activation as an obligatory intermediate step. Consequently, reactive oxygen species such as the superoxide anion are produced which may escape from the enzyme site and cause oxidative damage. Among the adverse effects of oxygen radicals is the initiation of lipid peroxidation, a process which as discussed previously, can have various toxic manifestations. Adrenocortical membranes seem particularly susceptible to peroxidative damage probably, at least in part, because of their high content of unsaturated fatty acids, substrates for lipid peroxidation. The high concentrations of antioxidants, especially ascorbic acid and α-tocopherol, normally found in adrenocortical cells may serve to protect against the oxidative stress created by normal physiological processes such as steroidogenesis. However the superimposition of exogenous oxidants or oxidant-generating substances may overwhelm the protective mechanisms and cause overt adrenal injury.

To provide specific examples of the actions and mechanisms of actions of adrenal toxins, the remainder of this chapter will focus on two compounds, the diuretic drug, spironolactone, and carbon tetrachloride. The studies described will serve to illustrate some of the more common experimental approaches employed to determine the sites and mechanisms of action of adrenal toxins as well as some of the problems unique to a complex endocrine organ such as the adrenal cortex. Although the discussion is limited to these two compounds, some of the observations are generally applicable to other adrenal toxins as well.

## Spironolactone-induced adrenocortical dysfunction

Spironolactone (SL) is an aldosterone antagonist that is used clinically in the treatment of edematous states, essential hypertension, and primary aldosteronism (Saunders & Alberti, 1978). The drug acts in the kidney by competitively inhibiting the binding of aldosterone to mineralocorticoid receptors, resulting in natriuresis, diuresis, and potassium retention. The results of some investigations suggest that part of the antimineralocorticoid action of SL is attributable to direct effects on the adrenal cortex (see Sherry *et al.*, 1986), inhibiting aldosterone production. In addition, diminished cortisol and/or testosterone secretion after treatment of patients with SL has been reported. Other clinical studies found changes in the pattern of corticosteroid secretion during SL treatment suggesting inhibition of some adrenal enzymes (Tuck *et al.*, 1981).

As a result of the studies indicating inhibitory effects of SL on adrenal and testicular hormone production, the mechanism of action of SL on steroid synthesis and secretion has been investigated. Owing to the importance of the cytochrome P-450-dependent steroid hydroxylation reactions for hormone synthesis, effects of SL treatment on the activities of these enzymes were evaluated. The results of several studies indicated that the administration of SL to experimental animals decreased cytochrome P-450 content in the adrenal cortex and testes, and consequently decreased the activities of cytochrome P-450-dependent steroid hydroxylases (Menard *et al.*, 1975; Greiner *et al.*, 1978). Other investigations demonstrated that the actions of SL to decrease cytochrome P-450 concentrations were apparently limited to steroidogenic organs since P-450 levels in liver and kidneys, for example, were not diminished by drug treatment *in vivo*.

To determine if SL acted directly on the adrenal cortex to inhibit steroidogenesis or if indirect effects involving other organs might be responsible, a number of *in vitro* investigations were done. Studies with intact adrenocortical cells were done to evaluate the direct effects of SL on steroid hormone synthesis from endogenous precursors (Fig. 8.8). Cells were preincubated with SL for varying lengths of time and cortisol secretion in response to ACTH stimulation was then measured. Preincubation with SL caused time-dependent decreases in cortisol secretion as well as in cellular cytochrome P-450 concentrations. In the absence of preincubation, SL had no effects on cortisol output, suggesting that metabolism was required for the inhibitory effects of SL. When the cytochrome P-450 inhibitor, SU-10'603, was included with SL during the preincubation period, the effects of SL on cortisol secretion were prevented (Fig. 8.9). The latter results, and those with various other P-450 inhibitors, implicate a cytochrome P-450 enzyme in the activation pathway for SL. Thus, cytochrome P-450 apparently participates in the conversion of SL to a toxic metabolite and is also a target for the metabolite.

Numerous studies with adrenal subcellular fractions localized the site

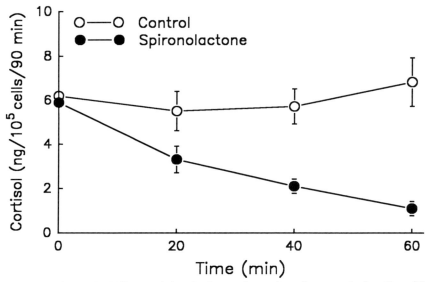

Fig. 8.8. Effects of incubating guinea-pig adrenocortical cells with spironolactone for varying lengths of time on subsequent cortisol secretion in response to ACTH (adrenocorticotrophin) stimulation.

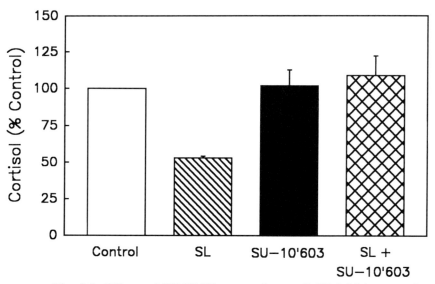

Fig. 8.9. Effects of SU-10′603, a cytochrome P-450 inhibitor, on the inhibition of cortisol production by spironolactone (SL) in guinea-pig adrenocortical cells.

Table 8.10. *Effects of incubating guinea-pig adrenal microsomes with spironolactone (SL) and/or NADPH on cytochromes P-450 and b$_5$ concentrations and steroidogenic enzyme activities*[a]

| | Incubation conditions | | | |
| --- | --- | --- | --- | --- |
| | Control | SL | NADPH | SL + NADPH |
| Cytochrome P-450 | 100 | 98 ± 7 | 102 ± 8 | 65 ± 5[b] |
| Cytochrome b$_5$ | 100 | 96 ± 4 | 96 ± 5 | 98 ± 6 |
| 17α-Hydroxylase | 100 | 95 ± 7 | 99 ± 6 | 38 ± 3[b] |
| 21-Hydroxylase | 100 | 103 ± 6 | 97 ± 5 | 93 ± 6 |

[a] Values expressed as mean % ± SE of corresponding control.
[b] $P<0.05$ (vs. corresponding control).

of SL activation to the microsomes. The data presented in Table 8.10 are indicative of the types of experiments done and the results obtained. Microsomal preparations from guinea pig adrenal cortices were incubated with SL in the absence or presence of NADPH and effects on cytochrome P-450 and steroid metabolism then determined. NADPH was included to promote SL metabolism and thereby evaluate the possible involvement of a metabolite in the actions of SL. As indicated in Table 8.10, incubation with SL plus NADPH effected a loss of cytochrome P-450 and decline in steroid 17α-hydroxylase activity. In the absence of NADPH, SL had no effect on any of the parameters measured. The need for NADPH to demonstrate the effects of SL further suggested that bioactivation of SL was required for the destruction of cytochrome P-450.

The apparent importance of local metabolism (activation) in the actions of SL on adrenal function led to investigations on the metabolic fate of SL in the adrenal cortex. Several of the proposed early steps in the overall metabolic pathway for SL are shown in Fig. 8.10. Of particular interest was the deacetylated derivative of SL, 7α-thio-SL, which like SL, catalyzed the degradation of adrenal cytochrome P-450, and in fact, was far more potent than SL (see Sherry *et al.*, 1986). However, 7α-thio-SL had never been definitively established as a tissue metabolite of SL; its formation was inferred on the basis of the structures of several urinary metabolites of SL.

Initial investigations on the tissue metabolism of SL were done with adrenocortical and hepatic microsomal preparations (Sherry *et al.*, 1986). The purpose of these comparative studies was to determine if differences in SL metabolism could account for the destruction of cytochrome P-450 in one organ (adrenal) but not the other (liver). The results of these studies revealed that in the absence of NADPH, both adrenal and hepatic

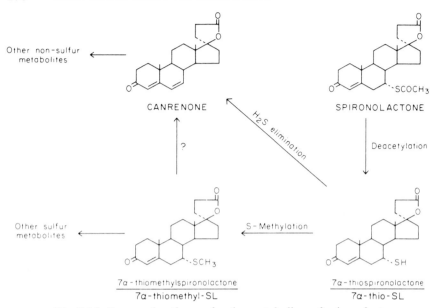

Fig. 8.10. Proposed pathways for the metabolism of spironolactone.

microsomal preparations converted SL to 7α-thio-SL as the only metabolite. This reaction is apparently catalyzed by non-specific tissue esterases, since esterase inhibitors block 7α-thio-SL formation.

In the presence of NADPH, conditions which cause the degradation of adrenal but not hepatic cytochrome P-450 (Sherry *et al.*, 1986), had no effect on hepatic SL metabolism but stimulated adrenal metabolism of SL. Very little 7α-thio-SL was recovered from the adrenal incubations, suggesting that the 7α-thio-SL was further metabolized by NADPH-dependent enzymes. The latter hypothesis was confirmed by incubating microsomal preparations with 7α-thio-SL as the substrate. 7α-Thio-SL was rapidly metabolized by adrenal but not by hepatic preparations. Under the same incubation conditions, there was rapid destruction of adrenal but not hepatic microsomal cytochrome(s) P-450, suggesting that the 7α-thio-SL was an obligatory intermediate in the degradation of adrenal cytochrome(s) P-450 by SL.

If the latter hypothesis were correct, blocking 7α-thio-SL production by inhibiting the deacetylation reaction should block the effect of SL on cytochrome P-450. A number of esterase inhibitors were tested and diethyl p-nitrophenyl phosphate (DPNP) was found to be the most potent inhibitor of SL deacetylation. A series of experiments was then done to assess the effects of DPNP on cytochrome P-450 degradation by SL. The

Table 8.11. *Effects of the esterase inhibitor DPNP on spironolactone (SL)- and 7α-thio-SL-mediated destruction of cytochromes P-450 in adrenal microsomes*

| Incubation conditions | Cytochromes P-450 concentration (% of control) |
|---|---|
| NADPH | 100 |
| NADPH + DPNP | 95.2 ± 1.9 |
| NADPH + SL | 74.5 ± 2.3[a] |
| NADPH + SL + DPNP | 92.8 ± 1.8 |
| NADPH + 7α-thio-SL | 47.0 ± 1.2[a] |
| NADPH + 7α-thio-SL + DPNP | 46.8 ± 1.5[a] |

[a] $p < 0.05$ (vs. NADPH alone).
(From Sherry *et al.*, 1986).

results are summarized in Table 8.11. Spironolactone, in the presence of NADPH, caused significant destruction of adrenal microsomal cytochrome P-450, as expected. When the esterase inhibitor was included in the incubation medium, the destruction of P-450 was prevented. However, when the deacetylation step was bypassed and incubations were done with 7α-thio-SL as substrate, the esterase inhibitor had no effect on the destruction of cytochrome P-450. The results proved that 7α-thio-SL was an obligatory intermediate in the actions of SL on adrenal cytochromes P-450 and indicated that the further NADPH-dependent metabolism of 7α-thio-SL was required for cytochrome P-450 destruction. It is likely that adrenal metabolism of 7α-thio-SL results in the production of a reactive metabolite which is responsible for the degradation of cytochrome(s) P-450 and decreases in steroidogenic enzyme activities. Further investigation is still needed to identify the reactive metabolite(s) produced, the enzymology involved in the production of the toxic metabolite(s), and the mechanism of cytochrome P-450 degradation by the metabolite.

## Carbon tetrachloride-induced adrenocortical toxicity

Another example of an adrenal toxin that requires metabolic activation is carbon tetrachloride ($CCl_4$). It has long been recognized that $CCl_4$ causes necrosis. In addition, zonal differences in detoxication pathways might similarly influence the extent of $CCl_4$ toxicity in various parts of the to $CCl_4$ also effects the degradation of adrenal microsomal cytochromes P-450, causing decreases in monooxygenase activities (Brogan *et al.*, 1984). Recent investigations indicate that adrenal metabolism plays an

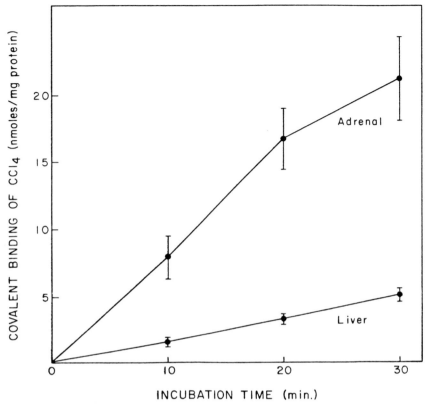

Fig. 8.11. Covalent binding of radioactivity to microsomal protein following the incubation of guinea-pig adrenal or hepatic microsomes with
$^{14}$C-carbon tetrachloride plus NADPH. (Brogan *et al.*, 1984.)

important part in the local toxicity of $CCl_4$. In experiments analogous to
those described above for spironolactone, incubation of guinea pig
adrenal microsomes with $CCl_4$ in the presence of NADPH was found to
result in the formation of reactive metabolites which initiated lipid peroxidation and bound covalently to adrenal microsomal protein (Fig.
8.11). The same incubation conditions caused destruction of cytochromes
P-450 (Brogan, Hinton & Colby, 1984), presumably mediated by the
reactive metabolite(s) produced. The results were similar to those
obtained previously with liver microsomes in studies addressing the
hepatotoxicity of $CCl_4$ (Recknagel *et al.*, 1989). In guinea-pigs, the rate of
activation of $CCl_4$ as indicated by covalent binding, was far greater with
adrenal than with hepatic microsomal preparations (Fig. 8.11). Although

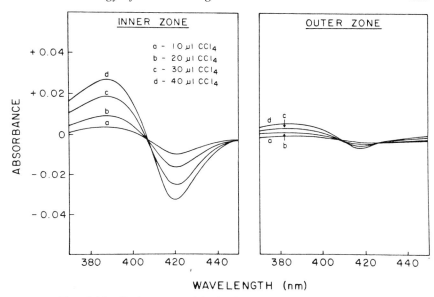

Fig. 8.12. Carbon tetrachloride-induced type I spectral changes in guinea-pig adrenocortical inner and outer zone microsomal preparations. (Brogan *et al.*, 1984.)

there are species differences in the relative rates of xenobiotic metabolism to toxic products by different organs, these observations further illustrate the potential for adrenal activation of foreign chemicals.

Since metabolic activation seemed to be required for the toxicity of $CCl_4$ it was assumed that the regional differences in $CCl_4$-induced adrenal necrosis were the result of differences in $CCl_4$ metabolism in different parts of the gland. However, differences in the intraadrenal distribution of $CCl_4$ *in vivo* might also have contributed to the localization of the necrosis. In addition, zonal differences in detoxication pathways might similarly influence the extent of $CCl_4$ toxicity in various parts of the adrenal gland. Therefore, studies were done in which guinea pig adrenal cortices were dissected into the chromatically distinct inner (zona reticularis) and outer (zona fasciculata plus zona glomerulosa) zones, and the activation of $CCl_4$ was evaluated using microsomes obtained from each zone. Direct addition of $CCl_4$ to the microsomal preparations produced typical type I spectral changes (Fig. 8.12), indicative of substrate binding to cytochrome P-450, an essential step in the metabolic activation of $CCl_4$ (Recknagel *et al.*, 1989). The magnitude of the $CCl_4$-induced spectrum was far greater in microsomes from the inner adrenal zone (Fig. 8.12), suggesting a higher concentration of the P-450 isozyme(s) involved in

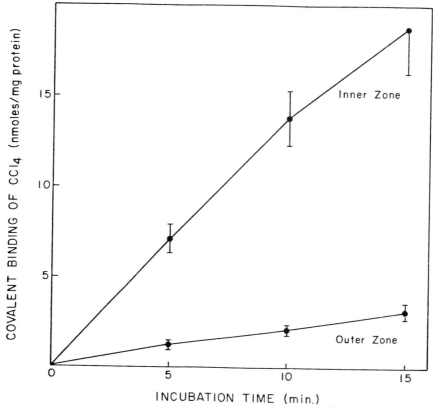

Fig. 8.13. Covalent binding of radioactivity to microsomal protein following the incubation of guinea-pig adrenal inner and outer zone microsomes with $^{14}$C-carbon tetrachloride plus NADPH. (Brogan et al.,
1984.)

CCl$_4$ metabolism in that zone. In addition, inner zone microsomes in the
presence of NADPH, catalyzed the conversion of CCl$_4$ to a metabolite(s)
that became covalently bound to the microsomal protein (Fig. 8.13). By
contrast, outer zone microsomes catalyzed very little binding. These
results support the hypothesis that regional differences in adrenal CCl$_4$
metabolism (activation) are responsible for the pattern of necrosis seen in
the gland.

## Summary and conclusions

As indicated previously in this chapter, the capacity for metabolic activation of xenobiotics contributes to the vulnerability of the adrenal gland to

chemical-induced toxicities. The studies described for spironolactone and carbon tetrachloride serve to illustrate this point. The actions of some other adrenal toxins are also known to be mediated by reactive metabolites, but for most chemicals that adversely affect the adrenal cortex, relatively little is known about their mechanisms of action. Differences in metabolic capabilities are known to account for organ-specific toxicities of some chemicals and, as described for carbon tetrachloride, may also explain region-specific toxicities within the adrenal gland. The role of metabolic activation in adrenal toxicities may be particularly important in the human foetus. Adrenal cortical xenobiotic-metabolizing activities are far greater in the foetus than in the adult (Juchau & Pedersen, 1973) and, in addition, foetal adrenals are proportionately much larger than adult glands. Thus, the production of reactive metabolites by various foetal tissues, including the adrenal cortex, may contribute to the sensitivity of the foetus to the toxic effects of many chemicals.

Although a large number of substances have been found to cause adrenal toxicities, there is little information available concerning the factors affecting the actions of adrenal toxins. For example, there is a paucity of information in the literature on the influence of physiological variables such as age, sex, and hormonal factors on chemical-induced adrenal lesions. In addition, although enzymatic activation of some adrenal toxins has been investigated, the roles of adrenal detoxification processes and other intra-adrenal protective mechanisms have received little attention. Studies in other organs have demonstrated the importance of the balance between activating and detoxifying pathways in controlling chemical toxicity. Pursuit of these and related areas should provide fruitful investigation and contribute to a fuller understanding of adrenal toxicology than is presently available.

## References

Almeida, H., Magalhaes, M. & Magalhaes, M.C. (1987). Nucleolar alterations induced by 4-aminopyrazolo(3,4-*d*)pyrimidine in adrenal cortex and liver cells of rats. *Cell and Tissue Research*, **248**, 231–4.

Ambrosio, S. & Mahy, N. (1989). Acute peripheral catecholaminergic changes in rat after MPTP and MPP$^+$ treatment. *Revista Española de Fisiologia*, **45**, 157–61.

Anderson, T.D. & Hayes, T.J. (1989). Toxicity of human recombinant interleukin-2 in rats. *Laboratory Investigation*, **60**, 331–46.

Baggett, J.McC., Thureson-Klein, Å. & Klein, R.L. (1980). Effects of chlordecone on the adrenal medulla of the rat. *Toxicology and Applied Pharmacology*, **52**, 313–22.

Barbeau, A., Dallaire, L., Buu, N.T., Poirier, J. & Rucinska, E. (1985).

Comparative behavioral, biochemical and pigmentary effects of MPTP, MPP$^+$ and paraquat in rana pipiens. *Life Sciences*, **37**, 1529–38.

Barbieri, R.L., Osathanondh, R., Canick, J.A., Stillman, R.J. & Ryan, K.J. (1980). Danazol inhibits human adrenal 21- and 11β-hydroxylation *in vitro*. *Steroids*, **35**, 251–63.

Barbieri, R.L., York, C.M., Cherry, M.L. & Ryan, K.J. (1987). The effects of nicotine, cotinine and anabasine on rat adrenal 11β-hydroxylase and 21-hydroxylase. *Journal of Biochemistry*, **28**, 25–8.

Boelsterli, U.A., Cruz-Orive, L-M. & Zbinden, G. (1984). Morphometric and biochemical analysis of adrenal medullary hyperplasia induced by nicotine in rats. *Archives of Toxicology*, **56**, 113–16.

Boelsterli, U.A. & Zbinden, G. (1985). Early biochemical and morphological changes of the rat adrenal medulla induced by xylitol. *Archives of Toxicology*, **57**, 25–30.

Brogan, W.C., Hinton, D.E. & Colby, H.D. (1984). Effects of carbon tetrachloride on adrenocortical structure and function in guinea pigs. *Toxicology and Applied Pharmacology*, **75**, 188–227.

Chan, M.Y. & Hung, F. (1983). A study on the effects of desipramine on rat adrenal steroidogenesis and cholesterol esterase activity. *Biochemical Pharmacology*, **32**, 1713–15.

Chowdhury, A.R., Deshmukh, M.B., Nashikkar, A.B., Raghuveeran, C.D. & Chatterjee, A.K. (1978). Cellular changes of adrenal under the acute stress of O-chlorobenzylidene malonitrile (CS). *Experientia*, **34**, 494–5.

Civen, M., Leeb, J.E., Wishnow, R.M., Wolfsen, A. & Morin, R.J. (1980). Effects of low level administration of dichlorvos on adrenocorticotrophic hormone secretion, adrenal cholesteryl ester and steroid metabolism. *Biochemical Pharmacology*, **29**, 636–41.

Colby, H.D. (1987a). The adrenal medulla. In *Clinical Endocrine Physiology*, ed. G.A. Hedge, H.D. Colby & R.L. Goodman, pp. 297–315. Philadelphia: W. B. Saunders.

Colby, H.D. (1987b). The adrenal cortex. In *Clinical Endocrine Physiology*, ed. G.A. Hedge, H.D. Colby & R.L. Goodman, pp. 127–59. Philadelphia: W.B. Saunders.

Colby, H.D. & Rumbaugh, R.C. (1980). Adrenal drug metabolism. In *Extrahepatic Metabolism of Drugs and Other Foreign Compounds*, ed T.E. Gram, pp. 239–66. New York: Spectrum Publications.

Cranmer, J.M., Cranmer, M.F. & Goad, P.T. (1984). Prenatal chlordane exposure: effects on plasma corticosterone concentrations over the lifespan of mice. *Environmental Research*, **35**, 204–10.

Cuellar, A., Escamilla, E., Ramirez, J. & Chavez, E. (1984). Adriamycin as an inhibitor of 11β-hydroxylase activity in adrenal cortex mitochondria. *Archives of Biochemistry and Biophysics*, **235**, 538–43.

Dexter, R.N., Fishman, L.M., Ney, R.L., Ney, R.L. & Liddle, G.W. (1967). Inhibition of corticosteroid synthesis by aminoglutethimide.

Studies of the mechanism of action. *Journal of Clinical Endocrinology and Metabolism*, **27**, 473–80.

DiBartolomeis, M.J., Moore, R.W., Peterson, R.E., Christian, B.J. & Jefcoate, C.R. (1987). Altered regulation of adrenal steroidogenesis in 2,3,7,8-tetrachlorodibenzo-*p*-dioxin-treated rats. *Biochemical Pharmacology*, **36**, 59–67.

Emorine, L.T., Marullo, S., Briend-Sutren, M.-M., Patey, G., Tate, K., Delavier-Klutchko, C. & Strosberg, A.D. (1989). Molecular characterization of the human $\beta_3$-adrenergic receptor. *Science*, **245**, 1118–21.

Eränkö, O. (1955). Nodular hyperplasia and increase of noradrenaline content in the adrenal medulla of nicotine-treated rats. *Acta Pathologica et Microbiologica Scandinavica*, **36**, 210–18.

Evans, H.M., Simpson, M.E. & Li, C.H. (1948). The gigantism produced in normal rats by injection of the pituitary growth hormone. I. Body growth and organ changes. *Growth*, **12**, 15–32.

Eroschenko, V.P. & Wilson, W.O. (1975). Cellular changes in the gonads, livers and adrenal glands of Japanese quail as affected by the insecticide Kepone. *Toxicology and Applied Pharmacology*, **31**, 491–504.

Feldman, D. (1986). Ketoconazole and other imidazole derivatives as inhibitors of steroidogenesis. *Endocrine Reviews*, **7**, 409–20.

Gowda, H., Uppal, R.P. & Garg, B.D. (1975). Effect of malathion on adrenal activity, liver glycogen and blood glucose in rats. *Indian Journal of Medical Research*, **63**, 126–9.

Grasso, R. (1963). Estudios citologicos y hisoquimicos en ratas albinas tratadas con la aloxana. *Archivos de Histologia Normal y Patologica*, **8**, 97–159.

Greiner, J.W., Rumbaugh, R.C., Kramer, R.E. & Colby, H.D. (1978). Relation of canrenone to the actions of spironolactone on adrenal cytochrome P-450-dependent enzymes. *Endocrinology*, **103**, 1313–20.

Hall, P.F. (1986). Cytochromes P-450 and the regulation of steroid synthesis. *Steroids*, **48**, 131–96.

Hallberg, E. (1990). Metabolism and toxicity of xenobiotics in the adrenal cortex, with particular reference to 7, 12-dimethylbenz-(a)anthracene. *Journal of Biochemical Toxicology*, **5**, 71–90.

Harris, C. (1968). The role of the adrenal in toxicity in rats caused by dimethylbenzanthracene. *Cancer Research*, **28**, 764–9.

Hart, M.M., Reagan, R.L. & Adamson, R.H. (1973). The effect of isomers of DDD on the ACTH-induced steroid output, histology and ultrastructure of the dog adrenal cortex. *Toxicology and Applied Pharmacology*, **24**, 101–13.

Hartmann, F. & Jentzen, F. (1979). Effect of Chlorphentermine on hormone content and function of the adrenal cortex in rats. *Hormone and Metabolic Research*, **11**, 158–60.

Hexum, T.D. & Russett, L.R. (1987). Plasma enkephalin-like peptide response to chronic nicotine infusion in guinea pig. *Brain Research*, **406**, 370–2.

Hoerr, N. (1931). The cells of the suprarenal cortex in the guinea pig. Their reaction to injury and their replacement. *American Journal of Anatomy*, **48**, 139–97.

Hopsu, V. (1960). Effects of experimental alterations of the thyroid function on the adrenal medulla of the mouse. *Acta Endocrinologica Supplementum*, **48**, 1–87.

Hornsby, P.J. (1989). Steroid and xenobiotic effects on the adrenal cortex: mediation by oxidative and other mechanisms. *Free Radical Biology and Medicine*, **6**, 103–15.

Huggins, C. & Morii, S. (1961). Selective adrenal necrosis and apoplexy induced by 7,12-dimethylbenz(a)anthracene. *Journal of Experimental Medicine*, **114**, 741.

Inao, S. (1970). Adrenocortical insufficiency induced in rats by prolonged feeding of kanechlor (Chlorobiphenyl). *Kumamoto Medical Journal*, **23**, 27–31.

Johannesson, J.N., Chieuh, C.C., Herkenham, M.A., Markey, S.P., Burne, R.S., Adams, J.D. & Schuller, H.M. (1986). Relationship of the *in vivo* metabolism of MPTP to toxicity. In *MPTP: A Neurotoxin Producing a Parkinsonian Syndrome*, ed. S.P. Markey, N. Castagnoli, Jr, A.J. Trevor & I.J. Kopin, pp. 173–89. New York: Academic Press.

Juchau, M.R. & Pedersen, M.G. (1973). Drug biotransformation reactions in the human fetal adrenal gland. *Life Sciences*, **12**, 193–204.

Kurokawa, Y., Hayashi, Y., Maekawa, A., Takahashi, M. & Kukubo, T. (1985). High incidences of pheochromocytomas after long-term administration of retinol acetate to F344/DuCrj rats. *Journal of the National Cancer Institute*, **74**, 715–23.

Landsberg, L. & Young, J.B. (1980). Catecholamines and the adrenal medulla. In *Metabolic Control and Disease*, 8th edn, ed. P.K. Bondy & L.E. Rosenberg, pp. 1621–93. Philadelphia: W.B. Saunders Company.

Langston, J.W., Irwin, I., Langston, E.B. & Forno, L.S. (1987). 1-methyl-4-phenylpyridinium ion (MPP+): identification of as metabolite of MPTP, a toxin selective to the substantia nigra. *Neuroscience Letters*, **48**, 87–92.

Lullman, H. & Lullman-Rauch, R. (1981). Tamoxifen-induced generalized lipidosis in rats subchronically treated with high doses. *Toxicology and Applied Pharmacology*, **61**, 138–46.

Marine, D. & Baumann, E.J. (1945). Hypertrophy of adrenal medulla of white rats in chronic thiouracil poisoning. *American Journal of Physiology*, **144**, 69–73.

Marzotko, D. & Pankow, D. (1987). Effect of single dichloromethanehane administration on the adrenal medulla of male albino rats. *Acta Histochemica (Jena)*, **82**, 177–83.

Mazzocchi, G. & Nussdorfer, G.G. (1985). Effects of chloramphenicol on the long term trophic action of ACTH on rat adrenocortical cells: a combined stereological and enzymological study. *Journal of Anatomy*, **140**, 607–12.

McComb, D.J., Kovacs, K., Horner, H.C., Gallagher, G.T., Schwedes, U., Usadel, K.H. & Szabo, S. (1981). Cysteamine-induced adrenocortical necrosis in rats. *Experimental and Molecular Pathology*, **35**, 422–34.

Menard, R.H., Martin, H.F., Stripp, B., Gillette, J.R. & Bartter, F.C. (1975). Spironolactone and cytochrome P-450: impairment of steroid hydroxylation in the adrenal cortex. *Life Sciences*, **15**, 1639–48.

Mohammed, A., Hallberg, E., Rydstrom, J. & Slanina (1985). Toxaphene: accumulation in the adrenal cortex and effect on ACTH-stimulated corticosteroid synthesis in the rat. *Toxicology Letters*, **24**, 137–43.

Moon, H.D., Simpson, M.E., Li, C.H. & Evans, H.M. (1950). Neoplasms in rats treated with pituitary growth hormone. II. Adrenal glands. *Cancer Research*, **10**, 364–70.

Morgan, M.W.E. & O'Hare, M.J. (1979). Cytotoxic drugs and the human adrenal cortex. *Cancer*, **43**, 969–79.

Neafsey, E.J., Hurley-Giue, K., Cheng, B.Y., Ung-Chhun, N., Pronger, D.A. & Colline, M.A. (1986). Comparison of the effects of MPTP and an endogenous analog, n-methyl-tetrahydro-beta-carboline, on brain and adrenal monoamines and brain monoamine metabolites in the owl monkey. In *MPTP: A Neurotoxin Producing a Parkinsonian Syndrome*, ed. S.P. Markey, N. Castagnoli, Jr, A.J. Trevor & I.J. Kopin, pp. 495–501. New York: Academic Press.

Nishiyama, S. & Nakamura, K. (1984). Effect of cadmium on plasma aldosterone and serum corticosterone concentrations in male rats. *Toxicology and Applied Pharmacology*, **76**, 420–5.

Panesar, N.S., Herries, D.G. & Stitch, S.R. (1979). Effects of cyproterone and cyproterone acetate on the adrenal gland in the rat: Studies *in vivo* and *in vitro*. *Journal of Endocrinology*, **80**, 299–338.

Preziosi, P. & Vacca, M. (1988). Adrenocortical suppression and other endocrine effects of etomidate. *Life Sciences*, **42**, 477–89.

Rebuffat, P., Kasprzak, A.A., Andreis, P.G. Mazzochi, G., Gottardo, G., Coi, A. & Nussdorfer, G. (1989). Effects of prolonged cyclosporin-A treatment on the morphology and function of rat adrenal cortex. *Endocrinology*, **125**, 1407–13.

Recknagel, R.O., Glende, E.A., Dolak, J.A. & Waller, R.L. (1989). Mechanisms of carbon tetrachloride toxicity. *Pharmacology and Therapeutics*, **43**, 139–54.

Reinhard, J.F. Jr, Dilberto, E.M. Jr, Viveros, O.H. & Daniels, A.J. (1987). Subcellular compartmentalization of 1-methyl-4-phenylpyridinium with catecholamines in adrenal medullary chromaffin vesicles may explain the lack of toxicity to adrenal chromaffin cells. *Proceedings of the National Academy of Sciences (USA)*, **84**, 8160–4.

Ribelin, W.E. (1984). Effects of drugs and chemicals upon the structure of the adrenal gland. *Fundamental and Applied Toxicology*, **4**, 105–19.

Rivera-Calimlim, L., Bosmann, H.B., Penney, D.P. & Karch, F.E. (1978). Biochemical, morphologic and physiologic changes in the adrenal glands of rats chronically treated with phenobarbital. *Research Communications in Chemical Pathology and Pharmacology*, **21**, 1–14.

Roe, F.J.C. & Bär, A. (1985). Enzootic and epizootic adrenal medullary proliferative disease of rats: influence of dietary factors which affect calcium absorption. *Human Toxicology*, **4**, 27–52.

Salsburg, D. (1980). The effects of lifetime feeding studies on patterns of senile lesions in rats and mice. *Drug and Chemical Toxicology*, **3**, 1–33.

Saunders, F.J. & Alberti, R.L. (1978). *Aldactone (Spironolactone): A Comprehensive Review*. New York: Searle, Inc.

Sherry, J.H., Flowers, L., O'Donnell, J.P., LaCagnin, L.B. & Colby, H.D. (1986). Metabolism of spironolactone by adrenocortical and hepatic microsomes: Relationship to cytochrome P-450 destruction. *Journal of Pharmacology and Experimental Therapeutics*, **236**, 675–83.

Simpson, M.E., Evans, H.M. & Li, C.H. (1949). The growth of hypophysectomized female rats following chronic treatment with pure pituitary growth hormone. I. General growth and organ changes. *Growth*, **13**, 151–70.

Szabo, S., Hütter, I., Kovacs, K., Horvath, E., Szabo, D. & Horner, H.C. (1980). Pathogenesis of experimental adrenal hemorrhagic necrosis ('apoplexy'). Ultrastructural, biochemical, neuropharmacologic, and blood coagulation studies with acrylonitrile in the rat. *Laboratory Investigation*, **42**, 533–46.

Szabo, S. & Lippe, I.Th. (1989). Adrenal gland: chemically induced structural and functional changes in the cortex. *Toxicologic Pathology*, **17**, 317–29.

Szabo, S., McComb, D.J., Kovacs, K. & Hütter, I. (1981). Adrenocortical hemorrhagic necrosis. *Archives of Pathology and Laboratory Medicine*, **105**, 536–9.

Thompson, S.W., Rac, V.S., Semonick, D.E., Antonchak, B., Spaet, R.H. & Schellhammer, L.E., Jr (eds) (1981). *The Adrenal Medulla of Rats. Comparative Physiology, Histology, Pathology*. Illinois: Charles C. Thomas.

Tischler, A.S. (1989). The rat adrenal medulla. *Toxicologic Pathology*, **17**, 330–2.

Tischler, A.S. & DeLellis, R.A. (1988). The rat adrenal medulla. II. Proliferative lesions. *Journal of American College of Toxicology*, **7**, 23–44.

Tuck, M.L., Sowers, J.R., Fittingoff, D.B., Fisher, J.S., Berg, G.J., Asp, N.D. & Mayes, D.M. (1981). Plasma corticosteroid concentrations during spironolactone administration: Evidence for adrenal biosynthetic blockade in man. *Journal of Clinical Endocrinology and Metabolism*, **52**, 1057–61.

United States Department of Health, Education, and Welfare (1978). *Bioassay of 1,1,2-trichloroethane for possible carcinogenicity.* DHEW Publication No. (NIH) 78-1324.

United States Department of Health and Human Resources (1982). *Third Annual Report on Carcinogens. Reserpine.* pp. 257.

Veltman, J.C. & Maines, M.D. (1986). Regulatory effect of copper on rat adrenal cytochrome P-450 and steroid metabolism. *Biochemical Pharmacology*, **35**, 2903–9.

Warner, W., Harris, L.S. & Carchman, R.A. (1977). Inhibition of corticosteroidogenesis by delta-9-tetrahydrocannabinol. *Endocrinology*, **101**, 1815–20.

Zaagsma, J. & Nahorski, S.R. (1990). Is the adipocyte β-adrenoceptor a prototype for the recently cloned atypical $\beta_3$-adrenoceptor? *Trends in Pharmacological Sciences*, **11**, 3–7.

# V  *Reproductive toxicology*

D.A. GARSIDE AND P.W. HARVEY

# 9 Endocrine toxicology of the male reproductive system

## Introduction

This chapter deals with the fundamentals of male reproductive endocrinology and toxicity. The general anatomy and physiology of the male reproductive system is reviewed, together with the toxicology of the testes (the most common target organ within the male reproductive system). The adult reproductive system will be the focus of attention (see Nalbandov, 1976 for information concerning endocrine control in the prepubertal male).

### The anatomy of the testis

The testis is surrounded by a dense connective tissue capsule, the tunica albuginea, from the internal surface of which extend connective tissue septa towards the mediastinum. This area consists of connective tissue which houses a network of ducts, that is the rete testis. The testis is divided into lobules, the number of which varies between species. Within these lobules lie the seminiferous tubules, the location for both Sertoli and germ cells, and therefore spermatogenesis. The seminiferous tubules make up over 90% of the testicular mass, and all drain into the rete testis and thus to the epididymis. The organization of the intertubular tissue varies between species, but all contain blood vessels, lymphatics, nerve fibres and the Leydig cells (Fig. 9.1).

The anatomical configuration within the seminiferous tubule (Fig. 9.2) and in particular, the presence of a basal lamina supporting the Sertoli cells, tight junctions between Sertoli cells and their biochemical activity, essentially forms a blood–testis barrier. This barrier protects and assists in the regulation of the chemical environment within the tubule to provide optimum conditions for spermatogenesis. As with other physiological barriers (e.g. brain and placenta) substances can cross by diffusion, and molecular weight is a fundamental limiting factor. An appreciation of the blood–testis barrier is important in considering structure–activity rela-

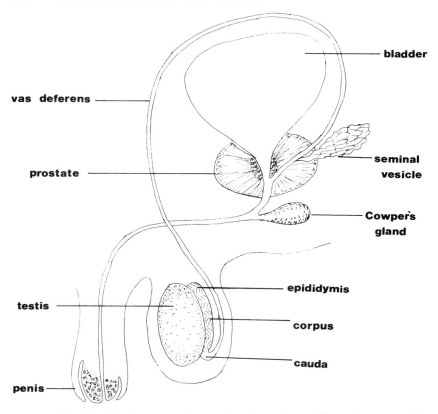

Fig. 9.1. The human male reproductive system. All species possess the organs represented by the human, other than the cat and dog where the seminal vesicles are absent.

tionships of testicular toxins (e.g. Bernstein, 1984). The anatomy and physiology of the blood–testis barrier is reviewed elsewhere (Jackson & Schnieden, 1982; Sever & Hessol, 1985).

The accessory glands include the paired seminal vesicles, the prostate and the paired bulbo-urethral or Cowpers glands. The size and anatomy of these glands vary considerably between species, indeed in the cat and dog, seminal vesicles are absent. Sperm produced within the seminiferous tubules is non-motile, undergoes a maturation process in the epididymis and only becomes motile and metabolically active on contact with the seminal plasma.

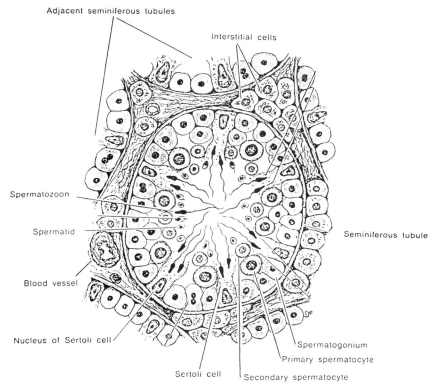

Adjacent seminiferous tubules

Interstitial cells

Spermatozoon

Spermatid

Seminiferous tubule

Blood vessel

Nucleus of Sertoli cell

Spermatogonium

Primary spermatocyte

Sertoli cell

Secondary spermatocyte

Fig. 9.2. Seminiferous tubule. A diagrammatic transverse section through the seminiferous tubule showing stages in development of a spermatozoa.

## Endocrine control of the testis

The testis performs two main functions that are largely complementary, namely the production of spermatozoa and the production of hormones, principally testosterone from the interstitial or Leydig cell (Figs. 9.2 and 9.3).

The Sertoli cell was originally described by Enrico Sertoli in 1865. These are individual cells that extend from the basement membrane to the lumen of the seminiferous tubule and envelope many germ cells associated with spermatogenesis. The Sertoli cells are often termed 'nurse cells', providing support for the germ cells throughout spermatogenesis (Kretser & Ker, 1988).

The Leydig cell is the principal hormone producing cell in the testis. In

1902, Ancel first offered convincing evidence that the Leydig cell provided the hormonal stimulus for production of sperm and for maintenance of secondary sexual characteristics (Ancel & Bouin, 1902). Testosterone was finally identified in 1965 as the chief androgen and the Leydig cell as its source (Christensen & Mason, 1965).

The hormonal control of the testis is apparently relatively simple, probably only because it has not been investigated thoroughly as yet. For the purpose of this chapter, it is probably simplest to consider the endocrine control of spermatogenesis (Sertoli cell) and steroidogenesis (Leydig cell) separately.

## Spermatogenesis

The pituitary gonadotrophins, follicle stimulating hormone (FSH) and luteinizing hormone (LH) are both important to the continuation of spermatogenesis, as pituitary gland removal results in testicular regression and cessation of spermatogenesis. Exogenous LH can restore some degree of spermatogenesis in hypophysectomized male and, therefore, can be considered to be the most important of the two hormones. However, the main action of LH on spermatogenesis is not a direct effect but is mediated through the Leydig cell and testosterone.

FSH acts synergistically with LH, since the effects of the two hormones in combination are greater than those of either alone. FSH effects are confined to a direct action on the Sertoli cells, the major site of FSH binding in the testis (Mears & Vaituleaitis, 1972). The actions of FSH on the Sertoli cell, such as energy metabolism, protein secretion and cell division are all mediated by several second messengers, including cAMP and $Ca^{++}$ (Bardin et al., 1988). FSH has been shown to affect the Sertoli cell secretion of several proteins which may be involved directly with spermatogenesis, the production of androgen binding protein (ABP) (Vernon, Kopec & Fritz, 1974) and a Leydig cell stimulating factor (Verhoeven & Cailleau, 1985). In addition, FSH influences Sertoli cell lactate production, the preferential germ cell energy source, thereby affecting their nourishment.

## Steroidogenesis

With regard to the endocrine activity of the testis, the effect of LH on spermatogenesis is via testosterone and testosterone receptors located on Sertoli cells (Tindall, Miller & Means, 1977). Some of the effects of testosterone mimic those already ascribed to FSH. There is evidence that androgens play a role in regulating the number of FSH receptors (Tsutsui

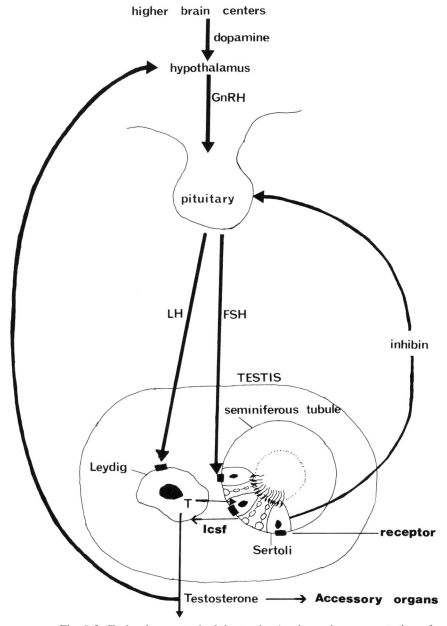

Fig. 9.3. Endocrine control of the testis. A schematic representation of the endocrine controlling mechanism of spermatogenesis.

& Ishii, 1978) thereby enhancing the effect of FSH, however in the adult, Sertoli cell function can be maintained by testosterone alone.

Testosterone is synthesized and released by the Leydig cell in response to LH (Dufau *et al.*, 1983). In the hypophysectomized male, the synthesis of androgens by the testis proceeds, but at a greatly reduced rate (Li & Evans, 1948), only being restored by injections of LH. The levels of LH are controlled by a functional negative feedback system and testosterone, progesterone and oestrogen decrease the release of LH from the pituitary. Similarly, oestrogen and inhibin (secreted by the Sertoli cell) depress FSH levels. Generally the pattern of gonadotrophin release in the male is relatively constant, however, in most species, sexual excitement may provoke a discharge of LH (Katangole, Naftolin & Short, 1971); whether this has any functional significance is not yet clear.

The Leydig cell is able to respond to changes in LH secretion within half an hour. This response represents an increase in the rate of biosynthesis of testosterone rather than a release of preformed stores. This response of the Leydig cell to LH involves biochemical membrane events involving LH binding to a specific receptor resulting in stimulation of a cellular response via a second messenger, cAMP. This in turn stimulates the transport of cholesterol (the steroid precursor) to the mitochondria where it is converted to testosterone (Hall *et al.*, 1979). The other androgen produced by the Leydig cell is androstenedione. This is a weak androgen and is mainly secreted prior to puberty. However, in some species (e.g. deer) the adult male undergoes a period of sexual quiescence, during which the testes regress and spermatogenesis ceases and the main androgen secreted at this time is androstenedione.

Other hormones which may increase testosterone synthesis are luteinizing hormone releasing hormone (LHRH) (Sharpe, 1984) and prostaglandins, however, these are both areas of recent research and the ideas too new for judgement.

The final level of endocrine control of the testis is that exhibited at a local level – within the testis itself, i.e. between the Sertoli and Leydig cell only. This is known as paracrine control and is believed to be an important means of cell-to-cell communication (Parvinen & Ruokonen, 1982). Leydig cells show a cyclic variation in size which is dependent on the stage of spermatogenesis of the tubules adjacent to them (Bergh, 1983). Also, in both the rat (Garside *et al.*, 1985) and the pig, Sertoli cells secrete a product that can stimulate Leydig cell production of testosterone, according to the needs of the stage of spermatogenesis. It has also been shown recently that Leydig cells can produce oxytocin which probably influences seminiferous tubule contractions. Figure 9.3 is a simplified diagram of endocrine interactions.

## Hormone regulation of the epididymis and accessory organs

Testosterone also influences accessory sex organs, and the anatomy and physiology of these structures will be briefly reviewed with emphasis on the rat.

### The epididymis

Generally, the maturation of spermatozoa begun in the seminiferous tubules is continued and completed in the epididymis. This extra-testicular maturation of spermatozoa (sperm) is not a rapid process, and it is important that the duct where it occurs should be long (3–4 m in man and 80 m in the horse). The epididymis, therefore, is a single highly convoluted duct divided into three main segments – the head (caput), body (corpus) and tail (cauda). There are three well established sperm related functions taking place in the epididymis, namely the transport of sperm from the testis to the vas deferens, the acquisition of fertilizing ability and the storage of spermatozoa. The acquisition of fertilizing ability is the process most under endocrine control and appears to occur in the caput and corpus sections. For reviews on the maturation of sperm in the epididymis see Orgebin-Crist (1969) and Courot (1981).

This process is androgen dependent (Brooks, 1981) and removal of the testis results in epididymal atrophy. However, it appears that dihydrotestosterone (DHT) is essential for sperm to acquire their fertilizing potential (Cohen, Ooms & Vreeburg, 1981), as shown by an inhibitor of 5α-reductase causing a decrease in the number of motile sperm.

Transport of sperm seems to be only indirectly dependent on the presence of androgens, since neuronal input is the apparent driving force. The storage of sperm is again directly dependent on androgen. Although it is clear that androgens regulate epididymal function, the mechanism by which they do so has yet to be defined (Coffey, 1988).

Earlier it was mentioned that the Sertoli cell produced androgen binding protein (ABP), which has been shown to enter the epididymis via the efferent ducts (Pelliniemi *et al.*, 1981). The function of this protein is unresolved but it has been proposed that it acts as an androgen concentrator in seminiferous tubules, transports androgens to the epididymis or is a regulator of epididymal 5α-reductase (Robaire, Sheer & Hachey, 1981). In the rat, a correlation between the amount of epididymal ABP and the fertilizing capacity of sperm has been established.

In addition to androgens there are a number of other hormones (e.g. prolactin, oestrogen) and vitamins A and D which affect epididymal function. Of these, the most studied is oestrogen which has been shown to increase the rate of transport through the epididymis (Meistrich, Hughes & Bruce, 1975).

## Prostate gland, seminal vesicles and bulbo-urethral gland

The secretions from the prostate, seminal vesicles and bulbo-urethral (Cowpers) glands constitute most of the volume and chemical composition of the seminal plasma. The sex accessory organs produce high concentrations of important biological substances such as prostaglandins (from the seminal vesicles), fructose, spermine, zinc and proteases; the physiological functions of which are not clear. Although the seminal plasma may not contain factors that are essential to fertilization, the constituents probably optimize conditions for sperm motility, survival and transport in both the male and female tracts.

As with the testis, it now appears that direct cell-to-cell communication as well as growth and endocrine factors, are responsible for the regulation of the sex accessory organs. The main controlling hormone is testosterone which is responsible for the growth of all the sex accessory organs (Bruchovsky & Wilson, 1985). There is little knowledge of the exact endocrine control of these organs, however, more is known about the prostate. For the purposes of this chapter, therefore only the prostate will be described and assumed to be similar for all accessory organs.

Only free testosterone enters the prostate cell by diffusion, where it is activated to DHT. DHT then binds to specific receptors and is translocated to the nucleus, thereby increasing transcription, expression and regulation of specific genes. As a result, DHT is responsible for the synthesis and storage of proteins in secretory granules, where they are then poised for secretion in the process of ejaculation. Adrenal androgens formed from androstenedione will also stimulate prostate growth and function, though this is only a small contribution, as castration in most animals leads to almost complete involution of the prostate.

Prolactin has been postulated to enhance androgen induced growth (Grayhock et al., 1955) although the actual mechanism has not yet been elucidated. Several protein-type growth factors may also play a role, including insulin and a paracrine prostatic growth factor. At the present time, however, it is unclear how the secretions from accessory sex organs specifically interact with sperm, and further evaluation of the secretory components is important in correlating glandular activity with fertility. Also we have little knowledge of the mechanisms and types of transport of ions, drugs, and natural products into and out of the sex accessory secretions. It is certain though that any inhibition of the endocrine factors

Table 9.1. *Compounds affecting the endocrine control of the male reproductive system*

| Compound | Effect |
|---|---|
| *Affecting peripheral control* | |
| Trifluorperazine HCl | Increase prolactin |
| Testosterone analogues | Reduces LH/FSH |
| Cimetidine | Anti-androgen |
| Naloxone | Decrease dopamine |
| Substituted triazoles | Anti-androgen/decreases LH/FSH |
| Progesterone analogues | Increase prolactin |
| *Affecting cellular interactions* | |
| Forskolin | Increase cAMP |
| Nicotine | Inhibits spermatogenesis |
| $Ca^{++}$ inhibitors | Interferes with hormone synthesis |
| Ethylene dimethane sulphate | Destroys Leydig cells |

LH = luteinizing hormone; FSH = follicle stimulating hormone

controlling their growth and function, especially testosterone, will impair fertility. Agents commonly used to influence endocrine control of the male reproductive system are given in Table 9.1.

## Common spontaneous lesions of the male reproductive system

The previous section has briefly outlined the endocrine control of the male reproductive organs, indicating the complexity of maintaining normal function. Obviously any abnormalities of the controlling system will lead to a malfunction of the reproductive process. These can occur spontaneously; common diseases and lesions being most prominent in the testis and prostate. As little is known about lesions in the other components of the male reproductive system, this section will deal only with the testicular and prostate abnormalities.

### The prostate

The diseases of the prostate are some of the most common and devastating in the male. Abnormal overgrowth (benign prostatic hyperplasia, BPH) of the human prostate occurs in about 80% of males before the age of 80, most requiring surgery to alleviate urinary obstruction as a result. However, it is surprising that there has been little research undertaken in this area, considering BPH is the second most common cause of surgery in the male.

Prostatic cancer is far less common than BPH but is the second leading cause of cancer deaths in man. Interestingly, the death rate is small considering that 30% of all males over 50 years of age have pathological evidence of latent cancer cells within the prostate at the time of death. The reason for dormancy of latent prostate cancer is not known, nor why there is so little prostate cancer clinically manifested in the Far East, where the same amount of latent cancer exists. These abnormalities of the prostate are common only to humans and dogs while all other mammalian species are essentially free from prostate diseases. Further questions have also yet to be answered concerning why in humans the prostate is the main site for lesions, while the seminal vesicles are almost devoid of any significant pathological abnormality. It appears that both receive the same endogenous hormones and are subjected to the same pathological insults, so should be prone to the same abnormalities.

Finally, with regard to both BPH and prostatic cancer, the main form of treatment, other than surgery, is physical or chemical castration. It is apparent, therefore, that androgens play a role in these diseases, possibly as a result of a breakdown in the fine control of androgens on growth. Treatment with a high dose of oestrogen may also be therapeutic, presumably indirectly, by acting on the testis to reduce testosterone output.

## The testis

The most common cancer of the testis is Leydig cell tumour, which arises from an over proliferation of Leydig cells and is accompanied by an increase in blood vessels and macrophages. This proliferation would normally occur in order to replace wasted Leydig cells, especially as a result of testicular damage. Elevation of LH is associated with the aetiology of Leydig cell tumours (Mori, 1988).

Such testicular damage may occur as a result of cryptorchidism. At puberty in some mammals (human, rat, dog), the testes descend from their original position in the abdomen to the scrotum. Cryptorchidism, or the failure of the testis/testes to descend is relatively common in the horse, pig and human, and results in a low androgen secretion. As spermatogenesis only occurs at 34°C (i.e. lower than body temperature), cryptorchidism results in a complete cessation of spermatogenesis and hyperplasia of the Leydig cells. Testicular tumours are more common among the lower mammals than among humans. More than half the number of dogs over seven years of age have testicular lesions, the most usual being Leydig cell tumours, which produce oestrogen. Leydig cell tumours have also been reported in the mule, bull and horse. Sertoli cell lesions frequently cause feminization due to secretion of large amounts of oestrogen, often also resulting in cystic hyperplasia of the mammary gland as well as atrophy of the testes. Testicular tumours spontaneously occur in both rats and mice, especially in the AC and JK strains of mice, indeed Leydig cell tumours can be induced in rodents by the use of LH, oestradiol, and stilboestrol but are inhibited by a simultaneous injection of testosterone.

Congenital lesions of the testis also occur. In guinea pigs, congenital spermatogenic hypoplasia is common, causing germinal aplasia of the seminiferous tubules; androgen secretion is unaffected. Another common example of a congenital lesion is in the mule which has a J-shaped chromosome contributed by the ass. Spermatogenesis does not proceed beyond meiotic prophase, thus no sperm cells are present and the testes become atrophic but the Leydig cells remain normal. Some types of inherited hypogonadism occur in bull and goats, resulting in idiopathic necrosis of the seminiferous tubule. It is interesting also to note here that often wild animals become sterile in captivity. Generally no cells of the germinal epithelium are found at necropsy except the occasional Sertoli cells, although again Leydig cells are normal. Whether this degenerative testicular lesion is caused by nutritional deficiency or the 'stress' of captivity is not known (adrenal–gonadal interactions are reviewed later in the toxicology of the xanthines).

Regarding the importance of the endocrine control of the testes by gonadotrophins from the pituitary, most lesions of the pituitary will result in testicular atrophy, for example pituitary dwarfism. In such cases the testes remain infantile for at least half, if not the entire lifespan of the mammal. In some selective types of gonadotrophic insufficiency, tubular maturation will proceed with differentiation of the Sertoli cell, but Leydig cells are not present. This is explained by the fact that FSH synthesis and secretion has occurred but that LH is absent from the pituitary. Generally, pituitary lesions before puberty result in immature testes while those incurred after puberty cause atrophy of the seminiferous epithelium and Leydig cells, but not immaturity.

Other abnormalities of the testis which should be noted are feminization and ageing. Testicular feminization usually occurs due either to a deficiency of the enzyme 5$\alpha$-reductase (where the males produce insufficient amounts of DHT) or to target organs that are insensitive to androgens (a receptor deficiency). In both cases the external genitalia are not fully masculinized and the animal may be mistaken externally as female (Austin & Short, 1984). The fate of Leydig cells with increasing age is still a topic for discussion (Shulze, 1984). It would appear, however, that in man and rats where spermatogenesis is normal, there is a significant negative correlation between age and total Leydig cell number (Soball, 1984), related perhaps to a decrease in LH and FSH secretion. The ageing stallion conversely shows a striking increase in Leydig cell number (Johnson & Neaves, 1981).

Vitamins E and A are important for testicular function, and spontaneous testicular abnormalities can occur as a function of diet. Degeneration of the testes in rats deficient in vitamin E was first reported in 1922 (Matill & Carman, 1922/3). The degeneration is complete and cannot be reversed by treatment with vitamin E and in this respect it differs from vitamin A deficiency, which responds to therapy. Vitamin E deficiency primarily affects spermatogenesis, but many of the water soluble vitamins are specific to the Leydig cell (e.g. biotin, riboflavin).

## Toxicology of the male reproductive system

The testes are the most significant sites of toxic damage affecting fertility within the male reproductive system. A variety of chemicals are known to be testicular toxins and this review will focus on two examples of compounds of pharmaceutical significance (anti-neoplastic agents and xanthines) and two examples of compounds of industrial importance (phthalates and cadmium compounds). Many agents that induce testicular toxicity and pathology inhibit protein synthesis (particularly the alkylating anti-neoplastic agents) where damage to rapidly dividing cell populations and cessation of spermatogenesis are common and predictable toxic endpoints. As the testes are major sites of DNA synthesis, protein synthesis and cell turnover, it is understandable that histopathological change is most readily observable here, although similar damage occurs elsewhere in the body. Not surprisingly, some compounds induce damage or change in the testes by alteration of the hormones of the pituitary–testicular axis (see Table 9.1). Further to this, a common finding in long-term rodent toxicity studies is Leydig cell tumours, and there is now strong evidence that these tumours are a result of excess LH production, Leydig cell hyperplasia and subsequent neoplasia (e.g. Mori, 1988). Given this example of excessive gonadotrophic hormone producing testicular pathology, it may be predicted that any compound chronically increasing LH concentration in the blood could also produce Leydig cell tumours. Thus there are two main recognized areas of endocrine toxicology (Mattison et al., 1990): the first concerns damage to an endocrine target organ by the direct action of a compound, and the second involves damage to an endocrine target organ by alteration of hormones within the local endocrine axis (e.g. gonadotrophins or sex steroids damaging the testes).

It is less obvious that there is scope for a third mechanism involving damage to an endocrine target organ by an agent that influences the secretion of hormones from an independent endocrine axis (e.g. adrenal products damaging the testes). Evidence is emerging that this may be the case for the xanthines, where testicular atrophy may be resulting from adrenocortical activity. As this mechanism is novel and has received relatively little previous attention, the endocrine toxicology of the xanthines will be reviewed first followed by anti-neoplastic agents (focusing on hormonal protection of testicular damage), cadmium and phthalates. This review has been written to cover more recent developments in the field of testicular toxicity, rather than list chemicals and their effects, and focuses on *in vivo* studies in the common laboratory species and man. Other comprehensive reviews of chemically induced testicular injury have been written relatively recently (e.g. Phillips, Foster & Gangolli, 1985, which is organized by cellular target site rather than compound class).

## Xanthines

Xanthines such as caffeine, theophylline and theobromine are constituents of coffee, tea, and cocoa. Such compounds have a number of pharmacological activities (e.g. adenosine antagonism, phosphodiesterase inhibition). Accordingly, theophylline has an important clinical application as a tracheal–bronchial relaxant in asthma and oxpentifylline is used as a blood flow improver in peripheral vascular disorders. Xanthines are also breakdown products of purines.

Caffeine, theophylline and theobromine administration to rats results in testicular atrophy characterized by degeneration of the seminiferous tubules (Tarka, Zoumas & Gans, 1979; Friedman *et al.*, 1979). Structure activity analysis of a range of novel xanthine derivatives has shown that 1-position-methylated compounds are more potent in inducing testicular atrophy (and indeed are more toxic) than analogues that are not methylated at the 1-position (Dahlback *et al.*, 1984). The most potent compound tested by Dahlback was approximately 100 times more potent as a testicular toxin than caffeine or theophylline, and characteristically resulted in seminiferous tubule atrophy. Thus, in the literature there are reports of at least seven xanthine analogues causing testicular atrophy in the rat.

There are a number of mechanisms via which xanthines may induce testicular atrophy. Xanthines are adenosine antagonists, and high concentrations of adenosine receptors have been found in the testes (Murphy & Snyder, 1981; Stiles, 1986). The physiological effects of these receptors in the testes are unknown but the effects of adenosine receptors in other tissues are well characterized (e.g. in the liver they are associated with gluconeogenesis, in the brain they are associated with sedation and modulation of neurotransmitter release – Stiles, 1986). It has been speculated (Stiles, 1986) that adenosine receptors in the testes may regulate adenylate cyclase and second messenger systems. This could in turn influence conventional hormonal control and support of the testes. Similarly, as adenosine is intimately involved in energy balance, interruption of such processes may be predicted to have an impact on cellular activity involving high metabolic energy demand, such as spermatogenesis. It is also possible that as xanthines are structurally related to purine nucleotides they directly interfere with nucleic acids and protein synthesis and hence spermatogenesis.

Another important action of xanthines is the inhibition of phosphodiesterase. This action is relevant to endocrine control mechanisms since phosphodiesterase breaks down cAMP, and its inhibition produces a state of biological amplification within endocrine systems resulting in excess hormone production and secretion.

There is growing evidence in the literature that an important action of xanthines is to alter hormone secretion. Dahlback et al. (1984) first noted that the toxicological profile of the xanthines resembles the stress syndrome in rats (atrophy of the thymus, spleen and testes, and most importantly hypertrophy of the adrenal). Recent studies have confirmed this observation, and have shown that caffeine increases corticosterone, and beta-endorphin, decreases growth hormone and thyroid stimulating hormone, but has no effect on prolactin in the rat (Spindel, Griffiths & Wurtman, 1983; Spindel, 1984). A novel xanthine, denbufylline, also causes testicular atrophy in rats, and it has been shown that a major endocrine effect of denbufylline treatment is the stimulation of adrenocorticotrophic hormone (ACTH) release from the pituitary (Hadley, Flack & Buckingham, 1990, 1991). It is interesting to note here a report that a 500 mg dose of caffeine (8 mg/kg) had no effect on plasma cortisol (or thyroid stimulating hormone, growth hormone, prolactin or triiodothyronine) in men (Spindel et al., 1984), and this may indicate species differences between rat and human in the hormonal effects of xanthines (although there may be other factors involving prior exposure to xanthines and dose considerations). Denbufylline was also shown to be without effect in a detailed clinical pharmacology study to examine pituitary-adrenal-testicular hormone secretion (W. Greb & H. Sourgen, SmithKline Beecham, unpub. data).

That range of xanthine structural analogues has been reported in the rat both to increase hormone secretion, particularly from the pituitary–

adrenal system, and to cause testicular atrophy, suggests a causal relationship. There is already evidence that glucocorticoids can affect testicular function, and given the well-documented physiological and toxicological effects of the xanthines it is a reasonable hypothesis that in the rat, xanthines increase corticosterone secretion which in turn affects the testes. Certainly, it has been known for nearly 25 years that the long-term administration of high doses of synthetic glucocorticoids (e.g. cortisone acetate) to immature rats inhibits spermatogenesis, whereas, there are no effects in adult rats or men (men being treated with up to 500 mg – Mancini *et al.*, 1966). However, there is an early report of ACTH (25 units) inducing azoospermia in men (see Mancini *et al.*, 1966) and this is likely to be a result of excessive endogenous glucocorticoids.

There is supportive evidence of how the adrenal influences the testis. Corticosterone inhibits LH secretion (Kamel & Kubajak, 1987). This would also reduce testosterone and influence all androgen dependent functions of the testes, including cell maintenance and spermatogenesis (see earlier sections of this chapter). Additionally, corticosterone in common with other glucocorticoids, inhibits protein synthesis in certain tissues (Gower, 1979), and this can also be envisaged to have a generalized detrimental effect in sites of high cell turnover such as the testes. Further, the natural stress of overcrowding in mice has been shown to decrease the number of seminiferous tubules and spermatids, and increase adrenal corticosterone (Gartner, Reznik-Schuller & Reznik, 1973). The significance of this study concerns the co-relation of endogenous adrenoglucocorticoids secreted in physiological concentrations, with testicular pathology, although extra-adrenal and indeed non-endocrine factors can also be argued as the mechanism of action of this apparent 'stress effect'.

## Anti-neoplastic agents

The two main groups of anti-neoplastic drugs are the alkylating agents and the anti-metabolites. The alkylating agents (e.g. chlorambucil, cyclophosphamide, carmustine, cisplatin) act by donating alkyl (e.g. methyl or ethyl) groups. These electrophilic groups readily bind to nucleophilic sites on DNA distorting the molecule such that DNA replication is arrested, and ultimately cell division ceases. This property is useful in the treatment of proliferating tumours, but other sites of rapid cell division are affected (e.g. bone marrow, gastrointestinal mucosa, testes). Similarly, the anti-metabolites (e.g. cytarabine, thioguanine, mercaptopurine) combine with the same enzymes as physiologically occurring cellular metabolites, thus preventing fundamental metabolic processes including the synthesis of nucleic acids. As with the alkylating agents, any effect on nucleic acids can be expected to impact on spermatogenesis, however, in practice anti-metabolites have relatively few effects on spermatogenesis, and in the case of one compound, methotrexate, impermeability of the blood–testis barrier has been suggested as a reason (Gradishar & Schilsky, 1988).

The clinical use of anti-neoplastic agents has been known for many years to be injurious to the testes. As drug regimes to treat cancer have become more successful, it has become more important to protect against chemotherapy-induced sterility. In the testes, the histological effects of using anti-neoplastic chemicals characteristically include loss of the germinal epithelium, but there is relative survival of Sertoli and Leydig cells (e.g. Waxman, 1983). In an early study of the progression of damage in the testes of mice treated with an alkylating agent (nitrogen mustard) germinal cell change (nuclear chromatin condensation, cytoplasmic eosinophilia and hyaline change) occurred within 24 hours, followed by germinal epithelium disruption, the appearance of abnormal germ cells (multi-nuclear giant cells) and finally germ cell lysis (Landing *et al.*, 1949). It has subsequently been determined that different types of anti-neoplastic drugs have different target sites in the germinal epithelium: essentially the alkylating agents (cisplatin, cyclophosphamide and nitrogen mustards) tend to affect spermatogonia, spermatocytes and spermatids, whilst Actinomycin-D and Doxorubicin affect stem cells (Gradishar & Schilsky, 1988). The degree of male sterility and the reversibility of the effects of anti-neoplastic agent exposure depends upon the compound, total dose and species and there are recent reviews of this elsewhere (Schilsky, 1989; Gradishar & Schilsky, 1988; Chapman, 1983).

Turning to the endocrine impact of chemotherapeutic testicular damage, the hormonal profile mirrors the histological events. In humans, LH and testosterone profiles are essentially normal when Leydig cells are preserved, whereas germ cell destruction raises FSH (Waxman, 1983). Although Leydig cells are not the proximal site of cytotoxicity, it has been reported that Leydig cell dysfunction is relatively common in men following chemotherapy and this is demonstrated by marked reductions in testosterone levels but normal LH levels (see Gradishar & Schilsky, 1988).

It has recently been postulated that deliberate suppression of hypothalamo-pituitary-testicular activity may protect the testes from cytotoxic damage. The rationale behind this approach is that a quiescent testis is less vulnerable to insult by cytotoxic, alkylating or anti-metabolite agents (Schilsky, 1989; Morris & Shalet, 1989; Morris & Shalet, 1990). There are currently two clinical strategies to protect the testes from chemotherapeutically-induced injury, the administration of sex steroids and the administration of a gonadotrophin releasing hormone (GnRH) analogue. The administration of androgens and other sex steroids decreases gonadotrophic support of the testes by negative feedback of the pituitary or hypothalamus, but their use is still the subject of research, and results in rodent models have been less than ideal (Morris & Shalet, 1989). GnRH analogues produce reversible testicular atrophy by reducing gonadotrophin output, presumably by blocking the action of endogenous GnRH.

Glode, Robinson & Gould (1981) first reported that a GnRH analogue (D-Leu[6] GnRH) could protect against testicular damage induced by cyclophosphamide in mice. In rats, GnRH agonists and antagonists have also been shown to protect against procarbazine-induced testicular damage (Karashima, Zalatnai & Schally, 1988). Similarly, in the dog, buserelin (a GnRH agonist) has been reported to afford some protection against cyclophosphamide-induced testicular damage (Nseyo *et al.*, 1985). However, other studies have failed to demonstrate protective effects of GnRH analogues in chemotherapeutic regimes in rodents (da Cunha, Meistrich & Nader, 1987) and there is one report of potentiation of gonadotoxicity in dogs (Goodpasture, Bergstrom & Vickery, 1988). Despite these apparently contradictory results (a situation not unusual in endocrinological investigation) it is clear that manipulation of pituitary–testicular hormones prior to chemotherapy does influence the degree of testicular damage, and continued future research will be required to elucidate which GnRH analogues and treatment regimes are likely to be beneficial to humans.

## Cadmium

Cadmium is a metal of major industrial importance. Cadmium is smelted from metal ores, and there is exposure both from industrial discharge into the atmosphere and from direct contact with diverse manufacturing processes and end products. It has been estimated that in the United States alone, over 1.5 million workers are exposed to this metal in its various forms (Ragan & Mast, 1990) and cadmium is regarded as one of the most hazardous air pollutants (Buell, 1975).

The toxicity of cadmium is well known, and whilst the adverse effects on the testes are the subject of this section, cadmium is highly systemically toxic, affecting most organ systems (e.g. Nath *et al.*, 1984). In the testes, the primary action of cadmium is on the testicular vasculature. Cameron & Foster (1963) administered cadmium chloride (9–18 mg/kg) subcutaneously to rabbits, and noted hyperaemia and interstitial haemorrhage within 5–12 days, accompanied by destruction of germ cells and

Leydig cells. Similarly, Gunn, Gould & Anderson (1963) administered a single dose of cadmium chloride (0.03 mmole/kg) subcutaneously to rats and mice, and reported testicular vascular damage. Gunn *et al.* (1963) also reported that whilst the testicular vascular damage repaired with time, both rats and mice developed interstitial (Leydig cell) tumours approximately one year later.

Although cadmium is a potent carcinogen and promotes tumour formation on contact, for example, at injection sites (IARC, WHO, 1973) it is not clear how testicular tumours develop so long after acute exposure in laboratory animals. Chronic cadmium exposure has been excluded as an aetiological factor in prostate cancer in men (Piscator, 1981). Indeed, the precise mode of action of the general testicular toxicity of cadmium is reportedly not fully understood (e.g. Singhal, Vijayvargiya & Shukla, 1985). Cadmium does not appear to penetrate the seminiferous tubules or become associated with sperm cells (e.g. Barlow & Sullivan, 1982). However, it is known that cadmium concentrates in the testes following subcutaneous administration (Johnson *et al.*, 1970) and this is an obvious pre-requisite for local, direct cytotoxic action. Thus, the primary effect of cadmium is on the testicular vasculature (hyperaemia and haemorrhage) resulting in ischaemia and finally necrosis within the testes.

The testicular effects of cadmium can be ameliorated by the co-administration of zinc and other metals. Gunn *et al.* (1963) noted that the administration of zinc to rodents treated with cadmium chloride prevented the development of testicular tumours. Additionally, selenium is reported to protect against cadmium induced testicular necrosis, and the interaction of cadmium with various metals and vitamins, and the influence of this on the testes, is reviewed elsewhere (see Nath *et al.*, 1984).

## Phthalates

The phthalate esters occur ubiquitously in products from the plastics industry and especially in polyvinyl chloride (PVC) formulations. The global production of one phthalate ester, di(2-ethylhexyl)phthalate (DEHP) is 3–4 million tonnes and this compound, together with other phthalate esters, are listed as priority pollutants (Wams, 1987). Whilst human exposure to phthalates occurring as environmental pollutants is of concern, there is even greater potential for phthalate exposure due to migration from PVC wrapping materials and containers. This has become particularly important because of their widespread use in the food industry, but concern is also being raised at the extent to which medical materials are employing plastics (e.g. blood storage bags, syringes). It has been established that the concentration of DEHP in blood stored in PVC blood bags is up to 10 mg/ml (an exchange transfusion procedure will yield a dose of 300 mg) and a patient receiving dialysis will be exposed to an average of 40 mg DEHP per day (Thomas & Thomas, 1984; Wams, 1987). It has also been established that the no-effect-level of phthalates based on animal data for the induction of liver damage, teratogenicity, testicular toxicity and carcinogenicity are 100 mg/kg, 70 mg/kg, 1 g/kg and 100 μg/kg, respectively, and as such, it can be appreciated why various regulatory agencies are concerned about potential health risks.

It is well known that phthalate esters cause testicular toxicity characterized by tubular atrophy, reduced testes weight and subsequent reduction in fertility, and that there are marked species differences in gonadotoxicity (rats and guinea pigs are more sensitive than mice, and hamsters are relatively unaffected; see Thomas & Thomas, 1984; Gray *et al.*, 1982). A number of studies have investigated the biochemical correlates of phthalate testicular toxicity. Foster *et al.* (1983) reported that a phthalate which caused testicular atrophy in rats (diphenyl phthalate) also decreased steroidogenic enzymes (17α-hydroxylase and 17–20 lyase) and reduced maximal binding of a natural substrate (progesterone) to testis microsomes, whilst a phthalate ester that did not cause testicular atrophy (diethyl phthalate) did not affect steroidogenic enzymes. These results suggest that an effect on androgen producing enzymes may mediate the induction of testicular damage. Certainly, a reduction of androgen production has been confirmed: administration of di-(2-ethylhexyl)phthalate to rats reduced serum testosterone, and was associated with decreased testes and accessory sex organ weights, testicular atrophy and reduced spermatogenesis (Oishi, 1985). The importance of androgens in mediating phthalate gonadotoxicity is also suggested by the finding that the co-administration of testosterone prevented the testicular injury normally resulting from di(2-ethylhexyl)phthalate treatment (Parmar *et al.*, 1987). Taken together, the results from these studies suggest that the phthalates affect Leydig cells and steroidogenesis, and the loss of androgenic support leads to testicular atrophy (possibly via a secondary action involving Sertoli cell dysfunction; Gray & Butterworth, 1980).

Direct evidence of an effect of phthalates on the Leydig cell has been provided by Garside in a scanning electron microscopy and cell ultrastructure study in rats (see also Liu *et al.*, 1988). Administration of di-(2-ethylhexyl)phthalate to rats produced Leydig cell mitochondrial swelling, smooth endoplasmic reticulum vesiculation and cisternal dilatation of the Golgi apparatus compared with controls (Figs 9.4 and 9.5). Further studies *in vitro* indicate that the monoester, mono-(2-ethylhexyl)

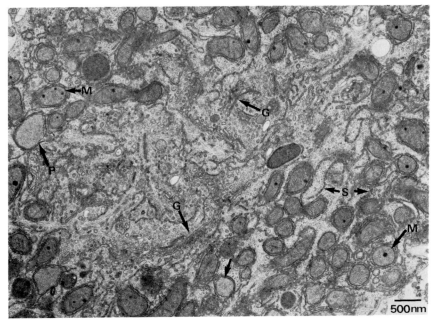

Fig. 9.4. Control (untreated) Leydig cell. High magnification electron micrograph (see scale bar) illustrating Leydig cell cytoplasmic ultrastructure. Note the abundance and uniquitous distribution of the smooth endoplasmic reticulum (S). Mitochondria contain relatively large electron-dense matrix granules (M). Peroxisome (P) and Golgi apparatus (G) are shown.

phthalate, which is metabolized from the di-ester, di-(2-ethylhexyl) phthalate, also damaged the Leydig cell. Mono-(2-ethylhexyl) phthalate caused a marked increase in the numbers and length of filopodia associated with the basal lamellar processes, which indicates cell compromise (Figs 9.6 and 9.7). Testosterone secretion was also inhibited.

Recent studies have also indicated an effect of phthalates on enzymes directly related to spermatogenesis and that testicular atrophy is associated with, or secondary to, these biochemical changes. Srivastava et al. (1990a,b) observed reductions in acid phosphatase and sorbitol dehydrogenase (enzymes associated with post-meiotic spermatogenic cells) activity and increases in lactate dehydrogenase, gamma-glutamyl transpeptidase, beta-glucuronidase and glucose-6-phosphate dehydrogenase (enzymes associated with pre-meiotic cells, Sertoli cells or Leydig cells) activity in rats treated with di-n-butyl phthalate. Although these studies are correlative in nature, they do show that phthalate esters are

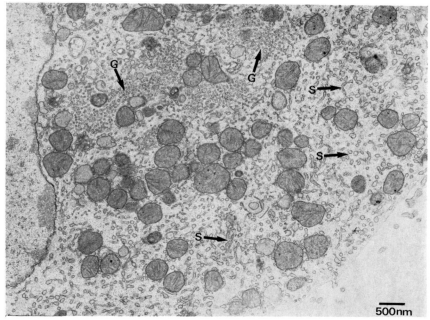

Fig. 9.5. Phthalate treated Leydig cell. Electron micrograph (see scale bar) illustrating dilation of the smooth endoplasmic reticulum (S). Mitochondria (M) are swollen and have lost their matrix granules. Vesicuolation of the Golgi apparatus (G) is noticed.

potentially toxic to a number of sites within the testes. Future work on structure activity analyses may reveal that different esters have different relative cytotoxic effects and target sites.

## Conclusion

The literature relating to chemicals known to have an adverse effect upon the male reproductive system is rapidly expanding. These agents are distributed throughout numerous chemical classes and include compounds developed as medicines (where a once acceptable side effect in clinical use is proving to be an unacceptable toxic effect), crop protection agents, veterinary and public health chemicals, or industrial materials. Bernstein (1984) has reviewed chemicals affecting the male reproductive system, focusing on structure–activity relationships and the multiple end points of testicular damage (e.g. sperm analysis, sexual behaviour, multi-generation and fertility studies). Despite the great range of compounds known to affect the testes, there are rules that can be applied to predict

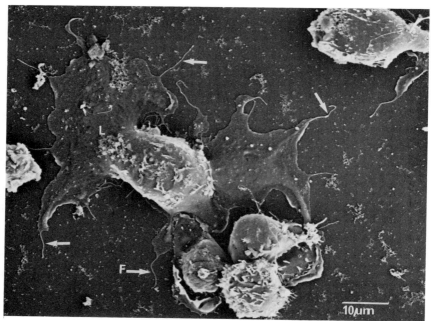

Fig. 9.6. Control (untreated) Leydig cell *in vitro*. Scanning electron micrograph (see scale bar). Leydig cell with flattened lamellar processes (L) in close association with the substratum. Note the raised central soma with few plasmalemmal ridges. F, filapodial projection.

testicular effects (e.g. low molecular weight compounds are likely to pass the blood–testis barrier; compounds affecting hormone secretion may interfere with hormonal support of the testes; alkylating agents are likely to affect spermatogenesis). However, it is impossible to predict testicular toxicity in all novel compounds because it is clear that the testes may be damaged in quite indirect ways, for example the possible involvement of the adrenal in the testicular toxicity of the xanthines.

The significance of testicular toxicity has not fully achieved the status afforded to other areas of target organ toxicity. This is possibly because the testes are not usually considered to be vital organs and their complexity of control and function has limited the pace of advancement. Despite this, interest in the testes as target organs is rapidly increasing, as evidenced by the recent research to develop clinical strategies for limiting testicular damage following cancer chemotherapy. Continued research is required to elucidate mechanisms of testicular toxicity, and especially to advance knowledge in the most fundamentally important area of testicu-

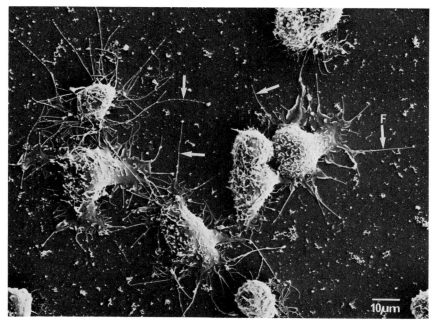

Fig. 9.7. Phthalate treated Leydig cell *in vitro*. Note the increase in length and abundance of filapodial projections (F) from lamellar processes and increased somal plasmalemmal ridges.

lar toxicity, namely to clarify the already questionable relevance of hormonal and pathological effects in laboratory rodents to humans.

### References

Ancel, P. & Bouin, P. (1902). The Leydig cell. *Arch. Zool.*, **1**, 437–523.

Austin, C. & Short, R. (Eds) (1984). *Reproductive Fitness*, Book 4, 2nd edn, p. 142. Cambridge: Cambridge University Press.

Bardin, C., Yan Cheng, C., Mustow, N. & Gunsalus, G. (1988). The Sertoli cell. In *Physiology of Reproduction*, ed. E. Knobil & J.D. Neill, pp. 946–8. New York: Raven Press.

Barlow, S. & Sullivan, F. (1982). *Reproductive Hazards of Industrial Chemicals*, p. 141. London: Academic Press.

Bergh, A. (1983). Paracrine regulation of Leydig cells by seminiferous tubules. *Int. J. Androl.*, **6**, 57–65.

Bernstein, M.E. (1984). Agents affecting the male reproductive system: Effects of structure on activity. *Drug Met. Rev.*, **15**, 941–96.

Brooks, D. (1981). Metabolic activity in epididymis and regulation by androgen. *Physiol. Rev.*, **61**, 516–55.

Bruchovsky, N. & Wilson, J. (1985). The conversion of testosterone to 5α-androstan–17β-ol-3 by rat prostate. *J. Biol. Chem.*, **243**, 2012–21.

Buell, G. (1975). Some biochemical aspects of cadmium toxicology. *J. Occup. Med.*, **17**, 189–95.

Cameron, E. & Foster, C.L. (1963). Observations on the histological effects of sub-lethal doses of cadmium chloride in the rabbit. *J. Anat.*, **97**, 269.

Chapman, R. (1983). Gonadal injury resulting from chemotherapy. *Am. J. Indust. Med.*, **4**, 149–61.

Christensen, A. & Mason, N. (1965). Comparative ability of seminiferous tubule of rat testis to synthesize androgens. *Endocrinology*, **76**, 646–56.

Coffey, D. (1988). In *Physiology of Reproduction*, vol. 1, ed. E. Knobil & J. D. Neill, p. 1081. New York: Raven Press.

Cohen, J., Ooms, M. & Vreeburg, J. (1981). Reduction in fertilising capacity of epididymal sperm by 5α steroid reductase inhibitor. *Experientia*, **37**, 1031–2.

Courot, M. (1981). Epididymal sperm maturation – a review. *Prog. Reprod. Biol.*, **8**, 67–79.

da Cunha, M.F., Meistrich, M.L. & Nader, S. (1987). Absence of testicular protection by a gonadotrophin-releasing hormone analogue against cyclophosphamide-induced testicular toxicity in the mouse. *Cancer Res.*, **47**, 1093–7.

Dahlback, M., Heintz, L., Ryrfeldt, A. & Stenberg, K. (1984). Toxic effects of some xanthine derivatives with special emphasis on adverse effects on rat testes. *Toxicology*, **32**, 23–35.

Dufau, M., Veldheis, J., Fraioli, F., Johnson, M. & Catt, K. (1983). Mode of bioactive LH secretion in man. *J. Clin. Endoc. Metab.*, **57**, 993.

Foster, P.M., Thomas, L.V., Cook, M.W. & Walters, D.G. (1983). Effect of di-n-pentyl phthalate treatment on testicular steroidogenic enzymes and cytochrome P450 in the rat. *Tox. Lett.*, **15**, 265–71.

Friedman, L., Weinberger, M.A., Farber, T.M., Moreland, F.M., Peters, E.L., Gilmore, C.E. & Khan, M.A. (1979). Testicular atrophy and impaired spermatogenesis in rats fed high levels of the methyl xanthines caffeine, theobromine or theophylline. *J. Environ. Pathol. Toxicol.*, **2**, 687–706.

Garside, D., Craig, P. & Cook, B.A. (1985). Evidence for a Sertoli cell factor(s) affecting Leydig cell functions *in vitro*. *J. Endoc.*, **107**, abs. 124.

Gartner, K., Reznik-Schuller, H. & Reznik, G. (1973). The influence of overcrowding on spermatogenesis, size of Leydig cell nuclei (histometrical investigation) and the adrenal corticosterone contents in mice. *Acta. Endocrinol.*, **74**, 783–91.

Glode, L.M., Robinson, J. & Gould, S.F. (1981). Protection from cyclophosphamide-induced testicular damage with an analogue of gonadotrophin releasing hormone. *Lancet*, **i**, 1132–4.

Goodpasture, J.C., Bergstrom, K. & Vickery, B.H. (1988). Potentiation of the gonadotoxicity of cytoxan in the dog by adjuvant treatment with a hormone luteinising releasing hormone agonist. *Cancer Res.*, **48**, 2174–8.

Gower, D.B. (1979). *Steroid Hormones*. London: Croom and Helm.

Gradishar, W.J. & Schilsky, R.L. (1988). Effects of cancer treatment on the reproductive system. *Crit. Rev. Oncol. Haematol.*, **8**, 153–71.

Gray, T.J. & Butterworth, K.R. (1980). Testicular atrophy produced by phthalate esters. *Arch. Tox. Suppl.*, **4**, 452–5.

Gray, T.J., Rowland, I.R., Foster, P.M. & Gangolli, S.D. (1982). Species differences in the testicular toxicity and phthalate esters. *Tox. Lett.*, **11**, 141–7.

Grayhock, J., Brume, P., Keorns, J. & Scott, W. (1955). Influence of pituitary on prostatic response to androgens in rat. *Bull. John Hopkins Hosp.*, **8**, 96–154.

Gunn, S.A., Gould, T.C. & Anderson, W. (1963). Cadmium-induced interstitial cell tumours in rats and mice and their prevention by zinc. *J. Nat. Cancer Inst.*, **31**, 745.

Hadley, A.J., Flack, J.D. & Buckingham, J.C. (1990). Modulation of corticotrophin release *in vitro* by methylxanthines and adenosine analogues. *Br.J.Pharmacol.*, **100** (Supl.), p. 337.

Hadley, A.J., Flack, J.D. & Buckingham, J.C. (1991). Selective phosphodiesterase inhibitors and the release *in vitro* of corticotrophin (ACTH) and luteinising hormone (LH). *Br.J.Pharmacol.* (Supl.), Proceedings of Glasgow Meeting, 10–12th July 1991. (In press.)

Hall, P., Charpannier, C., Nakamura, M. & Gabbioni, G. (1979). Role of microfilaments in response of Leydig cell to LH. *J. St. Biochem.*, **11**, 1361.

Hasson, V., Ritzen, E., French, F. & Nayfeh, S. (1975). In *Handbook of Physiology*, vol. 5, ed. E. Knobil & J.D. Neill, pp. 173–201. New York: Raven Press.

IARC (1973). *Monographs on the Evaluation of Carcinogenic Risk of Chemicals to Man*, volume 2. Lyon: WHO.

Jackson, H. & Schneiden, H. (1982). Aspects of male reproductive pharmacology and toxicology. *Rev. Pure Appl. Pharm. Sci.*, **3**, 1–81.

Johnson, A.D., Sigman, M.B. & Miller, W.J. (1970). Early actions of cadmium in the rat and domestic fowl testis. III. Subcellular localisation of injected $^{109}$cadmium. *J. Reprod. Fert.*, **23**, 201.

Johnson, L. & Neaves, W. (1981). Age related changes in Leydig cell population: sperm production. *Biol. Reprod.* **24**, 703–12.

Kamel, F. & Kubajak, C.L. (1987). Modulation of gonadotropin secretion by corticosterone; interaction with gonadal steroids and mechanism of action. *Endocrinology*, **121**, 561–8.

Karashima, T., Zalatnai, A. & Schally, A.V. (1988). Protective effect of luteinising hormone releasing hormone against chemotherapy-induced testicular damage in rats. *Proc. Nat. Acad. Sci. (USA)*, **85**, 2329–33.

Katangole, C., Naftolin, F. & Short, R. (1971). Relationship between LH and testosterone and effects on sexual stimulation. *J. Endoc.*, **50**, 457.

de Kretser D.M. & Ker, J.B. (1988). The testis: structure and function. In *Physiology of Reproduction*, p. 867. New York: Raven Press.

Landing, B.H., Goldin, A., Noe, H.A., Taylor, J.B., Fugmann, R.A., Goldberg, B. & Fisk, A.J. (1949). Testicular lesions in mice following parenteral administration of nitrogen mustard. *Cancer*, **2**, 1075–84.

Li, C. & Evans, H. (1948). In *The Hormones*, vol. 1, ed. G. Pincus & K. Thimann, p. 631. New York: Academic Press.

Liu, R., Garside, D., Jones, H., Roberts, J. & Gray, T. (1988). Characterisation of the effects of 4 phthalate esters on rat Leydig cells *in vitro*. *J. Endoc.*, **117** (Suppl.), Abst. 222.

Mancini, R.E., Lavieri, J.C., Muller, F., Andrada, J.A. & Saraceni, D.J. (1966). Effect of prednisolone upon normal and pathologic human spermatogenesis. *Fertil. Steril.*, **17**, 500–13.

Mattill, H. & Carman, J. (1922/3). Degeneration of the testis in vitamin E deficient rats. *Proc. Soc. Exp. Biol.*, **20**, 420.

Mears, A. & Vaituleaitis, J. (1972). Peptide hormone receptors; specific binding of FSH to testis. *Endocrinology*, **90**, 39–46.

Meistrich, M., Hughes, T. & Bruce, W. (1975). Alteration of epididymal sperm transport and maturation in mice by oestrogen and testosterone. *Nature*, **258**, 145–7.

Mattison, D.R., Plowchalk, D.R., Meadows, M.J., Al-Juburi, A.Z., Gandy, J. & Malek, A. (1990). Reproductive toxicity: male and female reproductive system as targets for chemical injury. *Med. Clinics. North. Am.*, **74**, 391–411.

Mori, H. (1988). Testicular interstitial cell tumours in experimental animals. *Exp. Pathol.*, **33**, 1.

Morris, I.D. & Shalet, S.M. (1989). Endocrine mediated protection from cytotoxic induced testicular damage. *J. Endocrinol.*, **120**, 7–9.

Morris, I.D. & Shalet, S.M. (1990). Protection of gonad function from cytotoxic chemotherapy and irradiation. *Baillieres Clin. Endocrinol. Metab.*, **4**, 97–118.

Murphy, K.M. & Snyder, S.H. (1981). Adenosine receptors in rat testes: labelling with $^{3}$H-cyclohexyl adenosine. *Life Sci.*, **28**, 917.

Nalbandov, A. (1976). In *Reproduction Physiology of Mammals and Birds*, pp. 220–40. Freeman & Co.

Nath, R., Prasad, R., Palinal, V.K. & Chopra, R.K. (1984). Molecular basis of cadmium toxicity. *Prog. Food Nutr. Sci.*, **8**, 109–64.

Nseyo, U.O., Huben, R.P., Klioze, S.S. & Portes, J.E. (1985). Protection of germinal epithelium with luteinising hormone releasing hormone analogue. *J. Urology*, **134**, 187–90.

Oishi, S. (1985). Reversibility of testicular atrophy induced by di-(2-ethylhexyl) phthalate in rats. *Environ. Res.*, **36**, 160–9.

Orgebin-Crist, M. (1969). Studies on the function of epididymis. *Biol. Reprod.*, **1**, 155–75.

Parmar, D., Srivastava, S.P., Singh, G.B. & Seth, P.K. (1987). Effect of testosterone on the testicular atrophy caused by di-(2-ethylhexyl) phthalate (DEHP). *Tox. Lett.*, **36**, 297–308.

Parvinen, M. & Ruokonen, A. (1982). Endogenous steroids in rat seminiferous tubule. *J. Androl.*, **3**, 211–20.

Pelliniemi, L., Dym, M., Gunsalas, G., Musto, N. & Hansson, V. (1981). Immunocytochemical localisation of ABP in the male rat. *Biol. Reprod.*, **108**, 925–31.

Phillips, J.C., Foster, P.M.D. & Gangolli, S.D. (1985). Chemically-induced injury to the male reproductive tract. In *Endocrine Toxicology*, ed. J.A. Thomas, K.S. Korach & J.A. McLauchlan, pp. 117–34. New York: Raven Press.

Piscator, M. (1981). Role of cadmium in carcinogenesis with special reference to cancer of the prostate. *Env. Health Perspectives*, **40**, 107–20.

Ragan, H.A. & Mast, T.J. (1990). Cadmium inhalation and male reproductive toxicity. *Rev. Env. Contam. Tox.*, **114**, 1–22.

Robaire, B., Sheer, H. & Hachey, C. (1981). In *Bioregulations of Reproduction*, ed. G. Jagillo & H. Vogel, pp. 487–98. New York: Academic Press.

Schilsky, R.L. (1989). Male fertility following cancer chemotherapy. *J. Clin. Oncol.*, **7**, 295–7.

Sertoli, E. (1865). Dell eristezia di particolai cellulae ramificate nai canalicoli seminiferi del testicolo. *Morgagni*, **7**, 31–9.

Sever, L.E. & Hessol, N.A. (1985). Toxic effects of occupational and environmental chemicals on the testes. In *Endocrine Toxicology*, ed. J.A. Thomas, K.S. Korach & J. McLachlan, pp. 211–48. New York: Raven Press.

Shalet, S.M. (1983). Disorders of the endocrine system due to radiation and cytotoxic chemotherapy. *Clin. Endocrinol.*, **19**, 637–59.

Sharpe, R. (1984). Intratesticular factors controlling testicular function. *Biol. Reprod.*, **30**, 29.

Shulze, C. (1984). Sertoli and Leydig cells in man. *Adv. Anat. Embryol. Cell Biol.*, **88**, 1–104.

Singhal, R.L., Vijayvargiya, R. & Shukla, G.S. (1985). Toxic effects of cadmium and lead on reproductive functions. In *Endocrine Toxicology*, ed. J.A. Thomas, K.S. Korach & J.A. McLachlan, pp. 149–80. New York: Raven Press.

Soball, Z. (1984). Morphology of human testis in various periods of life. *Folia Morphol.*, **23**, 102–11.

Spindel, E., Griffiths, L. & Wurtman, R.J. (1983). Neuroendocrine effects of caffeine. II. Effects on thyrotropin and corticosterone secretion. *J. Pharmacol. Exp. Ther.*, **225**, 346–50.

Spindel, E. (1984). Action of methylxanthines on the pituitary and pituitary-dependent hormones. *Prog. Clin. Biol. Res.*, **158**, 355–63.

Spindel, E., Wurtman, R.J., McCall, A., Carr, D.B., Conlay, L., Griffith, L. & Arnold, M.A. (1984). Neuroendocrine effects of caffeine in normal subjects. *Clin. Pharmacol. Ther.*, **36**, 402–7.

Srivastava, S., Singh, G.B., Srivastava, S.P. & Seth, P.K. (1990a). Testicular toxicity of di-n-butyl phthalate in adult rats; effect on marker enzymes of spermatogenesis. *Indian J. Exp. Biol.*, **28**, 67–70.

Srivastava, S.P., Srivastava, S., Saxena, D.K., Chandra, S.V. & Seth, P.K. (1990b). Testicular effects of di-n-butyl phthalate (DBP): biochemical and histopathological alterations. *Arch. Tox.*, **64**, 148–52.

Stiles, G.L. (1986). Adenosine receptors: structure, function and regulation. *Trends in Pharm. Sci.*, December 1986, 486–90.

Tarka, S.M., Zoumas, B.L. & Gans, J.H. (1979). Short-term effects of graded levels of theobromine in laboratory rodents. *Toxicol. Appl. Pharmacol.*, **49**, 127.

Thomas, J.A. & Thomas, M.J. (1984). Biological effects of di-(2-ethylhexyl) phthalate and other phthalic acid esters. *CRC Crit. Rev. Toxicol.*, **13**, 283–317.

Tindall, D., Miller, D. & Means, A. (1977). Characterisation of androgen receptor in Sertoli cell enriched testis. *Endocrinology*, **101**, 13–23.

Tsutsui, K. & Ishii, S. (1978). Effects of FSH and testosterone on receptors of FSH in the testis. *Gen. Comp. Endoc.*, **36**, 297–305.

Verhoeven, G. & Cailleau, J. (1985). A factor in spent media from Sertoli cell-enriched cultures that stimulate steroidogenesis in Leydig cells. *Mol. Cell. Endoc.*, **40**, 57–68.

Verhoeven, G., Kaninckx, P. & de Moor, P. (1982). *In vitro* culture of testicular cells. *J. St. Biochem.*, **17**, 319–30.

Vernon, R., Kopec, B. & Fritz, I. (1974). Observations of binding of androgen by rat testis, seminiferous tubule and testis extracts. *Mol. Cell Endoc.*, **1**, 167–87.

Wams, T.J. (1987). Diethylhexyl phthalate as an environmental contaminant – a review. *Sci. Total Environ.*, **66**, 1–16.

Waxman, J. (1983). Chemotherapy and the adult gonad: a review. *J. Royal Soc. Med.*, **76**, 144–8.

C.A. WILSON AND A.J. LEIGH

# 10 Endocrine toxicology of the female reproductive system

## Introduction

The endocrine control of the female reproductive system is complex, involving a wide variety of hormones and neuroendocrine factors that interrelate to effect the successful production of mature gametes in a benign propagative environment. Due to the delicate balance required to successfully co-ordinate these processes, any fluctuation in one aspect or factor can have far ranging consequences on the whole system. However, it should be noted that a number of agents appear to have similar or synergistic functions, and so there may be a physiological 'fail-safe' built into the regulatory mechanisms underlying the control of reproduction.

The first part of this review comprises a summary of the endocrinology and neuroendocrinology of normal female reproductive physiology, and is followed by some of the natural perturbations that can arise as a consequence of abnormal hormonal secretion. In the latter part of the review, the effects of drugs on the female reproductive system will be surveyed. These will include: (a) steroid hormones that are used to modulate reproductive function and have toxic effects on other systems; (b) toxic agents present as hazards in the environment and (c) drugs which have detrimental side-effects on the reproductive system.

Effects of these agents on embryonic and foetal development will not be included as they have been comprehensively covered elsewhere (Howard & Hill, 1979; Barlow & Sullivan 1982; Cetrulo & Sbarra, 1984; Kurzel & Cetrulo, 1985; Randall, 1987; Hawkins, 1987; Roubenoff *et al.*, 1988; Katter, 1988).

## Neuroendocrinology and endocrinology of the female reproductive system

### The hypothalamic-pituitary-gonadal axis

The pivot of the reproductive system is the gonad, which has two major functions: (i) to produce a viable gamete for fertilization, and (ii) to synthesize and secrete hormones which will maintain the remainder of the reproductive system, and stimulate the secondary sex characteristics. The reproductive system is controlled by the so-called 'hypothalamo-pituitary unit', where neurones within the basal hypothalamus secrete a decapeptide-gonadotrophin releasing hormone (GnRH) in a pulsatile fashion into the hypophyseal portal system to act on the specific receptors on the gonadotrophs in the anterior pituitary gland. The GnRH stimulates the release of the gonadotrophin hormones: luteinizing hormone (LH) and follicle stimulating hormone (FSH). These two hormones, together with prolactin, act in their turn on specific receptors in the ovary to stimulate the production of steroid hormones, and also to induce changes in the ovary leading ultimately to ovulation and gamete release.

Figure 10.1 depicts the inter-relationship of the hypothalamus, pituitary and ovary, and shows that the gonadal steroids can influence their own secretion by autoregulatory feedback effects at both the hypothalamic and pituitary levels. In most situations this is a negative feedback effect, either inhibiting the release of GnRH from the hypothalamus, or desensitizing the pituitary to the action of GnRH by reducing GnRH receptor density. Oestrogen and progesterone, however, can exert a positive feedback effect as well. This occurs only transiently under specific endocrine conditions. In general, a positive feedback stimulates a dramatic but transient increase in gonadotrophin release and occurs when circulatory oestradiol levels are above a critical concentration (200 pg/ml in women, 60 pg/ml in rats) for a critical length of time (48 hours in women). Progesterone antagonizes the stimulatory effect of the oestrogen if elevated concomitantly, but potentiates the positive feedback effect if it rises sequentially. In rodents and non-human primates the time of the positive feedback effect is influenced by the circadian light–dark cycle, probably mediated by melatonin from the pineal gland and/or serotonergic neuronal systems within the central nervous system (CNS).

The steroids exert their stimulatory effect on gonadotrophin secretion by enhancing the release of GnRH from the hypothalamus, and increasing the sensitivity of the pituitary gland toward GnRH. At the pituitary level, the steroids alter the $\beta$max (density) but not the Kd (affinity) of the GnRH receptors, and in this way modulate the response of the pituitary. Normally, GnRH receptors are only present on about 60% of the pituitary gonadotrophs, but in the presence of high levels of oestradiol (as on the day of proestrous in the rat), GnRH receptors can be detected on all of the gonadotrophs. At the hypothalamic level, it is unlikely that the steroids influence GnRH neurones directly, as there are no (or very low levels of) steroid receptors on either the perikarya or the nerve terminals; instead the steroids exert their effects via a variety of neuronal systems

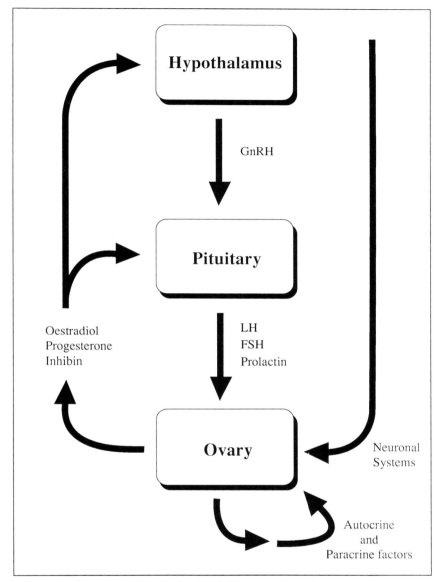

Fig. 10.1. The hypothalamic-pituitary-ovarian axis.

located in close anatomical proximity to the GnRH neurones. Examples of the transmitters in such systems include the amines (catecholamines, 5-hydroxytryptamine (5-HT), acetylcholine and histamine), amino-acids (Gamma-aminobutyric acid (GABA) and glutamate) as well as a number of peptide transmitter systems (vasoactive intestinal peptide (VIP), neuropeptide Y (NPY) and the endogenous opioids).

The positive feedback effect of the steroids is an important component of female reproductive function, since it forms the basis of the cyclical oestrus or menstrual changes seen in all female mammals (Johnson & Everitt 1988; Ojeda 1988).

## The ovary

The ovary is an ovoid mass of connective tissue (and stroma) situated dorsally in the peritoneal cavity and secured by a suspensory ligament. It is enveloped by the fallopian tube (or oviduct) which is a muscular tube continuous with the uterine lumen. Embedded within the tissue are spherical structures, called follicles, and within each follicle is a female gamete (oocyte, ovum or egg). All of the oocytes the female will ever possess are present in the ovary early in foetal development, and their nuclei exist arrested in the diplotene stage of the meiotic prophase. In the human, there are seven million oocytes at week 28 of foetal development. However, there are continuous losses, with the death of both the oocyte and its surrounding follicle, and thus, at birth the number is reduced to approximately two million, and by seven years of age a further substantial reduction to approximately 400,000 has occurred. Of these, only 0.1% (400) with the potential for fertilization will ever be released from the human ovary. The egg, together with its surrounding follicular tissue, is known as the primordial follicle, and in its most immature state, consists of a few rows of cells surrounding the egg. Cohorts of these structures develop spontaneously at intervals (a process designated recruitment) and pass into the pre-antral stage. At this point, stromal cells condense around the follicle forming a wall, the theca, which possesses LH receptors. Any further follicular development requires the presence of critical concentrations of LH and FSH, and if pre-antral follicles are formed when the gonadotrophins are below this critical value, then they become atresic, and both the follicles and the eggs within them degenerate. This accounts for the apparent wastage of gametes evident throughout the reproductive life of the female. Eventually, after about 40 years, all of the follicles are lost and the ovary ceases to function.

If the gonadotrophin levels are above the appropriate critical concentration at the time that a new wave of pre-antral follicles is developing, these will then continue to mature under the influence of the gonadotrophins, and will pass into the antral-preovulatory stage. The theca develops an inner and an outer wall, and becomes vascularized. The follicle enlarges and the cells within it, that is the granulosa cells, proliferate, but at no time do they receive a blood supply. Although proliferation continues, eventually the granulosa cells are unable to keep pace with the enlargement of the follicle, thus giving rise to a cavity, which becomes filled with the fluid secreted by the granulosa cells. As the follicle matures, developing into a Graafian follicle, it moves towards the periphery of the ovary, where it visibly protrudes. The oocyte, which has enlarged slightly, is now surrounded by a tough translucent shell called the zona pellucida, formed from secretions of the granulosa cells. At this time, the egg lies in the follicular lumen, and is surrounded by a thin layer of granulosa cells, which anchor it to the main bulk of the granulosa tissue in a stalk-like manner. Some of these cells in close proximity with the egg possess amoeboid-like processes which actually pass into the body of the egg and perform a supportive function, supplying it with nutrients. In the human, usually only one follicle is selected to progress to this stage, the dominant follicle, and it is this structure that is responsible for the secretion of oestradiol in the late follicular phase (in the rat, which is a multiovulator, a large number of follicles (8–12) reach this stage of maturation simultaneously).

Thus, an important function of the follicle is the maintenance of the oocyte. An additional important function is the production of steroids which prepare the remainder of the reproductive tract to support the egg in the event of fertilization occurring. Although both functions are primarily mediated by the pituitary gonadotrophins, a number of other agents are produced by granulosa cells under the influence of LH and FSH which act to modulate their activity; these include growth factors and peptide hormones. In addition, the ovary is innervated by a sympathetic, parasympathetic and peptidergic nervous supply, which also act to regulate follicular functions.

An oocyte is released from a mature Graafian follicle in each reproductive cycle in the process of ovulation, in which the follicle ruptures and the egg passes out of the ovary and into the peritoneum. It is now swept up in fluid movements caused by cilial movement of the oviductal fimbria, and in this way is conducted into the oviductal lumen. In the human, usually only one follicle ruptures in each cycle, whilst in rodents 8–12 ovulations occur concomitantly.

The granulosa cells in the ruptured follicle now differentiate into luteal cells (luteinization); they hypertrophy and become spherical with increased content of lipid, endoplasmic reticulum, and Golgi systems, and the structure as a whole takes on an opaque yellowish hue, giving rise to what is known as the corpus luteum (yellow body). The vascularization which was previously limited to the theca now penetrates through to supply the luteal cells. Like the follicle, it is capable of steroidogenesis, and the production of a number of peptides. If fertilization does not occur, the corpus luteum has only a limited life-span (of approximately 14 days in the human, 36 hours in the rat), after which time in humans, if hormonal support in the form of human chorionic gonadotrophin (hCG) is not forthcoming from a fertilized ovum, it becomes senescent and regresses (Austin & Short, 1982; Haney, 1985; Johnson & Everitt, 1988; Sakai & Hodgen, 1988; Cooper *et al.*, 1989b).

### Hormonal changes in the reproductive cycle

The pattern of plasma concentrations of the gonadotrophins and the gonadal steroids during the menstrual cycle in the human and the oestrous cycle in the rat are illustrated in Figs 10.2A and 10.2B, where it can be seen that the pattern of changes is similar, the major difference lying in the relative time-courses of the cycles.

Describing the menstrual cycle first, this has a normal duration of $28\pm7$ days, and in the first half, the steroids are produced by the follicles, hence this is known as the follicular phase of the cycle. At mid-cycle (around day 14), ovulation occurs, and in the second half of the cycle the role of steroid production devolves upon the corpus luteum, thus giving rise to the appelation of luteal phase. By convention, the first day of menstruation is taken as day 1 of the cycle, and at this time the plasma steroids are low. Thus, they exert only a weak negative feedback effect on pituitary gonadotrophin release, such that plasma concentrations of LH and FSH are marginally higher than at other times of basal release. These slightly elevated levels are of sufficient magnitude to stimulate the maturation of any wave of follicles that have spontaneously passed from the primordial to the pre-antral stage of development. The follicles therefore start to grow, and under the influence of the gonadotrophins secrete oestradiol. LH receptors develop on the thecal cells, and, acting here, LH stimulates – via cyclic adenosine monophosphate (cAMP) – the relevant cytochrome P450 enzymes that cleave the cholesterol side-chain to produce androgens and progesterone (Johnson & Everitt, 1988; Richards & Hedin, 1988). LH receptor density is enhanced by prolactin (Advis, Aguado & Ojeda, 1983) which, therefore, sensitizes the follicle towards the action of LH. FSH receptors develop on the granulosa cells and acting here, FSH stimulates the aromatizing enzyme that effects the conversion of androgens to oestradiol. This oestradiol induces the proliferation of the granulosa cells and as these all possess further FSH receptors, the structure as a whole becomes sensitized to FSH. Thus, although the rising levels of oestradiol exert a negative feedback effect on gonadotrophin release, the follicles still retain the capacity to respond to the reduced circulating concentrations. Oestradiol also induces the production of its

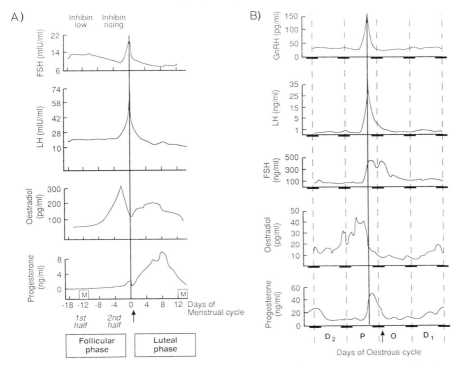

Fig. 10.2. Serum hormone levels during (A) the human menstrual cycle, (B) the rat oestrous cycle. The arrows indicate the time of ovulation. Fig. 10.2A. Day 0 taken as day of the pre-ovulatory surge. M, menstruation. Fig. 10.2B. Day of the oestrous cycle: proestrus (P); oestrus (O); first day of dioestrus (D1); second day of dioestrus (D2).

own receptors on the granulosa cells, and at this point, oestradiol and FSH act in unison to induce a new set of LH receptors on the granulosa cells (Richards & Farookhi, 1978; Erickson, 1986). The proliferative and differentiating effects of FSH and oestrogen on granulosa cells may be mediated, at least in part, by insulin-like growth factor (IGF-I), since the two hormones stimulate the secretion of the latter by the granulosa cells. IGF-I, acting via specific receptors on the granulosa cells, promotes replication of the cells, and enhances the activity of FSH in stimulating cAMP, progesterone and oestrogen production and inducing LH receptors. It also enhances LH activity on the thecal cells in stimulating androgen and progesterone synthesis (Hammond *et al.*, 1985; Davoren *et al.*, 1986; Adashi *et al.*, 1986; 1989).

Other growth factors may also act to modulate these effects, for instance, epidermal growth factor (EGF) is produced by the thecal cells, and there are EGF receptors present in thecal, granulosa and luteal cells. FSH increases EGF receptor numbers, and EGF stimulates IGF-I production and protein synthesis in granulosa cells; it is, however, inhibitory to steroidogenesis (Hsueh, Welsh & Jones, 1981; Chabot et al., 1986; Feng, Knecht & Catt, 1987). Transforming growth factor β (TGF-β) has a dual effect on FSH activity, potentiating low concentrations of FSH and inhibiting high concentrations in the stimulation of cAMP, steroidogenesis and LH receptor induction, TGF-β also inhibits LH-induced progesterone and androgen production by thecal cells (Dodson & Schomberg, 1987; see Tonetta & diZerega, 1989).

The granulosa cells produce a further range of peptidergic agents that influence follicular differentiation and steroidogenesis. These include:

(a)  Gonadocrinin – a GnRH-like peptide. Exogenous GnRH or its agonist analogues stimulate the basal secretion of prostaglandin E (PG-E) and progesterone in follicular tissue; the PG-E mediates the steroidogenic action of GnRH. The peptide also stimulates oocyte meiosis, and ovulation by a direct ovarian action, as it can act in hypophysectomized rats in vivo (Ekholm et al., 1982). In situations in which ovarian function is stimulated by gonadotrophin preparations, however, administration of GnRH either in vivo or in vitro inhibits the formation of LH and prolactin receptors on the granulosa cells and production of progesterone, androgens and oestrogen (Behrman, Preston & Hall, 1980; Magoffin, Reynolds & Erickson, 1981). Both the stimulatory and inhibitory effects are exerted via specific GnRH receptors. The stimulatory effect is mediated via protein kinase C (PKC) and calcium ion mobilization, and the inhibitory effect by functional uncoupling of the LH-receptor complex from adenyl cyclase (Kawai & Clark, 1986). In the normal physiological state, the circulating levels of GnRH are too low to exert an ovarian effect. The fact that ovarian GnRH receptors exist (at least in the rat, and human luteal cells) is indicative of the fact that GnRH may be produced locally. A small peptide (<3500 daltons) called gonadocrinin has now been isolated in rat, bovine, porcine, and human follicular fluid with GnRH-like activity, but an immunological and physical structure distinct from that of hypothalamic GnRH (Ying et al., 1981).

(b)  Inhibin, activin, and follistatin – inhibin is a heterodimer with the α and β subunits linked by disulphide bonds. There are two forms of the β subunit; β-A and β-B, either of which may be coupled to an α subunit to give rise to inhibin A or B, respectively. They are synthesized by the granulosa cells, and production is stimulated by FSH and oestradiol. In the human menstrual cycle, levels are constant in the follicular phase, and increase slightly over the period of ovulation, following which they rise further (by approximately three fold) to a peak in the mid-luteal phase, and finally decline as the corpus luteum regresses. Both inhibin A and B act similarly at the level of the pituitary, where they have an inhibitory action on the release of FSH, and are thus implicated in the modification of follicular maturation. Inhibin may also have a role in the process of ovulation, since it has been shown to enhance LH activity. The function of inhibin in the luteal phase is as yet unknown. Dimers of the β subunit, that is β-A–β-A and β-B–β-B, have been identified and are called Activin A and Activin B, respectively. These are antagonistic to inhibin in that they have a stimulatory effect on pituitary FSH release, and reduce LH activity. Another component of follicular fluid recently isolated is a protein which has been called follistatin. This is distinct from inhibin, but acts in a similar fashion, generating an inhibitory input to pituitary FSH release (Tonetta & diZerega, 1989).

(c)  Gonadotrophin surge attenuating factor (GnSAF) – this is a peptide produced mainly by small ovarian follicles. It acts at the level of the pituitary to attenuate the response to GnRH. There is a possibility that GnSAF may be involved in the 'fine tuning' of the timing of the preovulatory LH surge since it has been found to antagonize the positive feed-back effect of oestrogen and the self-priming action of GnRH, thus suppressing pituitary responsiveness in the presence of high oestradiol concentrations in the follicular phase. This suppressive effect is overcome when oestrogen levels surpass a threshold value for a critical period of time (see section *The hypothalamic-pituitary-gonadal axis* and below) (Fowler, Messinis & Templeton, 1990; Whitehead, 1990).

There are numerous other regulators controlling ovarian and oocyte function and response. These include oocyte maturation inhibitors (which

322  C.A. WILSON AND A.J. LEIGH

may be hypoxanthene and/or a phosphoprotein), meiosis promoting factors (which may be two proteins of 34 and 45 Kd), inhibitors of FSH and LH binding, a luteinizing stimulator and an inhibitor (Tsafriri, 1988).

At mid-cycle, circulating levels of oestradiol rise rapidly, and when plasma concentrations rise above 200 pg/ml, and are sustained for a critical period of 48 hours, the oestradiol ceases to exert a negative feedback input on pituitary gonadotrophin release, and instead actually stimulates a transient LH release, and to a lesser degree, FSH release. Throughout the menstrual cycle, GnRH and thus LH are released in a pulsatile manner at a frequency of approximately one pulse per hour. At mid-cycle the pulse amplitude and frequency increases. This change in signal output is essential to ovulation, and the high levels of LH acting on the newly induced LH receptors in the granulosa cells cause a number of important changes in the follicle and egg (Johnson & Everitt, 1988).

Firstly, as soon as the LH binds to its receptors on the granulosa cells, the FSH and oestradiol receptors disappear, causing a cessation of oestradiol production and a subsequent precipitous fall in plasma levels. Activation of the LH receptors on the granulosa cells, however, stimulates progesterone production, which is immediately detectable as a small rise in the circulation. According to a recent review (Smith, 1989), this LH-induced progesterone elicits the resumption of meiosis in the oocyte by reducing the activity of the meiosis-inhibitory-phosphoprotein (via reduction of both cAMP and inositol triphosphate activity), and thus allowing the meiosis promoting factor to induce completion of the first meiotic division and formation of the first polar body. Alternatively, the LH-induced maturation of the oocyte may be mediated by one of a number of growth factors, since IGF-I, TGF-$\beta$ and EGF can all stimulate meiosis (Dekel & Sherizly, 1985; Tsafriri, 1988).

Secondly, the LH surge stimulates an increase in plasminogen activator, both of the tissue type (tPA) produced by the granulosa cells, and of the urokinase type (uPA) produced by the theca. Both types are required for successful ovulation, and their function is to activate collagenase and thus bring about a weakening of the thecal wall (Reich, Miskin & Tsafriri, 1986; Canipari & Strickland, 1986). Thirdly, the LH activates prostaglandin synthetase (cyclo-oxygenase) and stimulates the production of prostaglandin F2-$\alpha$ (PGF2-$\alpha$) which acts on the thecal cells, causing them to contract (Lindner et al., 1980; Hedin et al., 1987). Preliminary data suggest that LH also stimulates phospholipase $A_2$ (Wilson & Bonney, 1990) which causes the release of the prostaglandin precursor, arachidonic acid, thus also facilitating prostaglandin production. (Summarized in Table 10.1.)

Ovulation has been compared to an inflammatory process, in that there

Table 10.1. *Actions of the pre-ovulatory luteinizing hormone (LH) surge*

| Effect of LH surge | | Result of change |
| --- | --- | --- |
| (1) FSH and oestradiol receptors on granulosa cells disappear | → | Cessation of oestradiol synthesis |
| (2) Progesterone synthesis increased | → | Stimulates resumption of meoisis of ovum |
| | → | Increased vascularization from theca to granulosa cells |
| (3) Increase in levels of IGF-I, TGF-β, EGF | → | Stimulates resumption of meoisis of ovum |
| (4) Increase in tPAF (from granulosa cells) and uPAF (from theca) | → | Weakens the thecal wall of the follicle |
| (5) Stimulates prostaglandin synthetase and possibly phospholipase $A_2$ | → | Stimulates prostaglandin production which causes contraction of the thecal wall |

FSH = follicle stimulating hormone; IGF = insulin-like growth factor; TGF-β = transforming growth factor; EGF = epidermal growth factor; tPAF = tissue platelet activator factor; uPAF = urokinase platelet activator factor.

is a rise in the ovary of many of the classical mediators of inflammation, such as prostaglandins, histamine and bradykinin, and there is also an influx of monocytes and lymphocytes (Espey, 1980). These cells also produce inflammatory mediators – the cytokines – and there is a rise in plasma levels of interleukin 1 (IL-1) at the time of follicular rupture (Cannon & Dinarello, 1985). It is possible that these agents are all involved in the process of ovulation, perhaps as back-up mechanisms. Histamine, for instance, can cause follicular rupture, acting on Histamine 1 and Histamine 2 receptors independently of the prostaglandins (Schmidt, Owman & Sjoberg, 1986).

After ovulation, the corpus luteum is formed from proliferating and enlarged granulosa cells, and the theca becomes highly vascularized. This may be under the autocrine control of fibroblast growth factor (FGF), which is secreted by luteal cells and has both mitogenic and angiogenic properties (Tonetta & diZerega, 1989). Blood vessels extend from theca into the granulosa cells and this is the first step in their conversion to luteal cells. Recent evidence suggests this vascularization is induced by the increase in progesterone at the time of the LH surge (Collins, pers. comm.).

The corpus luteum produces high levels of progesterone and also oestradiol, although oestradiol levels in the luteal phase never reach those seen in the first half of the cycle. Low levels of LH and prolactin are responsible for the maintenance of the corpus luteum. If fertilization does not take place, the corpus luteum regresses. The exact mechanism by which this occurs is not clear, but it has been suggested that the corpus luteum synthesizes oxytocin, which, in low concentrations, enhances steroidogenesis, but in higher concentrations stimulates the *in situ* production of PGF2-α (Flint & Sheldrick, 1982; Whathes, Swann & Pickering, 1984; Geenen *et al.*, 1985). In many species (including rodents), PGF2-α produced by the uterine endometrium is known to be the prime luteolytic factor; in humans it may also play a luteolytic role, but is produced locally within the ovary rather than the uterus. The PGF2-α acts by uncoupling the LH receptor complex from adenyl cyclase and prevents the usual functional outcome (Lindner *et al.*, 1980).

The control of the ovary also involves a sympathetic neuronal component, and interruption of the afferent neural supply to the ovary induces alterations in follicular maturation, steroid levels, and ovarian blood flow. The ovary is innervated by the sympathetic system with the sympathetic nerve terminals surrounding the blood vessels of the external theca of the follicles. Noradrenaline (NA) from these terminals acting on β-2 receptors causes an increase in cAMP, progesterone and androgen production, but not oestrogen. FSH, corticosterone and prolactin can enhance the effect of NA at a site distal to cAMP on the activity of the enzyme 3-β-hydroxysteroid dehydrogenase. Levels of NA increase in the follicular fluid at mid-cycle, and may play a role in the rupture of the follicle, since NA causes contraction of the thecal walls (mediated by both α and β adrenoceptors). It may also mediate the luteinization of the granulosa cells (Spicer, 1986; Bahr & Ben-Jonathan, 1985; Perkins, Cronin & Veldhuis, 1986).

Cholinergic nerves innervate the follicular wall, and acting on nicotinic receptors, inhibit FSH-induced steroidogenesis, however, acting on muscarinic receptors, acetylcholine can stimulate progesterone and oxytocin secretion in luteinized granulosa cells *in vitro* (Kasson & Hsueh, 1985; Luck, 1990). There are also two peptidergic tracts influencing the ovary. A VIP tract entering via the superior ovarian nerve, and a substance P tract via the ovarian plexus. The former stimulates aromatase activity in granulosa cells, and the latter, which innervates the interstitial cells, theca and blood vessels, may be important for its vasodilator effects (Dees, Ahmed & Ojeda, 1986; Ojeda, Urbanski & Ahmed, 1986).

Experiments in which hypothalamic stimulation has been used to induce steroidogenesis independently of the pituitary hormones indicate that there is a direct neural link between the hypothalamus and the ovary (Burden *et al.*, 1986).

In the follicular phase of the menstrual cycle, oestradiol causes proliferation of the uterine endometrium and induces progesterone receptors. In the second part of the cycle, progesterone increases the vascularity of the endometrium and stimulates secretory glands to produce glycoprotein nutrients ready to maintain the fertilized ovum should it appear in the uterine lumen. In the absence of fertilization, the corpus luteum regresses, and there is a fall in steroid production, and the uterine endometrium is no longer maintained. The arteries supplying the tissue undergo alternate contractions and dilatations which weaken the walls. During the constrictory phase, the surrounding tissue becomes anoxic and dies, and during the dilatatory phase blood escapes from the vessels and sloughs off the dead tissue. The endometrium synthesizes prostaglandins at this time, which act on the myometrium causing contractions which facilitate expulsion of the debris. This passes out, together with the blood as the menstrual flow over a period of three to five days (Yen, 1986).

In comparison to the human, the rat oestrous cycle lasts only four or five days. The profiles of the reproductive hormones, however, are similar in many ways. Over dioestrus, a wave of follicles matures and begins to secrete oestradiol, thus causing a rise in plasma levels which reach a peak on the early afternoon of proestrus. This stimulates an LH surge, which occurs in the late afternoon of proestrus, the exact time being subject to the influence of the diurnal light–dark cycle. Ovulation of eight to twelve mature follicles occurs twelve hours later in the early hours of oestrus. Concomitant with the LH surge, there are rises in FSH, prolactin, and progesterone. The later may be important for maintaining the steroidal positive feedback effect, and is a relatively large surge compared to the mid-cycle rise seen in the human. The ruptured follicles give rise to corpora lutea which secrete some progesterone, but this is minor in comparison to the preovulatory progesterone surge, and only lasts for 12 hours on the day of metoestrus or designated first day of dioestrus ($D_1$). Rat corpora lutea do not secrete any oestrogen. In a normal rat cycle, the corpora lutea are 'inactive' and regress after 36–48 hours, so that on the second day of dioestrus there is a fall in circulatory progesterone, and a new wave of follicles begins to develop under the slightly higher basal gonadotrophin levels. If the corpora lutea are 'activated' without fertilization of the eggs, their life-span is similar to that in the unfertilized human, that is around 14 days (see Johnson & Everitt, 1988; Freeman, 1988). Stimulation of peptidergic sensory nerves (Substance P, CCK, etc.) in the cervix causes this activation which is mediated by a release of prolactin (Traurig, Papka & Rush, 1988).

Although there are differences between the human and the rat, there are also many similarities, for example the hormonal control of ovarian activity and pituitary hormone release, and the feedback effects of the steroids at pituitary and hypothalamic levels are so similar that it seems likely that they are exerted by the same basic mechanisms (see Fig. 10.2). It is for this reason that much of our understanding of reproductive processes has been derived from experiments carried out in the rat. Similarly, the mode of action of toxic agents that disrupt human female reproductive function may be elucidated by studies carried out in rodents.

## Pregnancy

If fertilization takes place, the corpus luteum does not regress, but continues secreting progesterone. In the rat, the corpora lutea become activated, and also continue to function. The high levels of steroids act on the uterine endometrium causing an increase in its vascularization and stimulation of secretory glands. The egg undergoes rapid cell division and gives rise to a blastocyst with two components: the inner mass which eventually develops into the foetus, and the trophoblast which functions to maintain the foetus, and eventually forms the chorion and placenta. From the 8-cell stage, the blastocyst is capable of producing a gonadotrophin-like hormone (chorionic gonadotrophin; CG) which has a similar structure and activity to LH, and it is this hormone that overcomes the luteolytic action of the prostaglandin and maintains the corpus luteum. CG is considered to play a role in the mechanism of the maternal recognition of pregnancy, but other agents produced by the blastocysts also serve this function including oestrogens and Interferon I (better known as an anti-viral agent and immunosuppressant) (Chard *et al.*, 1986; Trounson *et al.*, 1989).

The blastocyst enters the uterine lumen five to six days after fertilization in the human (three to four days in the rat), where it forms an association with the endometrial wall implanting itself. The process of implantation can only take place over a critical time-period, when the endometrium has been sensitized to receive the blastocyst. Numerous agents have been proposed as important in the preparation of the endometrium, such as oestradiol, and prostaglandin $E_2$. The oestrogen probably acts by increasing phospholipase $A_2$ activity in the endometrium, so stimulating local prostaglandin production (Pakrasi, Cheng & Dey, 1983). Other agents include catecholoestrogens, histamine, and platelet activating factor (PAF); all these factors facilitate decidualization (a change in the cells on the surface of the endometrium) and increase vascular permeability, both of which are prerequisites for successful implantation. With the advent of *in vitro* fertilization, it has become possible to study secretions of the blastocyst, and these include PAF and embryo-derived-histamine-releasor (EDHR) which may stimulate histamine release from the endometrium and/or mast cells in the uterine wall (Weitlauf, 1988). Decidual cells are also capable of synthesizing prolactin, probably stimulated by the rising levels of progesterone, and in turn the prolactin increases phospholipase $A_2$ and thence prostaglandin production. It also stimulates polyamine production (via ornithine decarboxylase) and expression of the casein gene. Since it appears at the time of decidualization it may be concerned with the implantation process. This uterine prolactin may have an important role later in pregnancy, regulating the osmolarity of amniotic fluid and permeability of the amniotic sac via specific prolactin receptors on the chorion (Bonney & Franks, 1989). Another protein induced by the decidualized endometrium is called pregnancy protein 14 (PP-14), this influences lymphocyte activity and thence the immune response in early pregnancy. It is also a binding protein for the IGF produced by the foetus (Julkunen *et al.*, 1986).

After implantation, the trophoblastic cells insinuate projections into the uterine wall, destroying the tissue and blood vessels. These projections grow, and extrude branches such that tree-like structures develop, giving rise to what are eventually known as cotyledons, with foetal blood vessels in each branch and branchlet of the structure. The cotyledons lie in the spaces (lacunae) they have made by destroying uterine tissue, and are bathed in maternal blood from the uterine arteries which have undergone a 'physiological reaction', widening at the junction with the lacunae. Thus, although the foetal and maternal circulations are distinct at all times, they are in close proximity with only a two cell layer of tissue (the wall of the cotyledon) separating them. This enables a rapid and efficient exchange between the two circulatory systems. Eventually, the decidual uterine cells form a smooth plate below the lacunae and the trophoblast or chorionic cells, a plate above the cotyledons forming between them a smooth disc-like structure, the placenta. The placenta functions as the lung, gastrointestinal tract and kidney of the foetus, enabling gaseous exchange, passage of nutrients into, and removal of waste products from the developing foetus. It also acts as a barrier, selectively preventing noxious and infective agents from entering the foetal circulation. Thus, the placenta protects the developing foetus from a variety of drugs, although there are numerous exceptions. In addition, agents that affect blood vessels may affect placental blood flow, and alter the nature of the foetal–maternal circulatory interchanges (Fox, 1989).

In the primate, the placenta also has an endocrine function, synthesizing progesterone and a larger number of peptide hormones. Together with the foetus, it forms what is known as the 'fetoplacental unit' (FPU), and produces oestrogens: the foetus is responsible for converting C-21 steroids (progestogens) to C-19 steroids (androgens), probably under the influence of CG, and the placenta possesses the aromatizing enzyme that effects the conversion of androgens and oestrogens. The numerous peptides produced by the placenta include, in addition to CG, placental lactogen (which has prolactin and growth hormone activity and stimulates foetal IGF production), relaxin (which modulates the activity of the myometrium), α-interferon (which may act to protect the foetus from viral infections and is involved in differentiation of foetal tissue), the pro-opiomelanocortin (POMC) peptides, that is β-endorphin, adrenocorticotrophin (ACTH), α-melanocyte stimulating hormone (α-MSH) and β-lipotrophin; GnRH, thyroid releasing hormone (TRH) and corticotrophin releasing factor (CRF), etc. (Patillo *et al.*, 1983; Petraglia *et al.*, 1990). There are also a number of placental proteins originally thought to be specific to the placenta, although some have now been identified in the non-pregnant ovary and uterus. Examples are pregnancy-specific B glycoprotein (SP$_1$; which appears about 14 days after fertilization); pregnancy-associated-plasma proteins A and B (PAPP A and PAPP B) which are produced by both trophoblastic and decidual tissue, placental protein 5, which like the PAPPs, is stored within the placenta. The functions of these proteins have not been elucidated as yet, but they are present in abnormal concentrations in high-risk pregnancies, for example in pre-eclampsia (Bohn, Dati & Luben, 1983).

## Hypothalamic control of gonadotrophin release

The previous section clearly illustrates that ovarian function and secretion are under gonadotrophin control, and these in turn are regulated by the hypothalamic decapeptide GnRH. Steroids can alter the sensitivity of the pituitary toward GnRH, and also act at the hypothalamic level by altering GnRH neuronal activity. However, none of the factors influencing GnRH release, including the steroids, exert their effects directly on the GnRH neurones but rather via the mediation of other neuronal systems. Many neurotransmitters have been shown to alter GnRH, and thus gonadotrophin release; and many neuronal tracts have been demonstrated to possess nerve terminals impinging either directly onto the GnRH cell bodies in the preoptic area (POA), or onto GnRH nerve terminals in the median eminence (ME). Some of these neuronal systems possess steroid receptors, and are thus strongly implicated in the mediation of feedback effects of the ovarian steroids.

Studies investigating the influence of neurotransmitters on GnRH and gonadotrophin release can be divided into two types: (a) those in which the neurotransmitter activity is altered, perhaps using pharmacological agents and noting changes in hormone release; and (b) taking models in which gonadotrophin release is significantly different, and noting any parallel changes in neurotransmitter activity. Based on these types of experimentation, a summary of the effects of neurotransmitters has been compiled (see Table 10.2).

## Hypothalamic control of prolactin release

Unlike the other hormones of the anterior pituitary, prolactin is under a tonic inhibitory control, exerted by an hypothalamic inhibitory 'releasing factor'. There is clear evidence that this prolactin inhibitory factor (PIF) is dopamine (DA), since DA is released from nerve terminals in the ME into the hypophyseal portal system in sufficient concentrations to activate the dopamine 2 ($D_2$) receptors present on the pituitary lactotrophs. GABA neurones are similarly situated in the ME, and there are also GABA receptors on the lactotrophs, which, when activated, also inhibit prolactin release (MacLeod, 1976; de Feudis, 1984). Both systems are regulated by prolactin itself so that enhanced prolactin levels in the circulation increase hypothalamic DA and GABA turnover (Moore, 1987; Nicoletti *et al.*, 1983). Acetylcholine (AcC) may also inhibit prolactin release at the pituitary level, acting via muscarinic receptors. Both GABA and AcC in some situations, however, stimulate prolactin release by antagonizing the DA system within the hypothalamus (McCann *et al.*, 1988). A peptide 'PIF' has always been hypothesized as well, and this may exist: Seeberg and colleagues (Nikolics *et al.*, 1985) elucidated the structure of pro-GnRH and found that the 56-amino acid structure at the C-terminal named 'gonadotrophin releasing hormone associated peptide' (GAP) inhibits prolactin release *in vitro* and *in vivo*; it also possesses some GnRH-like activity.

There has been a long search for the identity of a prolactin releasing factor (PRF), and at present there are several contenders, all of which are measurable in the hypophyseal portal system and have receptors on the lactotrophs. Possibly all of them have a physiological role in specific situations of enhanced prolactin release. For instance, oxytocin synthesized in the hypothalamus and released into the portal system appears to be particularly involved in stimulating the preovulatory prolactin surge (Johnston & Negro-Vilar, 1988). Another potential PRF is thyroid hormone releasing hormone (TRH) which is the most potent of the prolactin stimulators, and which seems to act in opposition to the dopaminergic system which normally exerts an inhibitory effect on TRH release. Other of these contenders are: VIP, galanin, cholycystokinin (CCK), substance P and neurotensin (Neill, 1988; McCann *et al.*, 1988; Mogg & Samson, 1990).

Table 10.2. *The effect of neurotransmitters on gonadotrophin (GT) release*

| Neurotransmitter | Effect on GT release | Receptor type | Site of action | Tract | Conditions required for effect |
|---|---|---|---|---|---|
| Noradrenaline (NA) | + | α-1, β-2 | POA & ME | Dorsal NA tract | Presence of steroids |
| | – | α-1, β-1 | | Ventral NA tract acts via inhibitory intra-neuronal system | |
| Dopamine (DA) | – | D-1 | ME | Tuberoinfundibular (T-I) tract | |
| | + | D-1 | ZI or POA | Incertohypothalamic (I-H) tract | Presence of steroids |
| | + | | ME | Acts to stimulate NA system | |
| Adrenaline (Ad) | + (more potent than NA) | | POA | | |
| 5-hydroxytryptamine (5-HT) | + | | POA & ME | Tract originating from dorsal raphe. May act by antagonism of β-adrenergic system | May depend on circadian rhythm of 5-HT rather than absolute levels. |
| | – | | VMN & ZI | Tract originating from medial raphe. May be mediated via pineal or GABA system. | |

| Neurotransmitter | Effect | Receptor type | Site | Action | Notes |
|---|---|---|---|---|---|
| Acetylcholine (AcC) | +<br>− | Muscurinic<br>Nicotinic | | May act by stimulating dopaminergic T-I tract | |
| Histamine | + | H$_1$ and H$_2$ | ME and pituitary | | More effect in females and in luteal phase. |
| Gamma-aminobutyric acid (GABA) | +<br><br>−<br><br>− | GABA A<br><br>GABA A & B<br>GABA B | ME<br><br>POA<br>ZI | May act to inhibit dopaminergic T-I tract<br>Acts to inhibit noradrenergic system<br>Acts to inhibit dopaminergic I-H system. | |
| Excitatory amino acid transmitters, e.g. glutamate aspartate | + | NMDA and non-NMDA type | | | |
| Opiates, e.g. β-endorphin and Dynorphin (not enkephalins) | − | μ, κ & σ types | | Act to inhibit NA/NPY systems and enhance 5-HT system | |
| α-melanotrophin (α-MSH) | −<br><br>+ | | | Enhances dopaminergic T-I tract | Seen in men and women in the luteal phase and in vitro |

Table 10.2. (*Cont.*)

| Neurotransmitter | Effect on GT release | Receptor type | Site of action | Tract | Conditions required for effect |
|---|---|---|---|---|---|
| Neuropeptide Y (NPY) | + | High affinity receptor (NPY-1) | Same sites as NA, i.e. POA & ME and also at pituitary level | Co-exists with NA. May act by modulating dopaminergic T-I tract. | |
| | − | Low affinity receptor (NPY-2) | | | |
| Prostanoids: | | | | | |
| Prostaglandin (PgI) $E_2$ and $F_{2\alpha}$ | + | | At hypothalamic level | Mediates stimulatory effect of NA | |
| PgI D and $I_2$ | − | | At pituitary level | May release β-endorphin | |
| Leukotrienes (LT) C4 (not B4) | + | | At pituitary level | May be second messenger for GnRH | |

Abbreviations and symbols:
+ Stimulatory effect; − inhibitory effect
POA = preoptic area; ME = median eminence; VMN = ventral medial nucleus; ZI = zona incerta;
NMDA = N-methyl-d-aspartate.
References:
Fuxe *et al.*, 1977; Wilson, 1979; Walker, 1980; Barraclough & Wise, 1982; Ramirez, Feder & Sawyer, 1984; Bicknell, 1985; Kalra, 1986; Taleisnik & Sawyer, 1986. (Further references supplied on request to authors.)

At the hypothalamic level, 5-HT, histamine (acting on H1 receptors) and NA (acting on $\alpha$-1 and $\beta$-receptors) may all be important in stimulating one or more of the potential releasing factors, in stressful situations, suckling or mediating oestrogen-induced prolactin release. The endogenous opiate system also enhances prolactin release, and may do so by increasing 5-HT and/or reducing DA activity. Naloxone reduces normal prolactin levels indicating that there is some tonic stimulatory control opposing the DA system all of the time (see Wilson, 1979; Donoso & Banzan, 1980; Martinez, de la Escalera & Weiner, 1988).

In addition to the hypothalamic control, there are intra-pituitary factors exerting local regulation. Angiotensin II (A II) is present in pituitary gonadotrophs, and released by GnRH to exert a paracrine effect on A II receptors present on the lactotrophs and enhance prolactin release. VIP exists within lactotrophs, and exerts a stimulatory autocrine effect on prolactin release. These agents act via the phosphoinositol pathway, which involves lipo-oxygenase metabolism of arachidonic acid and these products, as well as PG E, can all stimulate prolactin release (Denef, Baes & Schramme, 1986; Hinkle, 1988).

Oestrogen stimulates prolactin release at several sites; it uncouples DA receptors at the pituitary level, and so prevents DA from exerting its inhibitory effect, and also acts at the hypothalamic level inhibiting DA release from the tuberoinfundibular (T-I) tract, and enhancing TRF output (Thorner & MacLeod, 1980).

## Some endogenous causes of reproductive dysfunction

### Hyperprolactinaemia

The development of radioimmunoassays for human prolactin resulted in the finding that 20% of women with amenorrhoea also had hyperprolactinaemia, usually as a consquence of a micro- or macro-pituitary adenoma (Evans, Cronin & Thorner, 1982). Causes of infertility in hyperprolactinaemia are shown in Table 10.3.

### Stress

Adaption to stress involves facilitation of neural pathways that increase arousal and attention, and inhibit non-adaptive functions such as feeding, sexual behaviour, and reproduction. A wide range of conditions, both physical and psychological, can be stressful, and all are associated with reduced fertility; for example, in animals – overcrowding, subordinance in social hierarchy and intensive farm management; and in humans – war, famine, threat of execution, and on a more normal level – a new job,

Table 10.3. *Infertility in hyperprolactinaemia*

| Cause of infertility | Site of action | Mediators of effect |
|---|---|---|
| (1) Inhibition of GnRH and gonadotrophin release | Hypothalamus | Prolactin enhances the DA and opiate systems that inhibit GnRH release (Sarker & Yen, 1985; Moore, 1987). |
| | Adrenal | Prolactin stimulates progesterone and glucocorticoid synthesis which exert an inhibitory effect at the hypothalamic and pituitary level (Moberg, 1987) |
| (2) Reduction in ovarian steroidogenesis and plasminogen activator (PA) production | Ovary | Prolactin inhibits steroidogenesis at the post cAMP stage. Its inhibition of PA prevents ovulation. (Magoffin & Erickson, 1982; McNeilly, 1986; Yoshimura *et al.* 1990). |

GnRH = gonadotrophin releasing hormone.

examinations, moving house, and chronic exercise. All of these events have been reported to induce amenorrhoea and/or infertility in females. The principal effector of these changes appears to be the hypothalamic-pituitary-adrenal axis and the noradrenergic system within the CNS. Other 'stress hormones' include the endogenous opiates and prolactin (Rabin *et al.*, 1988; Tilders & Berkenbosch, 1986). Causes of infertility induced by stress are shown in Table 10.4.

## Weight related disturbances in reproduction

### Weight loss

In 1974, Frisch & McArther associated body fat content with reproduction. The results of their surveys in a sedentary population indicate that the proportion of body fat must be >17% for the occurrence of menarche and >22% for maintenance of menstrual cycles. If the proportion falls below those figures menarche is delayed and after menarche cycles become irregular and eventually amenorrhoea occurs, depending on the extent of the fat loss. This is an adaptive response of the reproductive system towards adverse conditions and comes into play with low energy

Table 10.4. *Stress-induced infertility*

| Cause of infertility | Site of action | Mediators of effect |
|---|---|---|
| (1) Inhibition of GnRH and gonadotrophin release | Hypothalamus | Stress induces a rise in NA which stimulates the hypothalamic opioid system that inhibits GnRH release. Stress also stimulates hypothalamic 5-HT and DA activity which enhances prolactin release (see hyperprolactinaemia) (Petraglia *et al.* 1987a,b). |
| | Anterior pituitary-adrenal cortex axis | Stress induces release of CRF which stimulates ACTH and pituitary opioid release. The latter acts at the hypothalamic level. The former stimulates the adrenal to produce glucocorticoids. Both ACTH and the steroids reduce pituitary sensitivity toward GnRH and the steroids also exert a negative feedback effect at the hypothalamic level (Moberg, 1987). |
| | Posterior pituitary-adrenal medulla axis | CRF stimulates adrenal adrenaline release which enhances β-endorphin release from the posterior pituitary (Tilders & Berkenbosch, 1986). |

GnRH = gonadotrophin releasing hormone; 5-HT = 5-hydroxytryptamine; DA = dopamine; CRF = corticotrophin releasing factor; ACTH = adrenocorticotrophin

intake (as in dieting or starvation) or high energy output (as after excessive exercise, e.g. athletic or ballet training). Menstrual dysfunction or amenorrhoea occurs in both dieters (with loss of total body weight) and athletes in training (often with normal body weight but low fat content). The relationship between weight loss and infertility is summarized in Table 10.5.

Table 10.5. *Causes of infertility induced by weight loss*

| Cause of infertility | Site of action | Mediators of effect |
|---|---|---|
| Low levels of oestrogens reduced positive feedback effect resulting in absence of the pre-ovulatory LH surge | Peripheral fat stores | Fat depots are important sites of conversion of androgens to oestrogens. If fat stores are low, oestrogen production is reduced. When body-weight is low, steroid-hormone-binding globulin is high and so will inactivate a larger proportion of the oestrogen (Frisch, 1985). |
| Inhibition of GnRH and thence LH release | Hypothalamus | The stress of exercise increases CRF and β-endorphin activity (see Table 10.4) (Prior, 1987). |

LH = luteinizing hormone; GnRH = gonadotrophin releasing hormone; CRF = corticotrophin releasing factor

### Anorexia nervosa

Anorexia nervosa is an affective disorder occurring mainly in young girls in which they are hyperactive, have a disturbed body vision image, a distorted attitude to food (particularly carbohydrates), and implacably refuse to eat. This illness is, therefore, accompanied by severe weight loss and is always associated with secondary amenorrhoea which in 80% of cases occurs before any significant weight loss (Eisenberg, 1981). Thus although the reproductive dysfunctions are similar to those seen in dieters, the basic causes are different and a return to normal levels of LH is only associated with a return to normal behaviour. If weight gain occurs without loss of behavioural symptoms, the LH pattern remains at the pubertal stage (de Rosa *et al.*, 1983).

### Obesity

There is an increased incidence of amenorrhoea or dysfunctional uterine bleeding in obese women. There are probably multiple causes but primarily it may be due to increased degradation of cortisol to oestrone in the fat depots and this in turn will enhance basal LH secretion, while inhibiting the preovulatory gonadotrophin surge. In addition, free and therefore active levels of oestrogens are higher in obese women, as they possess lower levels of sex hormone binding globulin. The raised basal LH will stimulate ovarian thecal cells to produce inter-ovarian androgens and this will also disrupt follicular development (Kopelman *et al.*, 1981; Kopelman, 1988).

## Polycystic ovarian syndrome (PCO)

PCO is the cause of 50% of anovulatory infertility, but the mechanism of action is not understood (Schaison, 1988). A whole spectrum of conditions are included in this syndrome extending from normal fertile cycles in spite of the state of the ovary with multiple immature follicles and dense stroma, to its more extreme form which is associated with obesity, and hirsutism as well as infertility (Hancock, Oakey & Glass, 1987). It is clear that PCO is the result of a number of different abnormalities and treatments will depend on the aetiology of each case. The causes of infertility associated with PCO are shown in Table 10.6.

## Cell-mediated immune response

The products of activated leucocytes, that is the soluble products mediating the cell-mediated immune response and the products of plasma cells – antibodies – may affect reproductive functions and fertility. Firstly, the relevant cells are present in the reproductive tract; the endometrial lining of the human uterus contains lymphocytes and macrophages especially in the late luteal phase of the menstrual cycle and in the decidua of early pregnancy. These cells can also be found in the oviduct and at intercourse, leukocytes can infiltrate the uterine lumen from the cervix and vagina. There are also immunoglobulin secreting plasma cells in the cervix. The presence of sperm and/or seminal plasma activates leukocytes to produce antibodies locally.

Secondly, cell-mediated immune (CMI) reactions toward sperm have been shown to occur in infertile women and experiments in female mice immunized with sperm have duplicated the situation seen in the human. Similarly, infertility due to intrauterine infections is associated with raised numbers of T cells in the endometrium and infertility may be due to the lymphocyte products secreted as a result of cell activation by microbial or viral antigens. Another example of anorexia CMI-induced infertility is that seen in cases of endometriosis in which there are increased numbers of activated macrophages and lymphocytes. The products of the activated cells include lymphokines (e.g. gamma-interferon and tumour necrosis factor (TNF)), monokines, and free oxygen radicals, and they may cause infertility by reducing sperm motility and preventing penetration of the oocyte by the sperm (e.g. gamma-interferon and tumour necrosis factor).

Table 10.6. *Infertility associated with polycystic ovarian syndrome*

| Cause of infertility | Site of action | Mediators of effect |
|---|---|---|
| The ratio of LH:FSH is higher than normal (Burger *et al.* 1985) | Increased sensitivity of pituitary toward LH releasing effect of GnRH | Increased LH induces excess ovarian androstanedione which is aromatized to oestrone ($O_1$) in fat depots. $O_1$ may enhance LH and suppress FSH release so forming a vicious circle of continued raised LH:FSH (Lobo *et al.* 1981; Schaison, 1988). |
| Production of androgens | Ovary | Excess androgens can prevent normal follicular maturation (Baird *et al.* 1977) and/or abnormal ovarian production of peptide factors (Franks *et al.* 1988) |

LH = luteinizing hormone; FSH = follicle stimulating hormone; GnRH = gonadotrophin releasing hormone

Gamma-interferon, granulocyte macrophage colony stimulating factor, and IL-1 also have inhibitory effects on embryo and foetal development and trophoblast proliferation. These actions would result in abortion or if occurring later in pregnancy, in intra-uterine growth retardation (Anderson & Hill, 1988). Recently reports have shown that the interleukins and TNF exert an inhibitory effect on GnRH and LH release, and do so via stimulating CRF and thence β-endorphin release (Rivier & Vale, 1989). Interleukins (IL-1 and 6) may have other modulatory paracrine effects at the pituitary level, since they can stimulate LH release from pituitary cells *in vitro*, and IL-6 is produced in large amounts by pituitary cell cultures. At the ovarian level, IL-1 is inhibitory and has a down-regulatory effect on LH receptors and inhibits hCG-induced steroidogenesis (Bazer & Johnson, 1989; Suda *et al.*, 1990; Spangelo, MacLeod & Isakson, 1990).

## Toxicity of gonadal steroids and oestrogenic xenobiotics

### Action of steroids

#### Receptors

Steroids exert their effects via specific receptors that are now considered to be primarily situated within the nucleus (the earlier hypothesis that free receptors were cytoplasmic proteins that only translocated to the nucleus when bound to steroids was based on artefactual experimental results). After binding, the steroid increases the affinity of the receptor for chromatin and the steroid-receptor complex binds to specific sequences of DNA which are adjacent to the steroid-regulated genes. The complex acts as a transcriptional enhancer, stimulating promoter regions of the genes and thus increasing the rate of their transcription. This results in the accumulation of mRNA which enters the cytoplasm and is translated into specific proteins by the ribosomes.

Despite differences in their size, the general structures of the receptors (i.e. oestrogen, progesterone, androgen, glucocorticoid, and also thyroid hormone and retinoic acid) are related in terms of their overall organization, and at their carboxy-terminal, where there is a high degree of homology. The amino-acid chain of the receptor structure is divided into functional domains. The steroid-binding domain is at the carboxy-terminal and is adjacent to the DNA binding domain which contains two units enriched in cysteine, lysine and arginine which are folded into finger-like structures held in place by a zinc ion; it is these 'zinc-fingers' that attach to the DNA. There is a short region between the steroid and DNA binding domains which may serve as a 'hinge' between them. It is in the steroid binding, and particularly the DNA binding domains that the receptor homologies exist. The amino-terminal position is variable in both structure and length, and accounts for differences in receptor size. This domain may act to modulate receptor function and binding, but it is the DNA binding domain that determines the specificity of function.

It is suggested that the receptors normally exist in association with a 90,000 dalton phosphoprotein called heat-shock protein. On steroid binding, this dissociates from the receptor, thus enabling transformation of the latter to a DNA-binding state; perhaps the DNA binding-domain is unmasked by the removal of the heat-shock protein. Alternatively, activation is dependent on a change in the hinge region between the steroid and DNA binding domains, allowing the exposure of the previous occluded DNA binding site (King, 1987; Parker, 1988; Mendelson, 1988, Evans, 1988).

### Toxicity due to steroid receptor activation

The carboxy-terminal region of steroid receptors have a high degree of homology with the so-called V-erb A protein of the oncogenic avian erythroblastosis virus, which is not oncogenic itself but increases the oncogenic potential of another viral protein, V-erb B, which is homologous with a portion of the EGF receptor. Oestrogen stimulates the growth of oestrogen receptor-positive mammary tumours and is implicated in the pathogenesis of human breast cancer, perhaps by stimulating EGF itself or EGF receptors, that is, the oestrogen-receptor complex may stimulate tumour growth by stimulating an oncogene in the same way as V-erb A stimulates V-erb B.

Another possible cause of toxic effects may be the alteration of the steroid domain such that there is a change in receptor configuration enabling it to bind to the DNA without activation by the steroid; this mutation in the receptor may lead to it being in a constantly activated state, perturbing the homeostatic balance and abetting tumour growth. This could be the cause of the conversion of steroid dependent tumours to hormone-independent growth (Evans, 1988; Mendelson, 1988).

### Action of the gonadal steroids

Steroids exert two types of effects, organizational and activational:

#### Organizational actions:

This type of effect is permanent and irreversible, and occurs only during the foetal and neonatal periods in rodents and humans.

1. *The reproductive system*: The embryo is sexually bipotential, and before the sixth week in the human, the gonadal ridge is indifferent. If the foetal genotype is XY, the gonadal ridge differentiates into the testes at the seventh week. The foetal testis then produces a protein (with homology to inhibin and activin) called anti-Müllerian hormone which causes the potential female Müllerian tract to regress. At the eighth week the testes secrete testosterone, which increases to a maximum between the 11th and 18th week. This testosterone acts on the potential male Wolfian tract and stimulates its development into the vas deferens, epididymis, prostate and seminal vesicles. Finally, differentiation of the foetal cloaca occurs with development of the male external genitalia – penis, urethra, and fusion of labioscrotum. This change is under the influence of dihydrotestosterone which is produced in the target tissue from its precursor, testosterone, by the enzyme 5 α-reductase. In the absence of testosterone or its receptors, an XY foetus will develop into a female phenotype, indicating that 'neutral' development of the body is of the female type and must be actively suppressed by secretions of the testis. The gonadal ridge in an XX foetus develops into an ovary and in the absence of testosterone, the Wolfian tract regresses and the Müllerian tract develops forming the uterus and vagina (George & Wilson, 1988).

2. *The brain*: Sexual differentiation also occurs within the CNS, where the steroids act organizationally to influence the pattern of neuronal interconnections, particularly in the hypothalamus and amygdala. In the human, this presumably occurs at the end of the first trimester when testosterone

production is at its height. In rodents, testosterone production and sexual differentiation of the CNS occur over the last few days *in utero* and the first 10 days of neonatal life. This period of change has been extensively studied, and based on the findings, it is hypothesized that in the male neonatal rodent, testosterone from the foetal testis passes to the brain and influences neuronal structures causing changes in the interconnections between neurones, that is, the number of dendritic and axo-axonal synapses. This in turn leads to sexual differentiation of a number of functions regulated by the CNS in adulthood (e.g. sexual behaviour, sexual preference, aggressive behaviour, exploration, and anxiety), and also to sexual differentiation of the control of gonadotrophin release (Joseph, Hess & Birecree, 1978; Stewart & Cygan, 1980; van de Poll, van Zanten & de Jonge, 1986; de Jonge *et al.*, 1988). For instance, in the male rodent, the steroids exert only a negative feedback effect on GnRH and thence gonadotrophin release, while in the female both negative and positive feedback controls exist, which generate the cyclical pattern of gonadotrophin release. Paradoxically, the testosterone only induces masculinization of the hypothalamus and probably other areas of the brain, after conversion to oestrogen within the CNS. The foetal brains of both sexes are protected from maternal oestrogens by $\alpha$-foeto-protein ($\alpha$-FP), which avidly binds circulating oestrogen rendering it inactive. $\alpha$-FP has no affinity for testosterone, and so can gain unimpeded access to the CNS, where it is aromatized to oestrogen *in situ*. This conversion may not occur in all species, and there is conflicting evidence whether or not it occurs in primates (Arnold & Gorski, 1984) (see Baum *et al.*, 1990).

3. *The liver*: Hepatic function is also subject to sexual differentiation with differences in certain liver proteins and particularly enzymes concerned with steroid metabolism – the steroid hydroxylases are lower and 5 $\alpha$-reductase is higher in females compared to males. Neonatal castration of male rats alters the levels to those seen in the female, while conversely, hypophysectomy (at any time of life) in females induces male levels. This sexual dimorphism in the liver is controlled by the pattern of release of growth hormone (GH) which in turn is controlled by the sexually differentiated hypothalamus. Thus in the male, GH is released in a pulsitile manner while in the female the amplitude of the pulses is smaller but the basal concentration is higher. Hepatic enzyme levels can be manipulated by administration of exogenous GH simulating the differences in the pattern of release (Gustafsson *et al.*, 1983; Jansson, Edan & Isaksson, 1985). Other sexually differentiated hepatic proteins include $\alpha2U$-globulin (which is only found in the male), hepatic prolactin receptors (which have a higher density in the female) and enzymes controlling degradation of cadmium, ethylmorphine, aniline, lidocaine, imipramine,

and alcohol. Most of these enzymes are controlled by the 'imprinting' effects of neonatal androgens on the hypothalamus (as described above) together with an androgen-dependency in adulthood as well. Some enzymes however, are only androgen-dependent, for example monoamine oxidases which are 50% higher in males and can be reduced to female levels by castration in adulthood (Roy & Chatterjee, 1983; Norstedt & Palmiter, 1984; Gustafsson *et al.*, 1983; Teschke & Wiese, 1982).

4. *Steroid toxicity in the foetal/neonatal period*: It is clear that any abnormalities in the circulating steroids, in particular of the androgenic type, during pregnancy can lead to abnormalities in the development of the foetus, and administration of steroids to pregnant females may cause abnormalities in the development of the genitalia in female foetuses, abnormalities in the cyclical pattern of hormone release, and abnormalities in behaviour in adulthood. Many of the toxic agents which are potentially oestrogenic in their action cause acyclicity when given over the foetal and/or neonatal period in rodents. In the past, steroids have been administered in cases of threatened miscarriage in humans, and certain of the first generation progestogens employed then had sufficient androgenic activity to cause masculinization of the external genitalia in female progeny.

### Activational actions

The gonadal steroids exert a reversible (and therefore activational) effect on a large number of systems in the body, and so when present in abnormal concentrations, or mimicked or inhibited by exogenous agents, a wide variety of toxic effects can ensue.

1. *Peripheral system*: The main physiological function of the gonadal steroids is the maintenance of reproductive system, where they stimulate growth (i.e. gene transcription and protein synthesis) and secretory activity. Thus oestrogen causes hypertrophy of both the uterine myometrium and endothelium with an increase in uterine proteins, cell proliferation and the induction of progesterone receptors. The progesterone then acts on the oestrogen-primed uterus and stimulates secretion by the endothelial glands. A similar interaction occurs in the cervical secretory glands and in the vagina (Clark & Markaverich, 1988; Johnson & Everitt, 1988). Oestrogenic activity in putative toxic agents (xenobiotics) are often first demonstrated by noting induction of uterine hypertrophy in immature rodents (Kupfer, 1988).

2. *Central nervous system*: Apart from the organizational effects of the steroids on neuronal circuitary in the limbic system, steroids can affect neurotransmitter activity reversibly by influencing synthesis, uptake,

catabolism, and receptor density of a large number of neurotransmitters. For instance, administration of steroids to rodents increases the mRNA for tyrosine hydroxylase and decreases it for glutamic acid decarboxylase (these are the synthetic enzymes for the catecholamines and GABA). Similarly, they increase β-adrenergic receptors and 5-HT$_1$ receptors, and decrease GABA A and GABA B receptors. Oestrogens have long been known to inhibit monoamine oxidase enzymes (the catabolic enzymes for biogenic amines), while progesterone has the opposite effect. Since there are no steroid receptors on GnRH neurones, while they *are* present on a wide variety of other neurotransmitter systems, for example catecholamine, GABA and opioid, it is assumed the steroids exert their feedback on GnRH and gonadotrophin release indirectly via the latter (see section *Hypothalamic control of gonadotrophin release*). As all the other releasing hormones are controlled by similar neurotransmitter systems, the steroids can affect the release of many of the other pituitary hormones, for instance, oestrogen stimulates growth hormone releasing hormone (GHRH), thyrotropin releasing hormone (TRH) and inhibits hypothalamic dopamine which in turn increases the release of growth hormone, thyroid stimulating hormone (TSH) and prolactin (see Wilson, 1979; McEwen, Jones & Pfaff, 1987).

The steroidal effect on the various neuronal systems can also influence behaviour. In rodents and some non-human primates the presence of steroids is essential for the occurrence of female sexual behaviour (Morali & Beyer, 1979). Oestrogen also stimulates motor activity, inhibits feeding and alters sensory functions (Gandelman, 1983).

3. *Pituitary*: The steroids also act at the pituitary level to influence hormone release. Oestrogen and progesterone can down-regulate GnRH receptors and so inhibit gonadotrophin release. Oestrogen can also enhance post-receptor second messenger activity thus exerting a positive feedback at the pituitary level. Oestrogen stimulates prolactin release at the level of the pituitary by uncoupling dopamine receptors from their second messenger system (Clayton & Catt, 1981; Drouva *et al.*, 1990; Thorner & MacLeod, 1980).

### Toxicity of the steroids on the reproductive system

Abnormal steroid levels and/or patterns of secretion lead to infertility as can be seen in such conditions as PCO, hyperprolactinaemia, and stress (see sections *Hyperprolactinaemia*; *Stress*; and *Weight-related disturbances*). Since the advent of orally active gonadal steroids, deliberately increasing oestrogen and progesterone levels is used as a means of contraception. Administration of an orally active oestrogen such as ethinyl oestradiol or mestranol in conjunction with a progestogen such as norethynodrel or gestodene acts mainly to inhibit the mid-cycle LH surge and so prevent ovulation. There are 15 to 20 'escape' ovulations per 100,000 cycles, but in addition, the high steroid concentrations act at the level of the ovary attenuating its sensitivity towards gonadotrophins and at the level of the oviduct, uterus, and cervix altering motility of the two former and glandular secretions at all three sites. In particular, the high levels of progestogens induce secretion of a thick impenetrable cervical mucous unsuitable for sperm passage. In addition the progestogens inhibit sperm capacitation. The progesterone-only-pill acts to inhibit fertility mainly via by the latter two mechanisms. High doses of oestrogen can prevent implantation of the fertilized egg and so form the basis of the 'morning after pill'. It acts either by preventing passage of the egg through the oviduct by causing spasm of the smooth muscle wall or inducing contractions of the smooth muscle which speeds the passage of the egg so that it enters the uterine lumen before the endometrium is prepared for implantation (Briggs & Briggs, 1976).

## Toxicity of the steroids on other systems

### Cancer

As described above (see section *Toxicity due to receptor activation*), the steroid receptor is homologous to certain viral oncogene stimulators and it is possible that either steroids may activate these viral agents, or steroid receptors can become altered and act as oncogene stimulators after steroid binding. This may be the basis of steroid dependent cancers in parts of the reproductive tract, that is breast, uterus, cervix, and vagina. Treatment of mothers in cases of threatened miscarriage with diethyl-stilboestrol (a synthetic oestrogen) led to the appearance of vaginal and cervical adenocarcinoma in a small percentage (0.04–0.14%) of the female off-spring which was manifest after puberty, presumably after sufficient exposure to endogenous steroids (Melnick *et al.*, 1987). Lower doses given to pregnant rhesus monkeys and to rodents did not cause neoplasia but did cause structural abnormalities of the uterus, vagina, and cervix in the female offspring, the changes in the latter two sites resembling those seen in humans; this was associated with a slightly lower pregnancy rate (Rothschild, Calhoon & Boylan, 1988; Hendrickx, Prahalada & Binkerd, 1988; Gorwill & Steele, 1988).

Older oral contraceptive preparations with a high ratio of oestrogen and progesterone activity can induce endometrial cancer, but the more recent preparations with lower concentrations of oestrogen and a higher proportion of progesterone, appear to be protective. Some reports show that use of an oral contraceptive at an early age (i.e. before 25 years and before pregnancy) increases the risk of breast cancer before the age of 40; this is not supported by other studies. Prolonged exposure to an oral contraceptive slightly increases the risk of cervical cancer. In older women there is also an increase in the incidence of hepatocellular adenomas (Vessey, 1989).

It should also be stated that steroids may protect against both benign and malignant tumour growth, perhaps by preventing oncogene activity. Thus use of an oral contraceptive is protective against benign breast tumours, endometrial cancer, uterine fibroids, and epithelial cancer in the ovary (Drife, 1989; Schlesselman, 1989).

### Cardiovascular and lipid metabolism

High dose oestrogen preparations are associated with a three to six-fold increase in venous thrombosis and thrombotic strokes; this is unrelated to smoking. Haemorrhagic stroke risk is doubled and this is related to smoking and hypertension. Oral contraceptives increase the risk of myocardial infarction, and this is related to age and smoking, and due to the progesterone component of the pill. The mechanism of action of the thrombotic effect is not understood because although oestrogen increases prothrombin and factors 2, 7, 9 and 10, by twelve-fold, as they are already present in excess this should not have much of an adverse effect. The cause of ischaemic heart disease (myocardial infarction) by oral contraceptives is better understood, and is due to the effect of progesterone on circulating lipoproteins.

Ischaemic heart disease is correlated with high levels of blood lipids. These lipids, produced by the liver and intestine, are present in the circulation with carrier apolipoproteins which form hydrophobic membranes around the triglycerides and cholesterol esters. Low density lipoproteins carry 70% of plasma cholesterol and can deposit it on vessel walls. There is a positive correlation between low density lipoprotein-cholesterol complex (LDC-C) concentration and myocardial infarction. High density lipoproteins (HDL) carry cholesterol from cell membranes to the liver, where they are excreted, and levels of this carrier are negatively associated with the risk of ischaemic heart disease. The ratio of low density lipoproteins (LDL) and HDL-cholesterol or total cholesterol:HDL-C are often taken as an indicator of risk. Oestrogen increases HDL and reduces LDL and therefore reduces the likelihood heart disease, while progestogens have the opposite effect.

Oral contraceptives cause a slight increase in blood pressure in most women which is reversible on cessation of treatment. The cause is not known, as although oestrogen increases renin and angiotensin II secretion, this is unrelated to changes in blood pressure (Drife, 1989; Gillmer, 1989).

### Carbohydrate metabolism

Oestrogens reduce glucagon secretion and inhibit hepatic glucogenesis, so high dose oestrogen oral contraceptives induce glucose intolerance and increase in the insulin:glucose ratio (Gillmer, 1989).

### Liver

Oestrogens increase hepatic mitotic activity which may lead to benign or possibly malignant hypertrophy. They also decrease mixed function oxidase activity in the liver and so may affect metabolic activation or de-activation of toxic agents, for example the half-life of carcinogenic agents such as diethyl nitrosamine and N-nitro-morphiline is prolonged.

Since oestrogens increase the passage of cholesterol to the liver, there is an increased risk of gall stone formation (which are composed of 60–90% cholesterol). The risk is increased by the oestrogen induced decrease in secretion of bile acids (Mastri & Lucier, 1985).

### Immune system

In women humoral mediated immunity (with increased IgM levels) is higher and cell mediated immunity is lower than for men, because of the action of oestrogen. Administration of oral contraceptives or other oestrogenic agents, that is diethylstilboesterol and the phytotoxic agents, causes atrophy of the thymus and reduces cell mediated immunity, and natural killer cell activity, and depresses lymphocyte reactivity (Luster, Pfeifer & Tucker, 1985).

## Oestrogenic toxic agents

There is a large structurally diverse group of xenobiotics (environmental pollutants and therapeutic agents) and naturally occurring plant sub-stances (phyto-oestrogens) that mimic the physiological and biochemical properties of the classical oestrogens. They are usually 1000 to 10,000-fold less potent than oestradiol, but as many of them have long half-lives and are often widely distributed in the environment, animals and humans may be exposed to them for long enough for an oestrogenic response to occur. Since they are weak oestrogens, their effects depend very much on endogenous oestrogen concentrations. Thus when endogenous levels are low the xenobiotics will exert an oestrogenic effect, but when endogenous levels are high, the toxic agents will act as anti-oestrogens (Bulger & Kupfer, 1985).

Pesticides

The best known examples of oestrogenic xenobiotics are the chlorinated hydrocarbon pesticides such as ppDDT (1,1,bis(p-chlorophenyl)-2,2,2-trichloroethane), methoxychlor (2,2 bis (p-methoxyphenyl)-1,1,1-trichlorethane), Kepone (chlordecone; decachloro-octahydro-1,3,4-methano-2,1,1-cyclobuta [cd] pentalene; withdrawn from production in 1975) and Mirex, a halogenated analogue of chlorodecone which is converted to chlorodecone *in vivo* and dibromochloropropane (DBCP) used as a fumigant and nematocide.

These agents have caused disruption of the reproductive system in farm animals and humans, and many have been tested extensively for their toxic and oestrogenic effects. In order to show that a compound is truly oestrogenic, a variety of tests must be carried out, since a single test may be mimicked by non-oestrogenic agents; for instance, like oestrogens, androgens and progestogens are uterotrophic, and anti-oestrogens can bind to oestrogen receptors (Kupfer, 1988). However, the main xenobiotic agents above have all been shown to mimic oestrogens in a wide number of physiological actions (see Bulger & Kupfer, 1985):

(a) after chronic consumption there is a reduction in number of litters and litter size, and an increase in intervals between litters in rodents (Reel & Lamb, 1985).

(b) they induce constant oestrus and inhibition of ovulation (Pinkston & Uphouse, 1988 for chlordecone; Barlow & Sullivan, 1982 for DBCP) and follicular development (Swartz & Mall, 1989), as shown in rodents.

(c) they advance puberty in rodents and pigs and if given neonatally, prevent sexual differentiation of gonadotrophin release leading to sterility in adulthood (Haney, 1985).

(d) they cause structural changes in the oviduct, uterus and vagina in rodents (Reel & Lamb, 1985).

(e) they cause uterine hypertrophy, endometrial hyperplasia, increase uterine DNA, uterine proteins, uterine enzymes and uterine progesterone receptors and prevent implantation (Pinkston & Uphouse, 1988; Haney, 1985).

(f) they exert a negative feedback effect on gonadotrophin release and some agents (not chlordecone), enhance the secretion of prolactin (Reel & Lamb, 1985).

(g) they increase sexual receptivity in rodents and pigs (Bulger & Kupfer, 1985; Uphouse & Williams, 1989).

(h) they reduce antibody production and induce thymic atrophy at near lethal doses (Luster *et al.*, 1985).

Some of the xenobiotic agents are themselves oestrogenic such as DDT, Mirex, and chlordecone, but in addition, DDT is metabolized to hydroxylated derivatives, some of which can be more potently oestrogenic. Methoxychlor is actually a pro-oestrogen, and only when it is 0-demethylated or bis-hydroxylated to form phenolic derivatives (NB: the main metabolite is the bihydroxy derivative HPTE), do the oestrogenic effects occur. In addition, methoxychlor contains phenolic contaminants, such as chlorotrianisene (TACE), which are oestrogenic and which can be metabolized to other oestrogenic phenolic products. Even high grade methoxychlor contains oestrogenic impurities (Bulger & Kupfer, 1985).

### Industrial agents

Polychlorinated biphenyls, for example the Arochlor analogues, are highly stable compounds used as heat exchange fluids in the plastic industry and for electrical insulation. Their oestrogenic activity is one millionth that of oestradiol but due to their high degree of stability they are only very slowly degraded in the environment. They are highly lipid soluble and so are easily absorbed through the gut, lung, and skin, and accumulate in adipose tissue of fish, mammals, and humans. Production was banned in 1976 after it was shown to have detremental effects on fertility causing menstrual disturbances and an increase in urinary androgens. It was thought to induce miscarriages and to cause low birth weight offspring. Chronic administration to monkeys and rodents reduces fertility without completely blocking it, and causes prolonged cycles and reduces progesterone levels. Neonatal administration in rats causes precocious puberty, constant oestrus and infertility, and in adulthood the compounds are uterotrophic (Barlow & Sullivan, 1982; Lione, 1988).

Organic solvents such as carbon tetrachloride, benzene, and xylene are hepatoxic and can accumulate in fat depots, which means that women are more susceptible to their toxic effects than men. Anaemia, menstrual disorders, and increased abortion rate have been reported, possibly due to (a) increased oestrogen activity since the hepatotoxicity may reduce metabolism of the steroids, or (b) a direct effect on the ovary reducing oestrogen production, or (c) it may be a stress effect as adrenal hypertrophy has been noted after carbon tetrachloride (Barlow & Sullivan, 1982). Organosiloxane fluids, used in cosmetics may be oestrogenic as they are uterotrophic and cause endometrial proliferation and stimulate oviduct movement and thence passage of the oocytes, thus preventing implantation in early pregnancy. However, they also induce constant dioestrus in rodents and so may be anti-oestrogenic as well (Bulger & Kupfer, 1985).

Phytoestrogens

These are found in a number of Leguminosa and grasses, and are structurally and functionally similar to oestrogen. Examples include isoflavones such as genistein and genistin, and coumestans such as coumestrol. In addition, mycotoxins derived from common field fungi (e.g. *Fusarium roseum*) produce oestrogenic metabolites of the resocyclic acid lactone group; zearalenone and zearalenol (zeranol). These agents have been shown to impair reproductive function in animals and humans. They can either act as oestrogens or anti-oestrogens depending on the endogenous endocrine environment, or even in a mixed manner binding to oestrogen receptors to (a) affect cervical mucus, uterine growth and implantation, (b) cause follicular retardation and inhibit ovulation, (c) induce degeneration of oocytes and abnormal fertilization, (d) reduce gonadotrophin release and the sensitivity of the pituitary toward GnRH, and (e) masculinize behaviour (noted in sheep). In humans, phytoestrogens can cause coronary heart disease and oestrogen-dependent neoplasms, although they may act as anti-oestrogens in certain situations, and could be the reason for the lower incidence of breast cancer in women on vegetarian diets.

As expected of oestrogenic agents, in the short-term they act reversibly either mimicking or antagonizing endogenous oestrogen activity. In the longer term, irreversible anatomical changes can take place, and in sheep and rodents they irreversibly disturb differentiation of the reproductive system and sexual behaviour of off-spring (Kaldas & Hughes, 1989; Hughes, 1988; Shoental, 1977).

Therapeutic agents

Tolbutamide (hypoglycaemic agent) phenolhpthalein and phthalein (cathartics in laxative preparations) are oestrogenic.

## Anti-oestrogens

Tamoxifen

Tamoxifen is widely used clinically in the treatment of oestrogen-dependent breast cancer. As would be expected, it antagonizes the oestrogen action on all parts of the reproductive tract causing in particular uterine atrophy (Scialli, 1988). Tamoxifen may also have direct effects on the reproductive tract unrelated to its anti-oestrogen action, since when given neonatally to mice, it causes permanent chondrification of the pelvis, expansion of the pubic ligament, bladder hernia, and inhibition of the uterine decidual response in adulthood. Similar anti-oestrogens such as MER 25 and clomiphene do not have these effects (Iguchi *et al.*, 1988; Ohta, Iguchi & Takasugi, 1989).

### Clomiphene

Clomiphene is a mixed oestrogen agonist/antagonist and is used to induce ovulation in infertile women. It is thought that this effect is mediated by its anti-oestrogen action reducing the negative feedback effect of endogenous oestrogen and so increasing gonadotrophin release. However, the 70–90% ovulatory rate induced by clomiphene is followed only by a 30–40% pregnancy rate and possibly an increased incidence of spontaneous abortion. This may be due to the anti-oestrogen effect of clomiphene impairing functions of the follicle, the corpus luteum, and the uterine endothelium. Clomiphene-induced ovulation has been associated with luteal phase deficiency, where progesterone levels and the endometrial response are attenuated. Clomiphene either inhibits steroidogenesis and induction of gonadotrophin receptors in the follicle leading to poor corpus luteum development after ovulation, and/or it directly inhibits progesterone production by the corpus luteum. The low level of progesterone may be the cause of spontaneous abortion and/or clomiphene may have a direct degenerative effect on the oocyte. Supporting the latter site as the cause, spontaneous abortion is more frequent in women given clomiphene for more than six months (Scialli, 1988).

### Xenobiotic anti-oestrogens

Lindane is an insecticide with a wide range of toxic effects on the neurological and behavioural systems and it also disrupts reproductive function. Studies suggest this is due to its anti-oestrogen properties causing uterine atrophy, reduced circulating gonadotrophin and prolactin levels, and delayed puberty (Cooper *et al.*, 1989a).

## The effect of metal ions on the reproductive system

The compounds containing metallic ions are mostly environmental hazards, in particular, organic mercury compounds and cadmium salts which have multiple toxic effects, both on the peripheral system and centrally controlled functions. Many of them have marked effects on female fertility and these are summarized below and in Table 10.7.

### Mercury Compounds

The organic mercury compounds are more toxic than the inorganic salts. In women they cause menstrual disturbances with either hyper- or hypomenorrhoea or oligomenorrhoea and an increase in anovulatory cycles.

Table 10.7. *The sites of action of the toxic effects of metal ions on the reproductive system*

| Metal ion | Site of action | | | |
|---|---|---|---|---|
| | Hypothalamus | Pituitary | Ovary | Uterus |
| Mercury | Inhibits GnRH release and thence GT and ovulation | | Accumulates in corpora lutea prolonging life span | |
| Cadimum | Prevents cyclical LH surge, inducing constant oestrus | | Causes necrosis of follicles | Reduces blood flow |
| Lead | | Inhibits FSH release (perhaps due to hypothal-amic action) | Inhibits steroidogen-esis as toxic to ovary | Hypotrophy and inhibits induction of oestrogen receptors |
| Selenium (chronic only) | | Reduces fertility in rodents | | |
| Zinc (deficiency is toxic) | Zinc deficiency stimulates prolactin release | | | |
| Copper (deficiency is toxic) | Copper deficiency inhibits GnRH release | | | |

GT = gonadotrophin; GnRH = gonadotrophin releasing hormone; LH = luteinizing hormone; FSH = follicule stimulating hormone

In a recent study on macaque monkeys, chronic treatment with methyl mercury did not disrupt cycles or conception rate, although it did reduce the number of viable young (Burbacher, Mohamed & Mottett, 1988).

In rodents, chronic treatment prolongs dioestrous periods, inhibits ovulation and increases follicular atresia. This may be a central effect inhibiting gonadotrophin release, but in addition, mercury has a direct ovarian effect as it accumulates in corpora lutea prolonging their life-span. When given over the neonatal period, methylmercury causes irregular cycles in adulthood indicating that it must affect the development of the CNS control systems on gonadotrophin release (Barlow & Sullivan, 1982; Mattison & Thomford, 1989).

## Cadmium

Cadmium salts are extremely embryotoxic, but are thought to have little effect on fertility in humans, although they may prolong cycles on chronic intake. In rodents, cadmium causes follicular necrosis, ovulation is inhibited, and the rats become acyclic and go into constant oestrus; this is reversible on cessation of treatment (unlike the toxic effects in males). Cadmium salts also damage the microcirculation in the uterus. When they are given neonatally cadmium compounds cause ovarian necrosis and in adulthood the rats remain in constant dioestrus with reduced ovarian, uterine, and pituitary weights (Barlow & Sullivan, 1982; Mattison & Thomford, 1989).

## Lead

Lead compounds cause enzyme dysfunction and this is probably the basis of their effects on the reproductive system. In adult rodents, treatment with lead salts inhibits FSH release and this together with a direct effect, causes ovarian atrophy and a reduction in progesterone secretion. This results in uterine hypotrophy and in addition there is a direct uterine effect as lead inhibits implantation perhaps by preventing the induction of uterine oestrogen receptors. Neonatal treatment causes delayed puberty (Mattison & Thomford, 1989).

## Selenium

At non-toxic concentrations, short exposure to selenium has no effect on fertility. However, in rodents chronic selenium reduces fertility and the number of viable young (Barlow & Sullivan, 1982).

## Zinc

At physiological concentrations zinc exerts an inhibitory effect on prolactin secretion, so zinc deficiency may be associated with hyperprolactinaemia and therefore suppression of the hypothalamo-pituitary-gonadal axis (see section Hyperprolactinaemia). Hypothalamic concentrations of zinc are higher on the day of proestrus in rats and after ovariectomy indicating a correlation between gonadotrophin release and zinc, but while zinc can stimulate GnRH release *in vitro*, this only occurs at supraphysiological concentrations (Merriam *et al.*, 1979; Lei, Abbasi & Prasad, 1976; Burrows & Barnea, 1982; Login, Thorner & MacLeod, 1983).

Copper

Copper salts, and more effectively copper complexed to an amino-acid or ATP, stimulate GnRH and so LH release and ovulation. The copper acts at a post-synaptic receptor site via the calcium/calmodulin pathway to stimulate PG-E production, which mediates its effects. Copper is the most effective of the metal ions tested on stimulating LH release (i.e. it is three-fold more effective than zinc and eight-fold more effective than magnesium) and is present in the brain, and accumulates in the hypothalamus, where the concentration is increased by raised oestrogen levels. Therefore, copper ions may have a physiological function in controlling GnRH release, especially since copper deficiency leads to infertility in guinea-pigs and rats (Hiroi, Sugita & Suzuki, 1965; Merriam *et al.*, 1979; Burrows & Barnea, 1982; Barnea, Cho & Colombani-Vidal, 1986a,b)

## Reproductive toxicity of CNS drugs

The CNS drugs can be sub-divided according to their clinical use, although some from each category may have similar mechanisms of action. Most of them are used for the treatment of affective disorders which include depression, mania, anxiety, and schizophrenia. There are also motor disorders associated with the mental disturbances, for example tardive dyskinesia as seen in Huntington's Chorea, and rigidity and tremor in Parkinson's disease. Epileptic seizures due to cerebral hyperexcitability can be included here. Based on the mechanism of action of the drugs that alleviate these illnesses and also based on the level of transmitter metabolites in the cerebrospinal fluid (CSF) and urine of affected patients, the hypothesis was put forward that all the disorders are due to abnormalities of brain neurotransmitter activity. At first, the theories were confined to the catechole and indole amines, but more recently the involvement of GABA transmission has been incorporated (Schildkraut, 1965; Garver & Davis, 1979; Bartholini, 1985). Table 10.8 indicates some of the suggested aetiologies of some of the affective disorders. Sections *Hypothalamic control of gonadotrophin release and Hypothalamic control of prolactin release* describe the effect of the catecholamines, 5-HT and GABA systems on gonadotrophins and prolactin release (see Table 10.9a for general overview) and so the same transmitter disturbances that cause affective disorders may well also affect the endocrine systems and affective disorders may be associated with infertility; for instance, depression has been associated with amenorrhoea (Ossofsky, 1974; Laakmann & Benkert, 1978). Gonadal hormones can alter brain neurotransmitter activity and response to drugs (see section *Action of steroids*) and changes

Table 10.8. *The aetiology of some affective disorders and motor disturbances*

| Disorder | Hypothesized cause |
|---|---|
| Depression | Reduced NA and/or 5-HT and/or GABA transmission |
| Anxiety | Increased NA/Ad and decreased GABA transmission |
| Mania | Increase in DA transmission |
| Schizophrenia | Increase in DA transmission in the limbic system |
| Epilepsy | Reduction in inhibitory GABA transmission |
| Tardive dyskensia (Huntingdon's Chorea) | Increase in DA activity in the basal ganglia and degeneration of the inhibitory GABA system |
| Extra-pyramidal tremor (Parkinson's disease) | Degeneration of the DA system and an increase in cholinergic activity in the striatum |

NA = noradrenaline; 5-HT = 5-hydroxytryptamine; GABA = gamma-aminobutyric acid; Ad = adrenaline; DA = dopamine

Table 10.9a. *The overall effect of some neurotransmitters on hormone release*

|  | Gonadotrophins | Prolactin |
|---|---|---|
| Noradrenaline | ↑ | ↑ |
| Dopamine | ↓ | ↓ |
| 5-HT | ↓ | ↑ |
| GABA | ↓ | ↓ |

5-HT = 5-hydroxytryptamine; GABA = gamma-aminobutyric acid

in their circulatory levels may influence centrally controlled functions, for example epileptic seizures occur more frequently pre-menstrually and when progesterone levels are low (Hamilton *et al.*, 1984; Rosciszewska *et al.*, 1986), and conversely drugs employed in the treatment of CNS disorders may affect the reproductive system by altering the release of hypothalamic and therefore pituitary hormones (see Table 10.9b).

## Antidepressants and tranquillizers

### The tricyclic antidepressants
These are tertiary amines of the imipramine type that inhibit the uptake of monoamine transmitters back into neurones effectively prolonging

Table 10.9b. *The effect of CNS drugs on hormone release*

| Drug | Effect on transmitter activity | Effect on GT | Effect on prolactin |
|---|---|---|---|
| *Tricyclic antidepressants* | | | |
| amitriptyline | ↑ 5-HT and | | ↑ (not all |
| clorimipramine | ↓ DA | | reports |
| desimipramine | ↑ NA and | | ↑ (not all |
| protriptyline | DA ↓ | | reports) |
| normofensive | ↑ DA | | ↑ |
| MAOIs | 5-HT, DA and | ↓ | ↑ |
| NB: phenelzines are anti-progesterone at uterine level and anti-GT at ovarian level. | ↑ NA | | |
| *Benzodiazapines and GABA agonists* | ↑ GABA and may be ↑ DA, NA and 5HT | ↓ LH only (Sod. valporate) | ↓ (not all reports) |
| *Hypnotics and sedatives* some are anti-GT at ovarian level | 5-HT and GABA ↑ and DA ↓ | ↓ basal and LH surge | ↑ (transient) |
| *Neuroleptics* | ↑ 5-HT and ↓ DA | ↑ LH surge, not basal | ↑ |
| *Nicotine* (as in cigarettes) | ↑ DA | ↓ | ↓ |
| *Alcohol* | ↑ 5-HT and opioids and ↓ NA | ↓ LH only | ↑ |
| *Cannabis* may have oestrogenic activity | ↑ 5-HT | ↓ | ↓ |
| *Cocaine* | ↑ 5-HT, NA & DA and ↓ AcC | ↓ LH only | ↑ (acute) ↓ (chronic) |
| *Narcotics* | ↓ DA, NA (Mimic endogenous opioids) | ↓ | ↑ |

5-HT = 5-hydroxytryptamine; DA = dopamine; NA = noradrenaline; GT = gonadotrophin; GABA = gamma-aminobutyric acid; LH = luteinizing hormone their synaptic life-span – and thus their action on the post-synaptic receptors. Their therapeutic effect may be due to the resultant increase in transmission or due to the subsequent down-regulation of the post-synaptic receptors (especially β-adrenergic receptors) and modulation of the presynaptic receptors (Asakura, Tsukamoto & Hasegawa, 1982; Enna & Duman, 1983). Examples are amitriptyline and clorimipramine which act preferentially to inhibit 5-HT uptake and imipramine, desimipramine, and protriptyline which inhibit NA uptake, examples in both groups additionally reducing DA turnover in the striatum and blocking 5-HT receptors (Carlsson et al., 1969a,b; Fuxe et al., 1978). Normofensive preferentially inhibits DA uptake and also increases DA release. It is possible that the clinical success of this group of drugs lies in their wide spectrum of activity on neuronal transmission.

These drugs do not have a marked effect on the reproductive hormones. High doses of desimipramine, amitriptyline, and chlorimipramine given chronically can stimulate prolactin levels in women (Laakmann, 1980) and this seems to correlate with their enhancement of 5-HT activity; however, this effect has not been confirmed by others (e.g. Meltzer et al., 1977). Normofensive reduces prolactin release in female rats and humans whether initial levels are normal or hyperprolactinaemic, and this is probably exerted via a DA agonist action (Genazzini et al., 1980; Laakmann, 1980).

Amitriptyline and clorimipramine do not alter gonadotrophin levels although another tricyclic compound, doxapam, raises LH, but not FSH levels in men (Linnoila et al., 1977) and imipramine treatment can reinstate menstrual cycles in amenorrhoeaic girls suffering from endogenous depression (Ossofsky, 1974).

### Monoamine oxidase inhibitors

Monoamine oxidase (MAO) is the enzyme that degrades the monoamine neurotransmitters by deamination. It exists in two forms, MAO A and MAO B, which have distinct substrates and inhibitors; 5-HT is the specific substrate for MAO A, while NA and DA are metabolized by both MAO A and B in the human. Monoamine oxidase inhibitors, therefore, prevent the degradation of the monoamines and elevate amine levels in the CNS, and it is either the enhanced neurotransmission or resulting changes in receptor sensitivity that mediate their clinical effects (Siever, Uhde & Murphy, 1982; Enna & Duman, 1983). Examples are iproniazid (non-specific inhibitor) pargyline and deprenyl (MAO B inhibitors) and clorgyline (MAO A inhibitor).

The effect of this group of compounds on the reproductive system has been studied extensively in rodents. They can delay puberty and sexual maturation in young animals, and in adults inhibit ovulation inducing acyclicity and constant dioestrus. They inhibit both gonadotrophin and prolactin release, the former associated with raised 5-HT activity and the latter with raised DA activity, in the hypothalamus (Jaitley *et al.*, 1968; Kordon, 1969; Keane, Menager & Strolin Benedetti, 1981). However, there may be some peripheral effects as well, phenalzine derivatives have an anti-gonadotrophin activity at the ovarian level and they antagonize the action of progesterone at the uterine level (Jaitley *et al.*, 1969). Phenalzine derivatives also interrupt early pregnancy: in the pre-implantation period by inhibiting prolactin release, and in the post-implantation period by antagonizing the action of progesterone (Jaitly *et al.*, 1968; Robson, Sullivan & Wilson, 1971).

### The benzodiazapines and GABA agonists
GABA is an inhibitory transmitter acting to increase membrane permeability to Cl ions which is associated with a hyperpolarizing response post-synaptically and a depolarizing response pre-synaptically (resulting in inhibition of pre-synaptic transmitter release). The pre-synaptic receptors are not only autoreceptors but are present on other neurotransmitter nerve terminals providing a pre-synaptic inhibitory input on other systems (Johnston, Allan & Skerritt, 1982).

Agents that mimic GABA such as progabide are anti-depressants. Currently it is unclear whether the anti-depressive activity of GABA agonists is due to an alteration in catecholamine and 5-HT activity or via a direct action on the GABA system. The possibility also exists that the tricyclic compounds do not act primarily by altering monoamine activity, but rather their effects are mediated by GABA-ergic systems (Bartholini, 1985).

Benzodiazapines act on specific receptors to induce allosteric modification of GABA receptors so that they are more effectively coupled to Cl-conductance, that is they potentiate GABA activity. The benzodiazapine receptor contains three recognition sites for three different ligands: (a) benzodiazapine agonists which are anxiolytic, hypnotic, anti-convulsant, and muscle relaxant, and these are agents used clinically and include chlordiazapoxide, diazepam, and fluorazepam, (b) inverse agonists, for example, β-carbolines, which have the opposite effects and uncouple GABA receptors from the regulation of Cl-channels, and (c) competitive antagonists which have no intrinsic activity, but prevent or reduce the effects of both the agonists and the inverse agonists (Tallman & Gallager, 1985; Richards *et al.*, 1986; Oreland, 1987).

Although benzodiazapines enhance GABA activity and therefore alter release of DA and other monoamines, their effects on reproductive hormones are slight and reports are conflicting. Some rodent experiments indicate that they have no effect on either normal or stress-induced pro-lactin release (Fekete *et al.*, 1981; Kane *et al.*, 1981), while others show that the benzodiazapines can inhibit both basal and enhanced prolactin release (as seen after treatment with 5-HT agonists or DA antagonists) (Lotz, 1982; Grandison, 1983). Benzodiazapines do not appear to affect gonadotrophin release.

Inverse agonists may affect reproductive hormones as they can increase circulating levels of β-endorphin-like-immunoreactivity, probably by enhancing CRF activity, which in turn will release the pro-opiomelano-corticotrophin (POMC) derivatives (β-endorphin and ACTH) from the anterior pituitary (Maiewski *et al.*, 1985).

Sodium valproate is an inhibitor of the enzyme that degrades GABA, that is GABA-transaminase. It therefore raises endogenous GABA levels and is used clinically as an anti-convulsant. In women it reduces prolactin levels whether these levels are initially normal or enhanced (Melis *et al.*, 1982). It also inhibits LH (not FSH) release, but only during the luteal phase of the menstrual cycle (Melis *et al.*, 1986). Whether chronic administration of this agent would interfere with reproductive function and fertility has yet to be elucidated.

## Hypnotics and anaesthetics

Anaesthetics are thought to have non-specific effects on the structure of cell membranes due to their lipophilic properties increasing cell membrane fluidity, thus enhancing passage of ions. Certain anaesthetics may produce the same effect by acting on specific receptors (Richards & Hesketh, 1975). In particular, barbiturates enhance the GABA-ergic system by a direct effect on Cl-channels and like GABA increase membrane permeability for Cl ions (Johnston *et al.*, 1982). Ketamine is used as an anaesthetic and acts by inhibiting N-methyl-d-aspartate (NMDA) receptors and possibly modulating 5-HT activity as well (Watkins, Krogsgaard-Larson & Honore, 1990). Examples of anaesthetics are ether, chloroform, halothane, alethesin, ketamine, and the barbiturates.

Extensive investigations in rodents, monkeys, and humans show that in rodents nearly all the anaesthetics stimulate a transient release of prolactin which returns to normal or below normal 30 minutes after administration (Subramanian & Gala, 1977, 1978; Piercy & Shin, 1980), but has longer duration in humans (Hagen, Brandt & Kehlet, 1980). They also inhibit LH release in both primates and rodents, whether the LH is released as surges, pulses or in the case of long-acting anaesthetics (i.e. phenobarbitone) basal levels (Everett & Sawyer, 1949; Blake, 1974).

Interestingly in male rats phenobarbitone can stimulate LH release (Bizzaro *et al.*, 1982). Ketamine is exceptional in that it does not affect LH levels (Puri, Puri & Anand Kumar, 1981). The general mechanism of action of the anaesthetic on hormone release is probably due to a reduction of hypothalamic DA activity and increase of 5-HT activity. Some anaesthetics also act to reduce pituitary responsiveness to GnRH (urethane), but others do not (barbiturates) (Dyer & Mansfield, 1980; Ondo & Pass, 1980). Anaesthetics may also act directly at the ovarian level reducing the steroidogenic response to gonadotrophins (Blake & Sawyer, 1972; Hagen *et al.*, 1980; Soules *et al.*, 1980).

## Neuroleptics

This group of drugs includes the phenothiazines, (e.g. chlorpromazine), butyrophenones (e.g. haloperidol, pimozide), and benzamides (e.g. sulphiride). All the compounds either act as dopamine antagonists, and/or enhance 5-HT activity. As would be expected, they stimulate prolactin release and in rodents this is shown by induction of psuedo-pregnancy, lactation, and raised circulating levels of prolactin (Beumont *et al.*, 1974; Hayes, Poland & Rubin, 1980). In humans the increased prolactin induces galactorrhoea (Clemens, Smalstig & Sawyer, 1974). The effects on prolactin release can be reversed by DA agonists (Spitz *et al.*, 1979) and in some cases (e.g. chlorpromazine) 5-HT antagonists (Board & Fierro, 1981). At the same time these agents inhibit the pre-ovulatory LH surge and thus ovulation causing amenorrhoea, although basal levels are unaffected (Beumont *et al.*, 1974; Spitz *et al.*, 1979).

## Reproductive toxicity of chemotherapeutic drugs

The number of young women in their reproductive years that become long-term survivors of cytotoxic chemotherapy is increasing, and so evaluation and an understanding of any toxic effects of the treatment on ovarian function has become important. This can be difficult to assess for individual drugs, as it is now common practice to employ combined treatment, thus retrospective human studies and animal toxicity tests on individual drugs have been carried out.

Studies of clinical cases indicate that methotrexate, vincristine, and actinomycin D have little effect on ovarian function whether given separately or in combination, although vincristine with actinomycin D reduces fertility (Shamberger *et al.*, 1981; Rustin *et al.*, 1984; Gershenson, 1988).

Alkylating agents such as busulfan, cyclophosphamide and chlorambucil are associated with irregular cycles and amenorrhoea in humans (Gershenson, 1988). The cause is destruction of the follicles resulting in a reduction in oestrogen secretion and a concomitant rise in gonadotrophin levels. The prepubertal ovary is more resistant to these agents than that of the adult, and there is a higher possibility of resumption of fertility after treatment ceases in younger women compared to older women, when the infertility may be irreversible (Sanders *et al.*, 1983; Roubenoff *et al.*, 1988).

Cyclophosphamide is the most commonly used immunosuppressant and cytotoxic agent and has been the most thoroughly studied. Its active form is 4-hydroperoxycyclophosphamide (CTX) produced by the hepatic cytochrome P450 enzyme system. As an alkylating agent it can suppress ongoing immune responses and it also interferes with DNA synthesis. *In vitro* studies on both rat and human granulosa cells show that CTX decreases basal and LH-induced progesterone and PG-E production, and *in vivo* studies show it reduces oestrogen production too. This is probably secondary to the direct cytotoxic effects of alkylation, reducing the number of viable granulosa cells or damaging the surviving cells by alkylation of macromolecules involved in steroidogenesis and prostaglandin production (Ramahi-Ataya *et al.*, 1988). CTX can also reduce fertilization of the oocyte by preventing dissolution of the cumulus and in addition it can affect early cleavage of the blastocyst (Ataya, Pydyn & Sacco, 1988). Animal studies show that when cyclophosphamide is given during pregnancy, it causes foetal death or growth retardation with a reduction in foetal and placental cell numbers rather than cell size, and this parallels the findings in the human where it induces a higher incidence of premature delivery and small for gestational age off-spring (Scott, 1977).

Azathioprine is another immunosuppressant agent. It acts after it is degraded to 6-mercaptopurine, an antimetabolite, and primarily inhibits the induction phase of the immune response; it may be cytotoxic too. It reduced the number of live births in three successive generations of mice treated with the drug and this correlated with a reduction in ovarian weight. In pregnant rats it can cause foetal death or growth retardation, however in humans it does not affect menses or pregnancy although there may be some premature births and small off-spring (Scott, 1977; Roubenoff *et al.*, 1988).

Summarizing the findings in humans, alkylating agents do appear to induce infertility which is influenced by the age of the women, the dose, duration of treatment, and the concomitant use of other immunosuppressant therapies. In younger patients, the infertility is usually reversible but this declines with age. Antimetabolite agents, for example azathioprine and methotroxate do not appear to have a strong effect on human reproduction and there is no evidence for any risk using hydroxy-chloroquine, gold or penicillamine (Roubenoff *et al.*, 1988).

Ionizing radiation causes sterility by destroying the oocytes in primodial follicles; gamates in the larger Graafian follicles are more resistant. The oocyte in the primate is more resistant than that in the rodent, but resistance decreases with age. For instance, 2000 rads over five to six weeks causes infertility in young women, but only 100 rads has such an effect in women over 40 years of age (Lione, 1987).

### Reproductive toxicity of anti-inflammatory drugs

This group of drugs exert their effects by reducing the production of prostaglandins, one of the main mediators of the inflammatory response. However, prostaglandins are also important mediators of a number of reproductive functions, namely:

(a)  Stimulation of GnRH release from the hypothalamus and thence gonadotrophins from the pituitary (see section *Hypothalamic control of gonadotrophin release*).

(b)  Stimulation of ovarian steroidogenesis (see section *Hormonal changes in the reproductive cycle*).

(c)  Stimulating rupture of the follicular wall in the ovulatory process (see section *Hormonal changes in the reproductive cycle*).

(d)  Prostaglandins are the luteolytic factors controlling the life-span of the corpus luteum. In many species they are produced by the uterine endometrium, but in the human they may be formed within the corpus luteum (see section *Hormonal changes in the reproductive cycle*).

(e)  It has been suggested that prostaglandins may be one of the factors involved in the process of implantation (see section *Pregnancy*).

(f)  Prostaglandins are important stimulators of uterine contraction at parturition and also at menstruation (see section *Hormonal changes in the reproductive cycle*).

The involvement of prostaglandins in these functions has often been demonstrated by applying prostaglandin synthesis inhibitors (which disrupted these functions) and then reversing their effects by administration of prostaglandins.

The non-steroidal anti-inflammatory (NSAI) group of drugs act primarily by inhibiting the enzyme, prostaglandin synthetase (also called cyclo-oxygenase), which normally forms prostaglandins from their precursor arachidonic acid (Flower *et al.*, 1972). Steroidal anti-inflammatory agents which are based on the glucocorticoid structure also inhibit prostaglandin production by preventing the release of arachidonic acid from its esterified stores. Glucocorticoids are known to stimulate the production of a number of proteins classed as lipocortins and the current hypothesis suggests that their main action is to inhibit phospholipase $A_2$, the enzyme that liberates arachidonic acid from its stores (Flower, 1989).

Obviously, if inhibition of prostaglandins interferes with gonadotrophin release, steroidogenesis, ovulation, implantation, and parturition, anti-flammatory agents would be expected to have unwanted side-effects on the reproductive system. In rodents, indomethacin and aspirin have been shown to inhibit ovulation and implantation, and reduce fertility (Yegnanarayan & Joglekar, 1978; Chatterjee & Chatterjee, 1982; Seeley, 1983) and more recently, *in vitro* studies on porcine granulosa cells show that the NSAI compounds acetaminophen, fenoprofen, and sulindec suppress progesterone production and cell protein levels. Butazolidin also reduces cell protein, but stimulates progesterone secretion (Haney, Hughes & Hughes, 1988). This may be important as these drugs are used for the relief of dysmenorrhoea (preventing uterine contraction at menstruation) and may be taken routinely at the expected time of the late luteal phase when women may be unknowingly pregnant.

In pregnant rodents, aspirin and the glucocorticoids can increase the rate of embryo resorption and increase the incidence of still births. If they are given over the last few days of pregnancy they can prolong gestation and their ability to exert this effect is directly related to their potency in inhibiting prostaglandin synthesis (Powell & Cochrane, 1982; Roubenoff *et al.*, 1988).

In spite of the physiological importance of prostaglandins in reproductive functions and evidence from experiments in rodents, the NSAI compounds have little or no obvious effects on fertility in humans (Roubenoff *et al.*, 1988). Perhaps their effect is so short-lived, or 'fail-safe' mechanisms come into play with other mediators taking over the role of prostaglandins.

## The effect of drugs of abuse on the reproductive system

### Caffeine

Caffeinated beverages include coffee, tea, colas and are associated with reduced fertility in women. Two recent surveys have shown that women drinking more than one cup according to Wilcox *et al.* (1988) or seven cups according to Christianson, Oechsli & van der Berg (1989) of coffee per day, will be half as likely to become pregnant per cycle as those drinking less than one cup per day. The mechanism of this action has not been elucidated, but reduced pregnancy rates and number of live pups per litter have also been noted in caffeine-treated female mice (Nolan, 1988). Coffee can be uterotrophic, but this is associated with phytoestrogens in the beans themselves, rather than the caffeine (Kaldas & Hughes, 1989).

There is evidence in rodents that caffeine is teratogenic, but this has not been noted in humans. However, there is evidence that intake in pregnancy causes intra-uterine growth retardation and low birth weight although this only occurs in women who also smoke (Brooke *et al.*, 1989). This may be due to a direct effect on the foetus since caffeine can penetrate the blastocyst, but it may also be due to constriction of the utero-placental circulation since caffeine induces the release of catecholamines (Kurzel, 1984; Nolan, 1988).

## Tobacco

Cigarette smoke contains approximately 2000 compounds, the main constituents of concern being nicotine, carbon monoxide, and polycyclic aromatic hydrocarbons (such as benzopyrine) which are carcinogenic. Reports in 1984 and 1986 state that 35% of women of reproductive age smoke an average of 10 cigarettes/day and 20–25% of pregnant women smoke (Kurzel 1984; Stillman, Rosenberg & Sachs, 1986).

There are several epidemiological studies showing that smokers are less fertile than non-smokers and that infertility may be correlated with the number of cigarettes smoked per day (see Stillman *et al.*, 1986). Smokers tend to have a higher incidence of amenorrhoea, irregular cycles, and lower levels of oestrogens. This latter finding is supported by the fact that smokers suffer less from oestrogen-dependent disorders such as breast cancer, endometrial cancer, and endometriosis and have a higher incidence of osteoporosis (Stillman *et al.*, 1986). There are at least three possible mechanisms of action causing menstrual disorders and infertility:

(a)    The nicotinic component of cigarette smoke probably acts to inhibit GnRH and thus gonadotrophin release. This is based on findings in rats after acute administration of nicotine (Blake *et al.*, 1973; see Wilson, 1979) and exposure of rats to cigarette smoke for nine days where LH, FSH, and prolactin levels were significantly reduced, without any tolerance developing. The effect could be prevented by the nicotine antagonist, mecylamine. Based on experiments using nicotine itself, it is suggested that the smoke increased DA turnover in the median eminence which then suppressed GnRH and prolactin release (Fuxe *et al.*, 1987).

(b) Nicotine stimulates adrenal catecholamine secretion as well as oxytocin and vasopressin release which in turn increases oviduct and uterine motility causing abnormal passage of the oocyte through the reproductive tract (Yoshinaga *et al.*, 1979; see Mattison & Thomford, 1989).

(c) Components of cigarette smoke exert a direct effect on the ovary accelerating the rate of oocyte atresia which eventually leads to early menopause (Mattison, 1982). This may be due to nicotine or to the polycyclic aromatic hydrocarbons. High concentrations of nicotine prevent normal meiotic maturation of oocytes, but concentrations found in the 'average' smoker do not affect meiosis (Racowsky, Hendricks & Baldwin, 1989), so perhaps in smokers this action is due to the aromatic hydrocarbons.

In pregnancy, the main effects of smoking include low birth weight, increase in spontaneous abortions, premature births, prenatal loss, and abnormal bleeding in late pregnancy; there do not appear to be any teratogenic effects. These effects may be due to nicotine which can cross the placenta and affect the foetal cardiovascular systems, although its main effect is more likely to be a vasoconstrictor action on uteroplacental blood flow resulting in reduction of the passage of oxygen and nutrients to the foetus. This action is exerted via ganglionic stimulation of maternal adrenal secretion of catecholamines (Kurzel, 1984).

Another toxic component of tobacco smoke is carbon monoxide which combines with haemoglobin to form carboxyhaemoglobin which reduces foetal oxygenation by reducing the oxygen carrying ability of haemoglobin and its ability to unload oxygen (Kurzel, 1984). While it was previously assumed that low birth weight was correlated with the number of cigarettes smoked per day (see Stillman *et al.*, 1986) a recent epidemiological study has found that the 'strength' of the cigarette (i.e. capacity to produce carbon monoxide) was more important, presumably inducing a critical concentration of carbon monoxide and/or nicotine in the circulation, after which any increase in number of cigarettes has no further effect (Anderson, Bland & Peacock, 1991). Hydrogen cyanide is also found in cigarette smoke and may reduce foetal growth by reducing Vitamin $B_{12}$ activity and combining with sulphur-containing amino-acids (Kurzel, 1984).

In an effort to counter foetal hypoxia caused by the reduced uteroplacental perfusion, relative hypertrophy of the placenta compared to the foetus may occur and this may be the cause of bleeding in late pregnancy (placenta previa and abruptio). Necrotic lesions of the placenta may also occur perhaps due to the vasoconstrictor action of nicotine or the toxic effect of cadmium which is a contaminant of tobacco (Kurzel, 1984). Placental hormone production is also affected by smoking with a decrease in oestriol and hCG secretion (Bernstein *et al.*, 1989) and smoking can also increase the mono-oxygenase activities of placental cytochrome P450 enzymes (Pasanen *et al.*, 1988). The effects of smoking on pregnancy are reversible, and cessation of smoking at any time can mitigate or prevent the deleterious effects (MacArthur & Knox, 1988).

The cardiovascular effects of nicotine in cigarette smoke synergize with the effects of high levels of steroids in inducing myocardial infarction in women on oral contraceptives (Drife, 1989). Tobacco smoking may have deleterious interactions with other agents for instance low birth weight correlates with alcohol and caffeine intake in smokers, but neither of these agents affect birth weight in non-smokers (Brooke *et al.*, 1989).

## Alcohol

The toxic effects of alcohol on the female reproductive system are currently being extensively investigated. It is well-known that chronic alcoholism can induce infertility with either irregular cycles with shortened luteal phases, or amenorrhoea. There is a reduction in LH and oestrogen levels and inhibition of the mid-cycle surge, but there is no effect on FSH release. Hyperprolactinaemia can also occur, but is not seen in all cases and is not the cause of the reduced LH secretion as in studies on rhesus monkeys the changes in levels of the two hormones were not correlated (Mello *et al.*, 1988a; Mendelson & Mello, 1988). Occasional drinking and acute administration of alcohol does not affect fertility, although a transient inhibition of LH release has been reported by some. Interestingly acute alcohol intake can raise steroid levels as the alcohol saturates the hepatic oxidative enzyme systems so that they are unavailable for other reactions such as oxidizing hydroxysteroids (e.g. oestradiol) to keto-steroids (e.g. oestrone) (Ellinboe 1987; Mendelson & Mello, 1988; Becker *et al.*, 1988).

Similar findings have been obtained in rats where chronic administration causes acyclicity, inhibition of ovulation, reduction in LH, and increase in prolactin release. Ovarian weight and steroid production are also reduced (van Thiel, Gavaler & Lester, 1978; Sanchis, Esquifino & Guerri, 1985; Rettori *et al.*, 1987; Budec *et al.*, 1990). As seen in humans, FSH release is not affected. Acute alcohol treatment also inhibits ovulation and LH release (Dees *et al.*, 1985; Mancebo *et al.*, 1984), but in some of these reports the effects may have been due to the stress of administration rather than the alcohol itself (Ellinboe *et al.*, 1987).

There is some controversy over the site of action of alcohol in its effects on the reproductive system. Much of the data indicate that it acts at the hypothalamic level inhibiting GnRH release (Dees *et al.*, 1985; Rettori *et al.*, 1987; Ching, Valenca & Negro-Vilar, 1988), but there are a few reports showing that alcohol can alter the responsiveness of the pituitary toward GnRH (Schade *et al.*, 1983; Mello *et al.*, 1986; Mello, 1988). In addition, alcohol can alter the ratio of isoforms of LH released from the pituitary. It is suggested that the isoforms have differing biological potencies due to minor differences in their structure and/or charge. Alcohol increases the proportion of acidic LH forms and also decreases the overall biological potency of LH (Emanuele *et al.*, 1986; Budec, Leigh & Wilson, unpublished results). However, these effects may be indirect and due to an alcohol-induced reduction in GnRH which normally controls LH synthetic processes (Wilson, Leigh & Chapman, 1990).

Alcohol may also act at the ovarian level as after chronic treatment (i.e. 6 weeks) in rats ovarian weight was reduced by 60%, there was an absence of corpora lutea and steroidogenesis was reduced. These effects were not the result of reduced gonadotrophins as in these experiments FSH levels were normal and LH above normal (van Thiel *et al.*, 1978; Mello, 1988).

As a lipid soluble agent, alcohol alters membrane fluidity which results in changes in transmitter release and receptor availability in many parts of the brain. In general, it increases NA and DA turnover, and opiate and GABA levels in various brain areas (Bannister & Losowsky, 1986; Alari, Lewander & Sjoquist, 1987). However, the systems mediating the inhibitory effect of alcohol on GnRH release in the hypothalamus have not been elucidated. It is unlikely to involve DA since the inhibitory effect of acute administration of alcohol on LH release is not reversed by haloperidol (Chapin, Breese & Mueller, 1980). Reduction in LH release, however, does correlate with a fall in NA levels in the whole hypothalamus and a rise in 5-HT activity in the zona incerta (Mancebo *et al.*, 1984; Budec *et al.*, 1990). It is suggested that alcohol inhibits a stimulatory noradrenergic system and enhances an inhibitory 5-HT system. Earlier findings in male rats indicate that alcohol exerts an inhibitory effect on LH release via the opiate system since its effect could be reversed by naloxone (Cicero, 1980). However, in women and monkeys, alcohol enhances the stimulatory effect of naloxone on LH release (Mello *et al.*, 1988b; Teoh *et al.*, 1988). In summary it seems most probably that alcohol affects female reproduction primarily through a central effect on neuronal systems (as yet to be elucidated) that normally control GnRH release.

Women are more susceptible to liver cirrhosis than men and this is due to sex-dependent differences in their liver enzymes. Alcohol is degraded to acetaldehyde by three enzyme systems: (1) alcohol dehydrogenase (ADH), (2) the microsomal ethanol oxidizing system (MEOS), which includes cytochrome P450 and NADPH-cytochrome C reductase, and (3) catalase. Studies in rats show that males possess lower levels of ADH and higher levels of catalase and MEOS especially cytochrome P450, compared to females. Administration of testosterone to females (in adulthood) induces a male pattern and reduces ADH and increases MEOS activity, but ovariectomy and oestradiol treatment have no effect (Teschke & Wiese, 1982), indicating that this sexual dimorphism of the liver is androgen-dependent.

Alcohol has a spectrum of serious teratogenic effects which are collectively designated the 'foetal alcohol syndrome', but it does not seem to have marked effects on the maternal system in pregnancy although it increases the deleterious effects of poor nutrition and smoking (Randall, 1987; Brooke *et al.*, 1989).

## Cannabis (marijuana, hashish)

Cannabis is derived from the female hemp plant (*Cannabis sativa*) and the active ingredients are cannabinol (Δ9-tetrahydrocannabinol; Δ9 THC) and cannabidiol (Δ8 THC). These compounds are very lipid soluble and accumulate in fatty tissue including the brain and gonads with a half-life of three to five days (Kurzel, 1984; Horowitz, 1988). In women, cannabis shortens the luteal phase of the menstrual cycle and reduces plasma LH concentrations. Similarly in monkeys and rodents, administration of Δ9 THC (in the follicular phase for primates) reduces LH, FSH, and prolactin release, inhibits ovulation and reduces steroid secretion and these effects can be overcome by administration of exogenous gonadotrophins or GnRH indicating that the Δ9 THC acts at the hypothalamic level (Hughes, Everett & Tyrey, 1981; Steger *et al.*, 1980; Smith & Asch, 1987). Δ9 THC may also have a direct ovarian effect as it inhibits progesterone synthesis by granulosa cells *in vitro* (Moon, Duleba & Jakubovic, 1982). Menstrual cycles and ovulation return to normal when cannabis is taken chronically in parallel with the development of tolerance to its CNS effects. But acute administration in monkeys seems to affect reproductive functions for several months after the treatment and this may be associated with high levels of prolactin seen after cessation of treatment (Smith & Asch 1987).

The mechanism of action of cannabis is not known, it may act by: (a) by raising 5-HT synthesis (Johnson, Dewey & Bloom, 1981) which could then inhibit GnRH release, or (b) it may act as an oestrogenic agonist or partial agonist since it can bind to oestrogen receptors (Rawitch et al., 1977) and has similar effects to oestradiol on the CNS (Foy, Teyler & Vardaris, 1982) and it is uterotrophic (Solomon et al., 1976).

In pregnancy, the foetus can be affected by cannabis as this easily crosses the placenta and has similar effects to those of alcohol (Kurzel, 1984; Horowitz, 1988). In addition, it can be harmful to the maternal system in pregnancy and cause premature labour, and in early pregnancy cause abortion which is associated with a reduction in placental secretion of chorionic gonadotrophin and progesterone (Smith & Asch, 1987).

## Cocaine

Cocaine is an alkaloid extracted from the leaves of the coca plant (*Erythroxylon coca*). It is both a local anaesthetic inhibiting nerve conductance and a CNS stimulant acting to enhance catecholamine activity by competitatively inhibiting NA and DA uptake back into the nerve terminals. At the same time it enhances release of the catecholamines and also 5-HT and inhibits release of acetylcholine (Kurzel, 1984; Horowitz, 1988; King et al., 1990).

While there are a number of reports on the effect of cocaine in pregnancy (Little et al., 1988; Mittleman, Cofino & Hearn, 1989; Kurzel, 1984) there is very little in the literature on its effect on the non-pregnant women except that it can cause irregular menstrual cycles, hyperprolactinaemia and reduce libido (Dackis et al., 1986). In rats, chronic administration of cocaine also causes irregular cycles with prolonged dioestrus, reduction in LH release and inhibition of ovulation. After six weeks of treatment there is a 44% decrease in ovulation rate (King et al., 1990). Acute administration of cocaine to rats also inhibits LH (but not FSH) release at high doses (40 mg/kg), while lower doses (10–20 mg/kg) stimulates LH release; both dose levels inhibited prolactin release (Steger et al., 1981). Presumably these effects are due to the relative proportion of increase in DA and NA activity. After chronic treatment, depletion of DA occurs which is probably the cause of the hyperprolactinaemia seen after long-term treatment (Dackis et al., 1986; King et al., 1990).

Chasnoff & Griffiths were the first to report that cocaine was teratogenic; it also affects the maternal system in pregnancy causing spontaneous abortion, placenta abruptio, uterine contractions in late pregnancy, and low birth weight babies due to reduced placental blood flow (see Chasnoff & Griffith, 1989; Little et al., 1988; Kurzel, 1984). It is likely all the effects are due to an increase in NA activity causing vaso-constriction leading to damage to the uteroplacental vascular system and also causing uterine contractions (Horowitz, 1988; Landy & Hinson, 1988; Chasnoff & Griffith, 1989).

### Narcotics

The opiate narcotics include morphine, heroin, and methadone. They all have sedative and analgesic properties as well as hallucinatory effects that make them drugs of abuse.

Female heroin addicts suffer from menstrual irregularities, reduced libido, and infertility and all of the narcotics suppress secretion of LH and FSH and raise prolactin levels (Bruni *et al.*, 1977; Smith & Asch, 1987; Wardlaw *et al.*, 1980). In rats heroin and morphine induce acyclicity and inhibit both the basal pulsatile release of LH and the preovulatory LH surge (Barraclough & Sawyer, 1955; Sylvester *et al.*, 1982). There is a large body of evidence showing that this effect on both inhibiting the gonadotrophins and stimulating prolactin release is exerted at the hypo-thalamic level via inhibition of the catecholamine systems which results in a reduction of GnRH release and enhanced prolactin release (Miller, Clifton & Steiner, 1985; Leadem *et al.*, 1985; Kalra & Kalra, 1984). *In vitro* and *in vivo* studies show that the opiates do not act directly on the pituitary, as they cannot alter pituitary responsiveness to GnRH or change the release of prolactin after pituitary stalk sectioning (Wardlaw *et al.*, 1980; Ferin *et al.*, 1982).

The opiate antagonist naloxone stimulates gonadotrophin and inhibits prolactin release in rodents and primates, indicating that the endogenous opiates exert a tonic inhibitory control over gonadotrophin secretion, and it is further suggested that steroids exert their negative feedback effect via an opiate system (Sylvester *et al.*, 1982; Kalra, 1983). In rodents, exogenous opiates also inhibit the positive feedback effect of steroids in inducing an LH surge and this is also an intra-hypothalamic action via a noradrenergic system (Akabori & Barraclough, 1986). However, in monkeys, morphine does not affect the oestradiol induced LH surge, presumably because in primates the positive feedback effect of steroids is exerted mainly at the pituitary level, where opiates have no action (Ferin *et al.*, 1982). Thus the menstrual irregularities seen in human addicts are probably initially due to defective control of follicular growth by reduced basal gonadotrophin levels and/or hyperprolactinaemia rather than a direct inhibition of the mid-cycle LH surge.

Narcotics in pregnancy do not have a tetragenic or lethal effect on the foetus, but they can cause premature labour and low birth weight. The

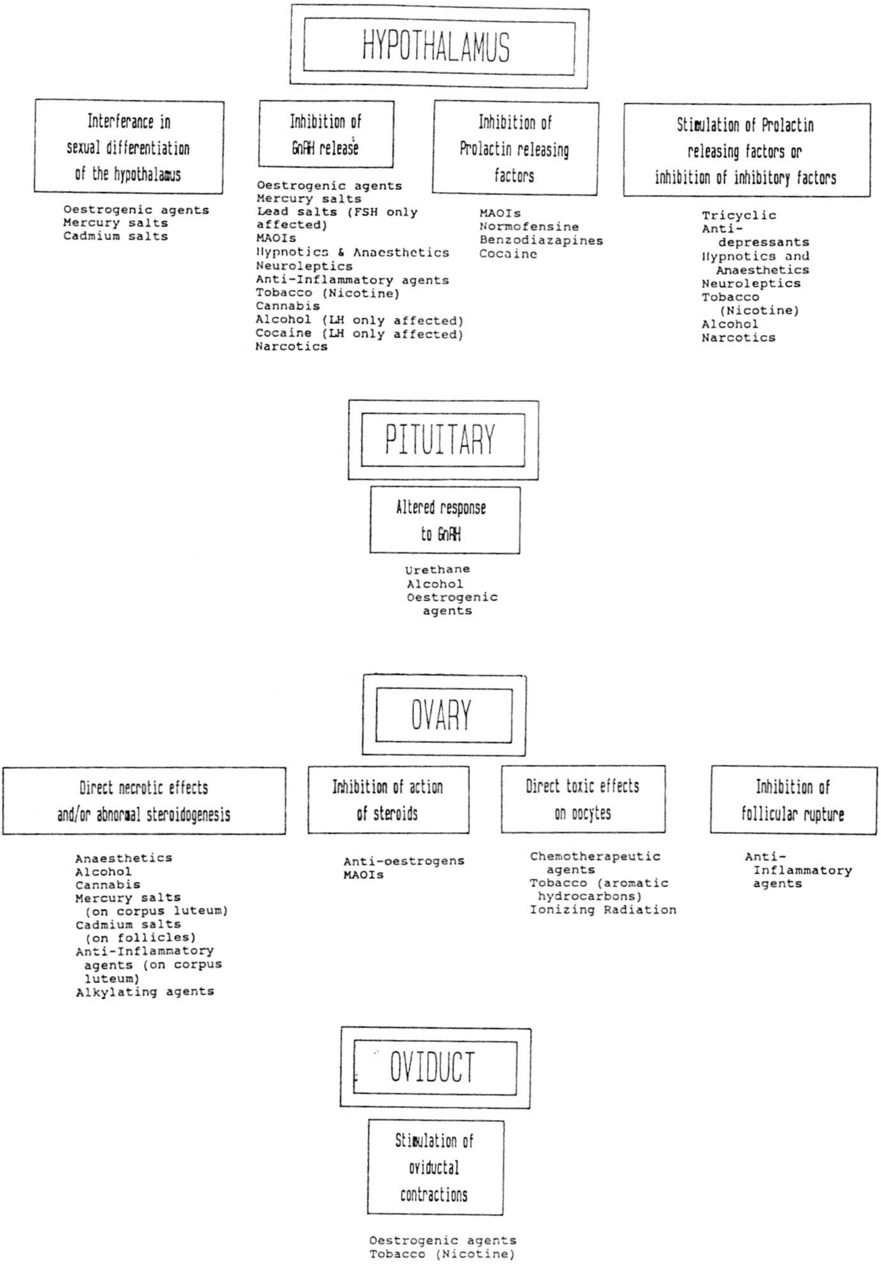

## HYPOTHALAMUS

**Interference in sexual differentiation of the hypothalamus**

Oestrogenic agents
Mercury salts
Cadmium salts

**Inhibition of GnRH release**

Oestrogenic agents
Mercury salts
Lead salts (FSH only affected)
MAOIs
Hypnotics & Anaesthetics
Neuroleptics
Anti-Inflammatory agents
Tobacco (Nicotine)
Cannabis
Alcohol (LH only affected)
Cocaine (LH only affected)
Narcotics

**Inhibition of Prolactin releasing factors**

MAOIs
Normofensine
Benzodiazapines
Cocaine

**Stimulation of Prolactin releasing factors or inhibition of inhibitory factors**

Tricyclic Anti-depressants
Hypnotics and Anaesthetics
Neuroleptics
Tobacco (Nicotine)
Alcohol
Narcotics

## PITUITARY

**Altered response to GnRH**

Urethane
Alcohol
Oestrogenic agents

## OVARY

**Direct necrotic effects and/or abnormal steroidogenesis**

Anaesthetics
Alcohol
Cannabis
Mercury salts (on corpus luteum)
Cadmium salts (on follicles)
Anti-Inflammatory agents (on corpus luteum)
Alkylating agents

**Inhibition of action of steroids**

Anti-oestrogens
MAOIs

**Direct toxic effects on oocytes**

Chemotherapeutic agents
Tobacco (aromatic hydrocarbons)
Ionizing Radiation

**Inhibition of follicular rupture**

Anti-Inflammatory agents

## OVIDUCT

**Stimulation of oviductal contractions**

Oestrogenic agents
Tobacco (Nicotine)

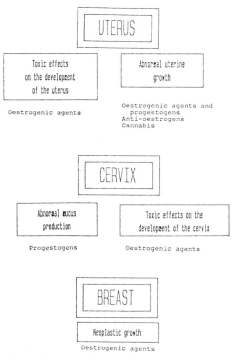

Fig. 10.3. Sites of action of xenobiotics in disruption of the reproductive system.

latter is associated with a reduction in cell numbers and reduced protein synthesis (Kurzel, 1984).

Exogenous morphine increases *in vitro* hCG synthesis by placental cells obtained in the first trimester of pregnancy. This may reflect the physiological action of endogenous opiates synthesized by the placenta (Cemerikic *et al.*, 1988). This is probably not at all harmful, but narcotics also reduce placental synthesis of oestradiol as they compete with the steroids for the microsomal mixed oxidases (Kurzel, 1984).

## Summary and conclusion

The above review has covered the effects of some hormones and xenobiotics on the female reproductive system and these are summarized in Figs 10.3 and 10.4. Where possible, we have included available information on the sites and mechanisms of action, necessitating a full survey of endo-

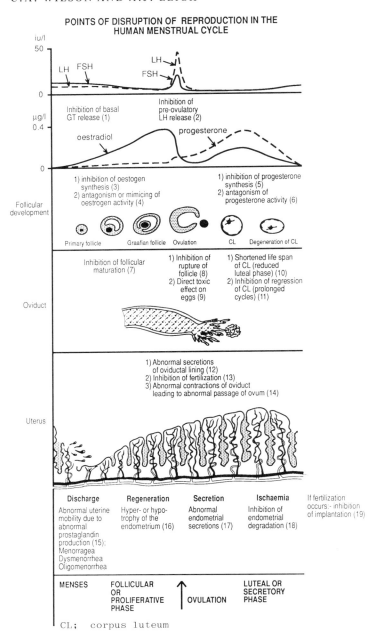

**POINTS OF DISRUPTION OF REPRODUCTION IN THE HUMAN MENSTRUAL CYCLE**

Fig. 10.4. Sites of toxic effects of xenobiotics in the menstrual cycle

genous mediators of normal reproductive function in the first part of the chapter. It is anticipated that as our knowledge of drug action becomes more comprehensive, it will become possible to identify the system(s) they affect, and thus to predict the induction of detrimental side-effects on the female reproductive system.

Fig. 10.4 (cont.)

| Drugs | Sites of toxicity (as shown in Fig. 10.4) |
|---|---|
| A. *Oestrogenic agents* | 1, 2, 7, 12, 14, 16, 17 |
| e.g. Pesticides | |
| Industrial agents | |
| Phytoestrogens | |
| B. *Anti-oestrogenic agents* | 3, 4, 5, 6, 10, 16, 19 |
| e.g. Phytoestrogens | |
| Clomiphene | |
| Tamoxifen | |
| Lindane | |
| C. *Metal ions* | |
| e.g. Mercury | 1, 11 |
| Cadmium | 7, 16, 17 |
| Lead | 1, 5, 19 |
| D. *CNS drugs* | |
| e.g. Tricyclics and | |
| Benzodiazapines | Not toxic |
| MAOIs | 1, 7, 17 |
| Sodium valproate | 1 |
| Hypnotics and anaesthetics | 1, 2, 3, 5 |
| Neuroleptics | 2 |
| E. *Chemotherapeutic agents* | 3, 5, 7, 9, 13 |
| and *ionizing radiation* | 9 |
| F. *Anti-inflammatory drugs* | 1, 2, 3, 5, 8, 11(?) 15, 19 |
| G. *Drugs of abuse* | |
| e.g. Tobacco | 1, 2, 3, 9, 14, 18 |
| Alcohol | 1, 2, 3, 10 |
| Cannabis | 1, 2, 4, 5, 10, 16 |
| Cocaine | 1, 2 |
| Narcotics | 1 |

# References

Adashi, E.Y., Resnick, C.E. & Rosenfeld, R.G. (1989). Insulin-like growth factor-I (IGF-I) and IGF-II hormonal action in cultured rat granulosa cells: mediation via type I but not type II IGF receptors. *Endocrinology*, **126**, 216–22.

Adashi, E.Y., Resnick, C.E., Svoboda, M.E. & Van Wyk, J.J. (1986). Somatomedin-C as an amplifier of follicle-stimulating hormone action: enhanced accumulation of adenosine 3′,5′-Monophosphate. *Endocrinology*, **118**, 149–55.

Advis, J.P., Aguado, L.I. & Ojeda, S.R. (1983). Hyperprolactinemia enhances ovarian estrogen responsiveness to gonadotropins in prepubertal rats: Antagonistic effect of adrenalectomy. *Biology of Reproduction*, **29**, 181–94.

Akabori, A. & Barraclough, C.A. (1986). Effects of morphine on luteinizing hormone secretion and catacholamine turnover in the hypothalamus of estrogen-treated rats. *Brain Research*, **362**, 221–6.

Alari, L., Lewander, T. & Sjoquist, B. (1987). The effect of ethanol on the brain catecholamine systems in female mice, rats and guinea pigs. *Alcoholism: Clinical and Experimental Research*, **11**, 144–9.

Anderson, D.J. & Hill, J.A. (1988). Review. Cell-mediated immunity in infertility. *American Journal of Reproductive Immunology and Microbiology*, **17**, 22–30.

Anderson, H.R., Bland, J.M. & Peacock, J.L. (1991). Effects of smoking on fetal growth: evidence for a threshold, the importance of brand of cigarette and inter-action with alcohol and caffeine consumption. Proc. Ciba Symposium on the effects of smoking on the fetus, neonate and child. (In press.)

Arnold, A.P. & Gorski, R.A. (1984). Gonadal steroids induction of structural sex differences in the central nervous system. *Annual Review Neuroscience*, **7**, 413–42.

Asakura, M., Tsukamoto, T. & Hasegawa, K. (1982). Modulation of rat brain $\alpha_2$- and $\beta$-adrenergic receptor sensitivity following long-term treatment with antidepressants. *Brain Research*, **235**, 192–7.

Ataya, K.M., Pydyn, E.F. & Sacco, A.G. (1988). Effect of 'Activated' cyclophosphamide on mouse oocyte in vitro fertilization and cleavage. *Reproductive Toxicology*, **2**, 105–9.

Austin & Short (eds) (1982). *Reproduction in Mammals* 1. Cambridge: Cambridge University Press.

Bahr, J.M. & Ben-Jonathan, N. (1985). Elevated catecholamines in porcine follicular fluid before ovulation. *Endocrinology*, **117**, 620–3.

Baird, D.T., Corker, C.S., Davidson, D.W., Hunter, W.M., Michie, E.H. & van Look, P.F.A. (1977). Pituitary-ovarian relationships in polycystic ovary syndrome. *Journal of Clinical Endocrinology Metabolism*, **45**, 798–809.

Bannister, P. & Losowsky, M.S. (1986). Cell receptors and ethanol.

*Alcoholism: Clinical and Experimental Research*, **10** (Suppl.), 50–4.

Barlow, S.M. & Sullivan, F.M. (1982). *Reproductive Hazards of Industrial Chemicals*. London: Academic Press.

Barnea, A., Cho, G. & Colombani-Vidal, M. (1986a). Extracellular calcium is required for copper-amplified prostaglandin $E_2$ stimulation of the release of gonadotropin-releasing hormone from median eminence explants. *Endocrinology*, **119**, 1262–7.

Barnea, A., Cho, G. & Colombani-Vidal, M. (1986b). Amplification of prostaglandin $E_2$ stimulation of luteinizing hormone-releasing hormone release from median eminence explants: a metal (II)-specific effect of chelated copper. *Brain Research*, **384**, 101–5.

Barraclough, C.A. & Sawyer, C.A. (1955). Inhibition of the release of pituitary ovulating hormone in the rat by morphine. *Endocrinology*, **57**, 329–37.

Barraclough, C.A. & Wise, P.M. (1982). The role of catecholamines in the regulation of pituitary luteinizing hormone and follicle-stimulating hormone secretion. *Endocrine Reviews*, **3**, 91–119.

Bartholini, G. (1985). GABA receptor agonists: Pharmacological spectrum and therapeutic actions. *Medicinal Research Reviews*, **5**, 55–75.

Baum, M.J., Carroll, R.S., Cherry, J.A. & Tobert, S.A. (1990). Steroidal control of behavioural, neuroendocrine and brain sexual differentiation: studies in a carnivore, the ferret. *Journal of Neuroendocrinology*, **2**, 401–18.

Bazer, F.W. & Johnson, H.M. (1989). Action of lymphokines and cytokines on reproductive tissue. *Progress in Neuroendocrine-immunology*, **2**, 50–4.

Becker, U., Gluud, C., Bennett, P., Micic, S., Svenstrup, B., Winkler, K., Christensen, N.J. & Hardt, F. (1988). Effect of alcohol and glucose infusion on pituitary-gonadal hormones in normal females. *Drug and Alcohol Dependence*, **22**, 141–9.

Behrman, H.R., Preston, S.L. & Hall, A.K. (1980). Cellular mechanism of the antigonadotropic action of luteinizing hormone-releasing hormone in the corpus luteum. *Endocrinology*, **107**, 656–64.

Bernstein, L., Pike, M.C., Lobo, R.A., Depue, R.H., Ross, R.G. & Henderson, B.E. (1989). Cigarette smoking in pregnancy results in a marked decrease in maternal hCG and oestradiol levels. *British Journal of Obstetrics & Gynaecology*, **96**, 92–6.

Beumont, P.J.V., Gelder, M.G., Friesen, H.G., Harris, G.W., MacKinnon, P.C.B., Mandelbrote, B.M. & Wiles, D.H. (1974). The effect of phenothiazines on endocrine function I. Patients with inappropriate lactation and amenorrhoea. *British Journal of Psychiatry*, **124**, 413–19.

Bicknell, R.J. (1985). Endogenous opioid peptides and hypothalamic neuroendocrine neurones. *Journal of Endocrinology*, **107**, 437–46.

Bizzarro, A., Di Martino, G., Iannucci, F., Verdoliva, A., Florion, A.,

Guarino, G. & Iacono, G. (1982). Effect of anaesthesia on serum levels of LH and FSH in man with and without GnRH test. *Acta Endocrinologica*, **99**, 14–17.

Blake, C.A. (1974). Localization of the inhibitory actions of ovulation-blocking drugs on release of luteinizing hormone in ovariectomised rats. *Endocrinology*, **95**, 999–1004.

Blake, C.A., Norman, R.L., Scaramuzzi, R.J. & Sawyer, C.A. (1973). Inhibition of proestrus surge of prolactin in the rat by nicotine. *Endocrinology*, **92**, 1334–8.

Blake, C.A. & Sawyer, C.A. (1972). Ovulation blocking actions of urethane in the rat. *Endocrinology*, **91**, 87–100.

Board, J.A. & Fierro, R.J. (1981). Effect of cyproheptadine on chlorpromazine stimulation of prolactin in women. *Am. Journal of Obstetrics and Gynaecology*, **139**, 160–3.

Bohn, H., Dati, F. & Luben, R. (1983). Human trophoblast specific products other than hormones. In *Biology of Trophoblast*, ed. Y. W. Lobe & A. Whyte, pp. 317–52. Amsterdam: Elsevier.

Bonney, R.C. & Franks, S. (1989). The role of prolactin in the uterus. In *Prolactin and Lesions in Breast Uterus and Prostate*, ed. H. Nagasarva, pp. 97–106. Florida: CRC Press.

Briggs, M.H. & Briggs, M. (1976). *Biochemical Contraception, Prospects for Human Development*. London: Academic Press.

Brooke, O.G., Anderson, H.R., Bland, J.M., Peacock, J.L. & Stewart, C.M. (1989). Effects on birth weight of smoking, alcohol, caffeine, socioeconomic factors, and psychosocial stress. *British Medical Journal*, **298**, 795–801.

Bruni, J.F., van Vugt, D., Marshall, S. & Meites, J. (1977). Effects of naloxone, morphine and methionine enkephalin on serum prolactin, luteinizing hormone, follicle stimulating hormone, thyroid stimulating hormones and growth hormone. *Life Sciences*, **21**, 461–6.

Budec, M., Hole, D.R., Wilson, C.A. & Slater, D.M. (1990). The effect of chronic alcohol consumption on gonadotrophin release in intact female rats. *Journal of Endocrinological Investigations*, **13**, Suppl. 2, p. 180.

Bulger, W.H. & Kupfer, D. (1985). Estrogenic activity of pesticides and other xenobiotics on the uterus and female reproductive system. In *Endocrine Toxicology*, ed. J.A. Thomas, K.S. Korach & J.A. McLachlan, pp. 357–92. New York: Raven Press.

Burbacher, T.M., Mohamed, M.K. & Mottett, N.K. (1988). Methylmercury effects on reproduction and offspring size at birth. *Reproductive Toxicology*, **1**, 267–78.

Burden, J.W., Leonard, M.J., Hodson, C.A., Louis, T.M. & Lawrence, I.E., Jr (1986). Effect of abdominal vagotomy at proestrus on ovarian weight, ovarian antral follicles, and serum levels of gonadotropins, estradiol, and testosterone in the rat. *Neuroendocrinology*, **42**, 449–55.

Burger, C.W., Korsen, T., van Kessel, H., van Dop, P.A., Caron, F.J.M. & Schoemaker, J. (1985). Pulsatile luteinizing hormone patterns in the follicular phase of the menstrual cycle, polycystic ovarian disease (PCOD) and non-PCOD secondary amenorrhea. *Journal of Clinical Endocrinology and Metabolism*, **61**, 1126–32.

Burrows, G.H. & Barnea, A. (1982). Copper stimulates the release of luteinizing hormone releasing hormone from isolated hypothalamic granules. *Endocrinology*, **110**, 1456–8.

Canipari, R. & Strickland, S. (1986). Studies on the hormonal regulation of plasminogen activator production in the rat ovary. *Endocrinology*, **118**, 1652–9.

Cannon, J.G. & Dinarello, C.A. (1985). Increased plasma interleukin-I activity in women after ovulation. *Science*, **227**, 1247–9.

Carlsson, A., Corrodi, H., Fuxe, K. & Hokfelt, T. (1969a). Effect of antidepressant drugs on the depletion of intraneuronal brain 5-hydroxytryptamine stores caused by 4-methyl alpha-ethyl-meta-tyramine. *European Journal of Pharmacol.*, **5**, 357–66.

Carlsson, A., Corrodi, H., Fuxe, K. & Hokfelt, T. (1969b). Effects of some antidepressant drugs on the depletion of intraneuronal catecholamine stores caused by 4-alpha-dimethyl-metatyramine. *European Journal of Pharmacol.*, **5**, 367–73.

Cemerikic, B., Genbacev, O., Sulovic, V. & Beaconsfield, R. (1988). Effect of morphine on hCG release by first trimester human trophoblast *in vitro*. *Life Sciences*, **42**, 1773–9.

Cetrulo, C.L. & Sbarra, A.J. (Eds) (1984). *The Problem-Orientated Medical Record for High-Risk Obstetrics*. New York: Plenum Medical Book Co.

Chabot, J.-G., St.-Arnaud, R., Walker, P. & Pelletier, G. (1986). Distribution of epidermal growth factor receptors in the rat ovary. *Molecular and Cellular Endocrinology*, **44**, 99–108.

Chapin, R.E., Breese, G.R. & Mueller, R.A. (1980). Possible mechanisms of reduction of plasma luteinizing hormone by ethanol. *Journal of Pharmacology and Experimental Therapeutics*, **212**, 6–10.

Chard, T., Craig, P.H., Menabawey, M. & Lee, C. (1986). Alpha interferon in human pregnancy. *British J. Obstetrics & Gynaecology*, **93**, 1145–9.

Chasnoff, I.J. & Griffith, D.R. (1989). Cocaine: clinical studies of pregnancy and the newborn. *Annals New York Academy of Sciences*, **562**, 260–6.

Chatterjee, A. & Chatterjee, R. (1982). Inhibition of ovulation by indomethacin in rats. *Prostaglandins Leukotrines and Medicine*, **9**, 235–40.

Ching, M., Valenca, M. & Negro-Vilar, A. (1988). Acute ethanol treatment lowers hypophyseal portal plasma luteinizing hormone-releasing hormone (LH–RH) and systemic plasma LH levels in orchidectomized rats. *Brain Research*, **443**, 325–8.

Christianson, R.E., Oechsli, F.W. & van der Berg, B.J. (1989). Caffeinated beverages and decreased fertility. *The Lancet*, **1**, 378.

Cicero, T.J. (1980). Common mechanisms underlying the effects of ethanol and narcotics on neuroendocrine function. In *Advances in Substance Abuse*, ed. W.K. Mello, pp. 201–54. Connecticut: J.A.I. Press.

Clark, J.H. & Markaverich, B.M. (1988). Actions of ovarian steroid hormones. In *The Physiology of Reproduction 1*, ed. E. Knobil & J.D. Neill, pp. 675–724. New York: Raven Press.

Clayton, R.N. & Catt, K.J. (1981). Regulation of pituitary gonadotropin-releasing hormone receptors by gonadal hormones. *Endocrinology*, **108**, 887–95.

Clemens, J.A., Smalstig, E.M. & Sawyer, B.D. (1974). Antipsychotic drugs stimulate prolactin release. *Psychopharmacologica*, **40**, 123–7.

Cooper, R.L., Chadwick, R.W., Rehnberg, G.L., Goldman, J.M., Booth, K.C., Hein, J.F. & McElroy, W.K. (1989a). Effect of lindane on hormonal control of reproductive function in the female rat. *Toxicology and Applied Pharmacology*, **99**, 384–94.

Cooper, R.L., Goldman, J.M. & Rehnberg, G.L. (1988b). Regulation of ovarian function. In *Toxicology of the Male and Female Reproductive Systems*, ed. P.K. Woking, pp. 15–29. New York: Hemisphere Publishing Corporation.

Dackis, C.A., Gold, M.S., Davies, R.K. & Sweeney, D.R. (1986). Bromocriptine treatment for cocaine abuse: the dopamine depletion hypothesis. *International Journal of Psychiatric Medicine*, **15**, 125–35.

Davoren, B., Kasson, B.G., Li, C.H. & Hsueh, A.J.W. (1986). Specific insulin-like growth factor (IGF) I- and II-binding sites on rat granulosa cells: relation to IGF action, *Endocrinology*, **119**, 2155–62.

Dees, W.L., Rettori, V., Kozlowski, G.P. & McCann, S.M. (1985). Ethanol and the pulsatile release of luteinizing hormone, follicle stimulating hormone and prolactin in ovariectomized rats. *Alcohol*, **2**, 641–5.

Dees, W.L., Ahmed, C.E. & Ojeda, S.R. (1986). Substance P- and vasoactive intestinal peptide-containing fibers reach the ovary by independent routes. *Endocrinology*, **119**, 638–41.

Dekel, N. & Sherizly, I. (1985). Epidermal growth factor induces maturation of rat follicle-enclosed oocytes. *Endocrinology*, **116**, 406–9.

Denef, C., Baes, M. & Schramme, C. (1986). Panacrine interactions in the anterior pituitary gland. Role in the regulation of prolactin and growth hormone secretion. In *Frontiers in Neuroendocrinology 9*, ed. W.F. Ganong & L. Martini, pp. 115–48. New York: Raven Press.

Dodson, W.C. & Schomberg, D.W. (1987). The effect of transforming growth factor-$\beta$ on follicle-stimulating hormone-induced differentiation of cultured rat granulosa cells. *Endocrinology*, **120**, 512–16.

Donoso, A.O. & Banzan, A.M. (1980). $H_1$- and $H_2$-histamine receptor antagonists and induced release of prolactin in male rats. *Neuro-endocrinology*, **30**, 11–14.

Drife, J. (1989). Complications of combined oral contraception. In *Contraception Science and Practice*, ed. M. Filshie & J. Guillebaud, pp. 39–51. London: Butterworths.

Drouva, S.V., Gorenne, E., Laplante, E., Derat, E., Enjalbert, A. & Kordon, C. (1990). Estradiol modulates protein kinase C activity in the rat pituitary in vivo and in vitro. *Endocrinology*, **126**, 536–44.

Dyer, R.G. & Mansfield, S. (1980). Relationship between duration of urethane and pentobarbitone anaesthesia in male and female rats and adenohypophyseal response to luteinizing-hormone releasing hormone. *British Journal of Pharmacology*, **69**, 139–43.

Eisenberg, E. (1981). Toward an understanding of reproductive function in anorexia nervosa. *Fertility and Sterility*, **36**, 543–50.

Ekholm, C., Clark, M.R., Magnusson, C., Isaksson, O. & LeMaire, W.J. (1982). Ovulation induced by a gonadotropin releasing hormone analog in hypophysectomized rats involves prostaglandins. *Endocrinology*, **110**, 288–90.

Ellinboe, J. (1987). Acute effects of ethanol on sex hormones in non-alcoholic men and women. *Alcohol and Alcoholism*, Suppl. 1, 109–16.

Ellinboe, J., Shaw, F.H., Skupney, A.S.T. & Sikorski, M.A. (1987). Does ethanol inhibit LH secretion in the rat? *Alcohol & Alcoholism*, Suppl. 1, 539–43.

Emanuele, M.A., Hojvat, S., Emanuele, N.V., Zelke, S., Kirsteins, L. & Lawrence, A.M. (1986). The effect of alcohol on quantitative and qualitative changes in luteinizing hormone (LH) in the female rat. *Endocrine Research*, **12**, 123–36.

Enna, S.J. & Duman, R.S. (1983). β-Adrenergic receptor regulation and antidepressants: the influence of adrenocorticotropin. *Journal of Neural Transmission*, **57**, 297–307.

Erickson, G.F. (1986). An analysis of follicle development in ovum maturation. *Seminars in Reproductive Endocrinology*, **4**, 233–54.

Espey, L.L. (1980). Ovulation as an inflammatory reaction – A hypothesis. *Biology of Reproduction*, **22**, 73–106.

Evans, R.M. (1988). The steroid and thyroid hormone receptor super family. *Science*, **240**, 889–95.

Evans, W.S., Cronin, M.J. & Thorner, M.O. (1982). Hypogonadism in hyperprolactinaemia and proposed mechanisms. In *Frontiers in Neuroendocrinology* 7, ed. W.F. Ganong & L. Martini, pp. 71–122. New York: Raven Press.

Everett, J.W. & Sawyer, C.H. (1949). A neural timing factor in the mechanism by which progesterone advances ovulation in the cyclic rat. *Endocrinology*, **45**, 581–95.

Fekete, M.I.K., Szentendrei, T., Kanyicska, B. & Palkovits, M. (1981). Effects of anxiolytic drugs on the catecholamine and DOPAC (3,4-dihydroxyphenylacetic acid) levels in brain cortical areas and on corticosterone and prolactin secretion in rat subjected to stress. *Psychoneuroendocrinology*, **6**, 113–20.

Feng, P., Knecht, M. & Catt, K. (1987). Hormonal control of epidermal growth factor receptors by gonadotropins during granulosa cell differentiation. *Endocrinology*, **120**, 1121–6.

Ferin, M., Wehrenberg, W.B., Lam, N.Y., Alston, E.J. & Vande Wiele, R.L. (1982). Effects and site of action of morphine on gonadotropin secretion in the female rhesus monkey. *Endocrinology*, **111**, 1652–6.

de Feudis, F.V. (1984). Review. Gaba and endocrine regulation-relation to neurologic-phychiatric disorders. *Neurochemistry International*, **6**, 1–16.

Fink, G. (1988). Gonadotropin secretion and its control. In *The Physiology of Reproduction*, ed. E. Knobil & J. Neill, pp. 1349–77. New York: Raven Press.

Flint, A.P.F. & Sheldrick, E.L. (1982). Ovarian secretion of oxytocin is stimulated by prostaglandins. *Nature*, **297**, 587–8.

Flower, R. (1989). Lipocortin. *Biochemical Society Transactions*, **17**, 276–8.

Flower, R., Gryglewski, R., Herbaczynska, C.K. & Vane, J.R. (1972). Effects of anti-inflammatory drugs on prostaglandin biosynthesis. *Nature*, **238**, 104–6.

Fowler, P.A., Messinis, I.E. & Templeton, A.A. (1990). Gonadotrophin surge-attenuating factor (GnSAF) is produced preferentially by small follicles in super-ovulated women. *J. Reproduction and Fertility. Abstract Series*, **5**, No. 6.

Fox, H. (1989). The placenta, membranes and umbilical cord. In *Obstetrics*, ed. K.A. Turnbull & G. Chamberlain, pp. 67–81. Edinburgh: Churchill Livingstone.

Foy, M.R., Teyler, T.J. & Vardaris, R.M. (1982). $\Delta^9$-THC and 17-β-estradiol in hippocampus. *Brain Research Bulletin*, **8**, 341–5.

Franks, S., Mason, H.D., Polson, D.W., Winston, R.M.L., Margara, R. & Reed, M.J. (1988). Mechanism and management of ovulatory failure in women with polycystic ovary syndrome. *Human Reproduction*, **3**, 531–4.

Freeman, M.E. (1988). The ovarian cycle of the rat. In *The Physiology of Reproduction* 1, ed. E. Knobil & J.D. Neill, pp. 1893–1928. New York: Raven Press.

Frisch, R.E. (1985). Fatness, menarche, and female fertility. *Perspectives in Biology and Medicine*, **28**, 611–33.

Frisch, R.E. & McArthur, J. (1974). Menstrual cycles: fatness as a determinant of minimum weight for height necessary for their maintenance or onset. *Science*, **185**, 949–51.

Fuxe, K.I., Lofstrom, A., Eneroth, P., Gustafsson, J.-A., Skett, P., Hokfelt, T., Weisel, F.-A. & Agnati, L. (1977). Involvement of central catecholamines in the feedback actions of 17β-estradiol benzoate on luteinizing hormone secretion in the ovariectomized female rat. *Psychoneuroendocrinology*, **2**, 203–25.

Fuxe, K., Ogren, S.-O., Everitt, B.J., Agnati, L.F., Eneroth, P., Gustaffson, J.A., Johsson, G., Skett, P. & Holm, A. (1978). Antidepressants and brain amine metabolism. In *Proceedings of the 13th Symposium on Medicine. Hoechst on Depressive Disorders*, ed. S. Garattini, pp. 67–91. New York: Schattauer.

Fuxe, K., Anderson, K., Eneroth, P., Harfstrand, A., Nordberg, A. & Agnati, F. (1987). Effects of nicotine and exposure to cigarette smoke on discrete dopamine and noradrenaline nerve terminal systems of the telencephalon and diencephalon of the rat: relationship to reward mechanisms and neuroendocrine functions and distribution of nicotinic sites in brain. In *Advances in Behavioral Biology* 31, *Tobacco Smoking and Nicotine*, ed. W.R. Martin, G.R. van Loon *et al.*, pp. 225–62. New York: Plenum Press.

Gandelman, R. (1983). Gonadal hormones and sensory function. *Neuroscience & Behavioural Reviews*, **7**, 1–17.

Garver, D.L. & Davis, J.M. (1979). Biogenic amines hypotheses of affective disorders. *Life Science*, **24**, 383–94.

Geenen, V., Legros, J.J., Hazee-Hagelstein, M.T., Louis-Kohn, F., Lecomte-Yerna, M.J., Demoulin, A. & Franchimont, P. (1985). Release of immunoreactive oxytocin and neurophysin I by cultured luteinizing bovine granulosa cells. *Acta Endocrinologica*, **110**, 263–70.

Genazzini, A.R., Camanni, F., Massara, F., Piccioilini, E., Cocchi, D., Belforte, L. & Muller, E.E. (1980). A new pharmacological approach to the diagnosis of hyperprolactinaemic states: the nomifensine test. *Acta Endocrinol.*, **93**, 139–48.

George, F.W. & Wilson, J.D. (1988). Sex determination and Differentiation. In *The Physiology of Reproduction* 1, ed. E. Knobil & J.D. Neill, pp. 3–26. New York: Raven Press.

Gershenson, D.M. (1988). Menstrual and reproductive function after treatment with combination chemotherapy for malignant ovarian germ cell tumours. *Journal of Clinical Oncology*, **6**, 270–5.

Gillmer, M.D.G. (1989). Metabolic effects of combined oral contraceptives. In *Contraception Science and Practice*, ed. M. Filshie & J. Guillebaud, pp. 11–38. London: Butterworths.

Gorwill, R.H. & Steele, H.D. (1988). The long-term effect of clomiphene citrate on vaginal epithelial differentiation in the mouse. *Reproductive Toxicology*, **1**, 263–6.

Grandison, L. (1983). Action of benzodiazepines on the neuroendocrine system. *Neuropharmacology*, **22**, 1505–10.

Gustafsson, J.-A., Mode, A., Norstedt, G. & Skett, P. (1983). Sex steroid induced changes in hepatic enzymes. *Annual Reviews in Physiology*, **45**, 51–60.

Hagen, C., Brandt, M.R. & Kehlet, H. (1980). Prolactin, LH, FSH, GH

& cortisol response to surgery and the effect of epidural analgesia. *Acta Endocrinol.*, **94**, 151–4.

Hamilton, J.A., Lloyd, C., Alagna, S.W., Phillips, K. & Pinkel, S. (1984). Gender, depressive subtypes, and gender-age effects on antidepressant response: Hormonal hypotheses. *Psychopharmacology Bulletin*, **20**, 475–80.

Hammond, J.M., Lino, J., Baranao, S., Skaleris, D., Knight, A.B., Romanus, J.A. & Rechler, M.M. (1985). Production of insulin-like growth factors by ovarian granulosa cells. *Endocrinology*, **117**, 2553–5.

Hancock, K.W., Oakey, R.E. & Glass, M.R. (1987). Treatment of polycystic ovary syndrome. In *Recent Advances in Obstetrics & Gynaecology* No. 15, ed. J. Bonnar, pp. 239–58. Edinburgh: Churchill Livingstone.

Haney, A.F. (1985). Effect of toxic agents on ovarian function. In *Endocrine Toxicology*, ed. J.A. Thomas, K.S. Korach & J.A. McLachlan, pp. 181–210. New York: Raven Press.

Haney, A.F., Hughes, S.F. & Hughes, C.L. Jr (1988). Effects of acetaminophen and nonsteroidal anti-inflammatory drugs on progesterone production by porcine granulosa cells in vitro. *Reproductive Toxicology*, **1**, 285–91.

Hayes, S.E., Poland, R.E. & Rubin, R.T. (1980). Prolactin releasing potencies of antipsychotic and related non-antipsychotic compounds in female rats. *Journal of Pharmacology Experimental Therapeutics*, **214**, 362–7.

Hawkins, D.F. (Ed.) (1987). *Drugs and Pregnancy; Human Teratogenesis and Related Problems*, 2nd edn. publ. Edinburgh: Churchill Livingstone.

Hedin, L., Gaddy-Kurten, D., Kurten, R., DeWitt, D.L., Smith, W.L. & Richards, J.S. (1987). Prostaglandin endoperoxide synthetase in rat ovarian follicles: content, cellular distribution, and evidence for hormonal induction preceding ovulation. *Endocrinology*, **121**, 722–31.

Hendrickx, A.G., Prahalada, S. & Binkerd, P.E. (1988). Long-term evaluation of the diethylstilbestrol (DES) syndrome in adult female rhesus monkeys (*Macaca mulatta*). *Reproductive Toxicology*, **1**, 253–61.

Hinkle, P.M. (1988). Regulation of prolactin synthesis by peptide hormones. In *Effects and mechanism of action* 3, ed. A. Negro-Vilar & P.M. Conn, pp. 143–54. Boca Raton: CRC.

Hiroi, M., Sugita, S. & Suzuki, M. (1965). Ovulation induced by implantation of cupric sulphate into the brain of the rabbit. *Endocrinology*, **77**, 963–7.

Horowitz, J. (1988). Anaesthetic implications of substance abuse in the parturient. *Journal of American Association of Nurse Anesthetists*, **56**, 510–14.

Howard, F.M. & Hill, J.M. (1979). Review. Drugs in Pregnancy. *Obstetrical & Gynaecological Survey*, **34**, 643–53.

Hsueh, A.J.W., Welsh, T.H., Jones, P.B.C. (1981). Inhibition of ovarian and testicular steroidogenesis by epidermal growth factor. *Endocrinology*, **108**, 2002–4.

Hughes, C.L. (1988). Effects of phytoestrogens on GnRH-induced luteinizing hormone secretion in ovariectomised rats. *Reproductive Toxicology*, **1**, 179–81.

Hughes, C.L., Everett, J.W. & Tyrey, L. (1981). $\Delta^9$-tetra-hydrocannabinol suppression of prolactin secretion in the rat: lack of direct pituitary effect. *Endocrinology*, **109**, 876–80.

Iguchi, T., Irisawa, S., Uchima, F.-D.A. & Takusugi, N. (1988). Permanent chondrification in the pelvis and occurrence of hernias in mice treated neonatally with Tamoxifen. *Reproductive Toxicology*, **2**, 127–34.

Jaitley, K.D., Robson, J.M., Sullivan, F.M. & Wilson, C.A. (1968). The effects of monoamine oxidase inhibitors on ovulation, implantation and pregnancy. *Journal of Reproduction Fertility*, Suppl. 4, 757–9.

Jaitley, K.D., Robson, J.M., Sullivan, F.M. & Wilson, C.A. (1969). Maintenance of pregnancy after implantation in hypophysectomised or ovariectomised mice treated with phenelzine derivatives. *Journal of Endocrinology*, **41**, 519–30.

Jansson, J.-O., Eden, S. & Isaksson, O. (1985). Sexual dimorphism in the control of growth hormone secretion. *Endocrine Reviews*, **6**, 128–50.

Johnson, K.M., Dewey, W.L. & Bloom, A.S. (1981). Adrenalectomy reverses the effects of delta-9-THC on mouse brain 5-hydroxytryptamine turnover. *Pharmacology*, **23**, 223–9.

Johnson, M. & Everitt, B. (1988). *Essential Reproduction*. Oxford: Blackwell Scientific Publications.

Johnston, C.A. & Negro-Vilar, A. (1988). Role of oxytocin on prolactin secretion during proestrus in different physiological and pharmacological paradigms. *Endocrinology*, **122**, 341–50.

Johnston, G.A.R., Allan, R.D. & Skerritt, J.H. (1982). Gaba Receptors. In *Handbook of Neurochemistry*, 2nd edn, vol. 6, *Receptors*, ed. A. Lajtha, pp. 1–24. New York: Plenum Press.

de Jonge, F.S.H., Muntjewerff, J.-W., Louweise, A.L. & van de Poll, N.E. (1988). Sexual behaviour and sexual orientation in the female rat as a function of hormonal treatment during various stages of development. *Hormones and Behaviour*, **22**, 100–16.

Joseph, R., Hess, S. & Birecree, E. (1978). Effects of hormone manipulations and exploration on sex differences in maze learning. *Behavioral Biology*, **24**, 364–77.

Julkunen, M., Koistinen, R., Sjoberg, J., Rutanen, E., Wahlstrom, T.

& Seppala, M. (1986). Secretory endometrium synthesises placental protein 14. *Endocrinology*, **118**, 1782–6.

Kaldas, R.S. & Hughes, C.L. (1989). Reproductive and general metabolic effects of phytoestrogen in mammals. *Reproductive Toxicology*, **3**, 81–9.

Kalra, S.P. (1983). Opioid peptides – inhibitory neuronal systems in regulation of gonadotropin secretion. In *Role of Peptides and Proteins in Control of Reproduction*, ed. S.M. McCann, D.A. Dhindsa, pp. 63–78. New York: Elsevier.

Kalra, S.P. (1986). Neural circuitry involved in the control of LHRH secretion: a model for preovulatory LH release. *Frontiers in Neuroendocrinology* 9, ed. W. F. Ganong & L. Martini, pp. 31–73. New York: Raven Press.

Kalra, S.P. & Kalra, P.S. (1984). Opioid-adrenergic-steroid connection in regulation of LH secretion in the rat. *Neuroendocrinology*, **38**, 418–26.

Kane, J.M., Cooper, T.B., Sachar, E.J., Halpan, F.S. & Bailine, S. (1981). Clozapine: plasma levels and prolactin response. *Psychopharmacology*, **73**, 184–7.

Kasson, B.G. & Hsueh, A.J.W. (1985). Cholinergic inhibition of follicle-stimulating hormone-induced progestin production by cultured rat granulosa cells. *Biology of Reproduction*, **33**, 1158–67.

Katter, H. (Ed.) (1988). *Issues and Reviews of Teratology*. New York: Plenum Press.

Kawai, Y. & Clark, M.R. (1986). Mechanisms of action of gonadotropin releasing hormone on rat granulosa cells. *Endocrine Research*, **12**, 195–209.

Keane, P.E., Menager, J. & Strolin Benedetti, M. (1981). The effect of monoamine oxidase A and B inhibitors on rat serum prolactin. *Neuropharmacology*, **20**, 1157–62.

King, R.J.B. (1987). Structure and function of steroid receptors. *Journal of Endocrinology*, **114**, 341–9.

King, T.S., Schenken, R.S., Kang, I.S., Javors, M.A. & Riehl, R.M. (1990). Cocaine disrupts estrous cyclicity and alters the reproductive neuroendocrine axis in the rat. *Neuroendocrinology*, **51**, 15–22.

Kopelman, P.G. (1988). Review. Neuroendocrine function in obesity. *Clinical Endocrinology*, **28**, 675–89.

Kopelman, P.G., White, N., Pilkington, T.R.E. & Jeffcoate, S.L. (1981). The effect of weight loss on sex steroid secretion and binding in massively obese women. *Clinical Endocrinology*, **14**, 113–16.

Kordon, C. (1969). Effect of selective experimental changes in regional monoamine levels on super-ovulation in the immature rat. *Neuroendocrinology*, **4**, 129–38.

Kupfer, D. (1988). Critical evaluation of methods for detection and assessment of estrogenic compounds in mammals: Strengths and limitations for application to risk assessment. *Reproductive Toxicology*, **1**, 147–53.

Kurzel, R.B. (1984). Substance abuse in pregnancy. In *The Problem-Orientated Medical Record for High-Risk Obstetrics*, ed. C.W. Cetrulo & A.J. Sbarra, pp. 29–84. New York: Plenum Medical Book Co.

Kurzel, R.B. & Cetrulo, C.L. (1985). Chemical Teratogenesis and Reproductive Failure. *Obstetrical and Gynecological Survey*, **40**, 397–424.

Laakmann, G. (1980). Effects of antidepressants on the secretion of pituitary hormones in healthy subjects, neurotic depressive patients and endogenous depressive patients. *Nervenarzt*, **51**, 725–32.

Laakmann, G. & Benkert, O. (1978). Effects of antidepressants on pituitary hormones. In *Proceedings of the 13th Symposium on Medicine. Hoechst on Depressive Disorders*, ed. S. Garrattini, pp. 255–66. New York: Schattauer.

Landy, H.J. & Hinson, J. (1988). Placental abruption associated with cocaine use: case report. *Reproductive Toxicology*, **1**, 203–5.

Leadem, C.A., Crowley, W.R., Simpkins, J.W. & Kalra, S.P. (1985). Effects of naloxone on catecholamine and LHRH release from the perifused hypothalamus of the steroid-primed rat. *Neuroendocrinology*, **40**, 497–500.

Lei, K.Y., Abbasi, A., Prasad, A.S. (1976). Function of pituitary-gonadal axis in zinc-deficient rats. *American Journal of Physiology*, **230**, 1730–2.

Lindner, H.R., Zor, U., Kohen, F., Bauminger, S., Amsterdam, A., Lahav, M. & Salomon, Y. (1980). Significance of prostaglandins in the regulation of cyclic events in the ovary and uterus. *Advances in Prostaglandin and Thromboxane Research*, **8**, 1371–90.

Linnoila, M., Leppaluoto, J., Seppala, T. & Ranta, T. (1977). Serum gonadotropin and TSH levels after tricyclic antidepressants in healthy males. *Acta Pharmacologica Toxicologica*, **41**, 285–8.

Lione, A. (1987). Ionising radiation and Human Reproduction. *Reproductive Toxicology*, **1**, 3–16.

Lione, A. (1988). Polychlorinated biphenyls and reproduction. *Reproductive Toxicology*, **2**, 83–9.

Little, B.B., Snell, L.M., Palmore, M.K. & Gilstrap, L.C. (1988). Cocaine use in pregnant women in a large public hospital. *American Journal of Perinatology*, **5**, 206–7.

Lobo, R.A., Granger, L., Goebelsmann, U. & Mischell, D.R. (1981). Elevations in gonadotrophins, serum estradiol and possible mechanism for inappropriate gonadotrophin secretion in women with polycystic ovarian disease. *J. Clinical Endocrinology & Metabolism*, **52**, 156–8.

Login, I.S., Thorner, M.O. & MacLeod, R.M. (1983). Zinc may have a physiological role in regulating pituitary prolactin secretion. *Neuroendocrinology*, **37**, 317–20.

Lotz, W. (1982). Benzodiazapine antagonist Ro15-178 counteracts the prolactin-lowering effects of other benzodiazepines in rats. *Neuroendocrinology*, **35**, 32–6.

Luck, M.R. (1990). Cholinergic stimulation, through muscarinic receptors, of oxytocin and progesterone secretion from bovine granulosa cells undergoing spontaneous luteinization in serum-free culture. *Endocrinology*, **126**, 1256–62.

Luster, M.I., Pfeifer, R.W. & Tucker, A.N. (1985). Influence of sex hormones on immunoregulation with specific reference to natural and environmental estrogens. In *Endocrine Toxicology*, ed. J.A. Thomas, K.S. Korach & J.A. McLachlan, pp. 67–84. New York: Raven Press.

MacArthur, C. & Knox, E.G. (1988). Smoking in pregnancy: effects of stopping at different stages. *British J. Obstetrics & Gynaecology*, **95**, 551–5.

MacLeod, R.M. (1976). Regulation of prolactin secretion. In *Frontiers in Neuroendocrinology* 4, ed. L. Martini & W.G. Ganong, pp. 169–94. New York: Raven Press.

Magoffin, D.A. & Erickson, G.F. (1982). Prolactin inhibition of luteinizing hormone-stimulated androgen synthesis in ovarian interstitial cells cultured in defined medium: Mechanisms of action. *Endocrinology*, **111**, 2001–7.

Magoffin, D.A., Reynolds, D.S. & Erickson, G.F. (1981). Direct inhibitory effect of GnRH on androgen secretion by ovarian interstitial cells. *Endocrinology*, **109**, 661–3.

Maiewski, S.F., Larscheid, P., Cook, J.M. & Mueller, G.P. (1985). Evidence that a benzodiazepine receptor mechanism regulates the secretion of pituitary β-endorphin in rats. *Endocrinology*, **117**, 474–80.

Mancebo, M.J., Alfonso, M., Duran, R. & Marco, J. (1984). Effects of ethanol administration in a preovulatory period on hypothalamic-pituitary-gonadal axis in female rats. *Research Communications in Substances of Abuse*, **5**, 221–31.

Martinez, G., de la Escalera, F. & Weiner, R. (1988). Dopamine removal: a selective signal for prolactin release and lactotroph responsiveness. In *The Brain and Female Reproductive Function*, ed. A.R. Genazzini, V. Montemagno, C. Nappi & F. Retraglia, pp. 145–56. Carnworth: The Panthenon Publishing Group.

Mastri, C. & Lucier, G. (1985). Actions of hormonally active chemicals in the liver. In *Reproductive Toxicology*, ed. R.L. Dixon, pp. 335–55. New York: Raven Press.

Mattison, D.R. (1982). The effects of smoking on fertility from gametogenesis to implantation. *Environmental Research*, **28**, 410–33.

Mattison, D.R. & Thomford, P.J. (1989). Mechanisms of action of reproductive toxicants. In *Toxicology of the male and female reproductive systems*, ed. P.K. Woking, pp. 101–29. New York: Hemisphere Publishing Corporation.

McCann, S.M., Yu, W., Khorram, O., Kentroli, S., Vijayan, E. & Arisawa, M. (1988). In *The Brain and Female Reproductive Function*, ed. A.R. Genazzani, U. Montemagno, C. Nappi & F. Petraglia, pp. 57–64. Carnworth: The Panthenon Publishing Group.

McEwen, B.S., Jones, K.J. & Pfaff, D.W. (1987). Hormonal control of sexual behaviour in the female rat: molecular, cellular and neurochemical studies. *Biology of Reproduction*, **36**, 37–45.

McNeilly, A.S. (1986). Prolactin. In *Neuroendocrinology*, ed. S. L. Lightman & B.J. Everitt, pp. 538–61. Oxford: Blackwell Scientific Publications.

Melis, G.B., Paoletti, A.M., Mais, V., Mastrapasqua, N.M., Strigini, F., Fruzzetti, F., Guarrieri, G., Gambacciani, M. & Fioretti, P. (1982). The effects of the GABAergic drug, sodium valproate on prolactin secretion in normal and hyperprolactinemic subjects. *Journal of Clinical Endocrinology and Metabolism*, **54**, 485–9.

Melis, G.B., Mais, V., Paoletti, A.M., Beneventi, F., Petacchi, F.D. & Fioretti, P. (1986). Involvement of endogenous gabaergic system in the modulation of gonadotropin secretion in normal cycling women. *Journal of Endocrinological Investigation*, **9**, 71–6.

Mello, N.K. (1988). Effects of alcohol abuse on reproductive function in women. *Recent Developments in Alcohol*, **6**, 253–76.

Mello, N.K., Mendelson, J.H., Bree, M.P. & Skupny, A. (1986). Alcohol effects on luteinizing hormone-releasing hormone stimulated luteinizing hormone and follicle-stimulating hormone in ovariectomised female rhesus monkeys. *Journal of Pharmacology and Experimental Therapeutics*, **239**, 693–700.

Mello, N.K., Mendelson, J.H., King, N.W., Bree, M.P., Skupny, A. & Ellinboe, J. (1988a). Alcohol self-administration by female macaque monkeys: A model for study of alcohol dependence, hyperprolactinemia and amenorrhea. *Journal of Studies on Alcohol*, **49**, 551–60.

Mello, N.K., Mendelson, J.H., Bree, M.P. & Skupny, A. (1988b). Alcohol effects on naloxone-stimulated luteinizing hormone, follicle-stimulating hormone and prolactin plasma levels in female rhesus monkeys. *Journal of Pharmacology and Experimental Therapeutics*, **245**, 895–904.

Melnick, S., Cole, P., Anderson, D. & Herbst, A. (1987). Rates and risks of diethylstilbestrol-related clear-cell adenocarcinoma of the vagina and cervix. An update. *New England Journal of Medicine*, **316**, 514–16.

Meltzer, H.Y., Fang, V.S., Simonovich, M. & Paul, S.M. (1977). Effect of metabolites of chlorpromazine in plasma prolactin levels in male rats. *European Journal of Pharmacology*, **41**, 431–6.

Mendelson, C.R. (1988). Mechanisms of hormone action. In *Textbook of Endocrine Physiology*, ed. J.E. Griffin & S.R. Ojeda, pp. 28–55. Oxford: Oxford University Press.

Mendelson, J.H. & Mello, N.K. (1988). Chronic alcohol effects on anterior pituitary and ovarian hormones in healthy women. *Journal of Pharmacology and Experimental Therapeutics*, **245**, 407–12.

Merriam, G.R., Nunnelley, L.L., Trish, J.W.V. & Naftolin, F. (1979). Sex-related and cyclic variation of trace elements in rat hypothalamus and pituitary. *Brain Research*, **171**, 503–10.

Miller, M.A., Clifton, D.K. & Steiner, R.A. (1985). Noradrenergic and endogenous opioid pathways in the regulation of luteinizing hormone secretion in the male rat. *Endocrinology*, **117**, 544–8.

Mittleman, R.E., Cofino, J.C. & Hearn, W.L. (1989). Tissue distribution of cocaine in a pregnant woman. Case Report. *Journal of Forensic Sciences*, **34**, 481–6.

Moberg, G.P. (1987). Influence of the adrenal axis upon the gonads. In *Oxford Reviews of Reproductive Biology* 9, ed. J.R. Clarke, pp. 456–96. New York: Raven Press.

Mogg, R.J. & Samson, W.K. (1990). Interactions of dopaminergic and peptidergic factors in the control of prolactin release. *Endocrinology*, **126**, 728–35.

Moon, Y.S., Duleba, A.J. & Jakubovic, A. (1982). Effect of cannabinoids on progesterone production by ovarian granulosa cells of pig and rat. *Life Sciences*, **31**, 315–18.

Moore, K. (1987). Interactions between prolactin and dopamine neurons. *Biology of Reproduction*, **36**, 47–58.

Morali, G. & Beyer, C. (1979). Neuroendocrine control of mammalian oestrous behaviour. In *Endocrine Control of Sexual Behaviour*, ed. C. Beyer, pp. 33–75. New York: Raven Press.

Neill, J.D. (1988). Prolactin secretion and its control. In *The Physiology of Reproduction* 1, ed. E. Knobil & J.D. Neill, pp. 1379–92. New York: Raven Press.

Nicoletti, F., Clementi, G., Prato, A., Canonico, P.L., Rampello, L., Patti, F., Di Giorgion, R.M. & Scapagnini, U. (1983). Effects of hyper- and hypoprolactinemia on glutamate decarboxylase activity in medial basal hypothalamus of male rat. *Neuroendocrinology*, **36**, 13–16.

Nikolics, K., Mason, A.J., Szonyi, E., Ramachandran, J. & Seeberg, P.H. (1985). A prolactin-inhibiting factor within the precursor for human gonadotrophin-releasing hormone. *Nature*, **316**, 511–17.

Nolan, G.A. (1988). The developmental toxicology of caffeine. In *Issues and Reviews of Teratology*, ed. H. Kater, pp. 305–50. New York: Plenum Press.

Norstedt, G. & Palmiter, R. (1984). Secretory rhythms of growth hormone regulates sexual differentiation of mouse liver. *Cell*, **36**, 805–12.

Ohta, Y., Iguchi, T. & Takasugi, N. (1989). Deciduoma formation in rats treated neonatally with the anti-estrogens tamoxifen and Mer-25. *Reproductive Toxicology*, **3**, 207–13.

Ojeda, S.R. (1988). Female Reproductive Function. In *Textbook of*

*Endocrine Physiology*, ed. J.E. Griffin & S.R. Ojeda, pp. 129–64. Oxford: Oxford University Press.

Ojeda, S.R., Urbanski, H.F. & Ahmed, C.E. (1986). The onset of female puberty: studies in the rat. *Recent Progress in Hormone Research*, **42**, 385–442.

Ondo, J.G. & Pass, K.A. (1980). Pituitary LH response to LHRH in male rats following pentobarbital anesthesia. *Life Sciences*, **27**, 2071–4.

Oreland, L. (1987). The benzodiazepines: a pharmacological overview. *Acta Anaesthesia Scandanavia*, **32**, Suppl. 88, 13–16.

Ossofsky, H.J. (1974). Amenorrhea in endogenous depression. *International Pharmacopsychiatry*, **9**, 100–8.

Pakrasi, P., Cheng, H.C. & Dey, S.K. (1983). Prostaglandins in the uterus: modulation by steroid hormones. *Prostaglandins*, **26**, 991–1009.

Parker, M.G. (1988). The expanding family of nuclear hormone receptors. *Journal of Endocrinology*, **119**, Suppl. 2, p. 180.

Pasanen, M., Stenback, F., Park, S.S., Gelboin, H.V. & Pelkonen, O. (1988). Immunohistochemical detection of human placental cytochrome P-450-associated mono-oxygenase system inducible by maternal cigarette smoking. *Placenta*, **9**, 267–75.

Patillo, R.A., Hussa, R.O., Yorde, D.E. & Cole, L.A. (1983). Hormone synthesis by normal and neoplastic human trophoblast. In *Biology of the Trophoblast*, ed. Y.W. Lobe & A. Whyte, pp. 283–316. Amsterdam: Elsevier.

Perkins, S.N., Cronin, M.J. & Veldhuis, J.D. (1986). Properties of β-adrenergic receptors on porcine corpora lutea and granulosa cells. *Endocrinology*, **118**, 998–1005.

Petraglia, F., Sulton, S., Vale, W. & Plotsky, P. (1987a). Corticotropin releasing factor decreasing LH levels in female rats by inhibiting gonadotrophin releasing hormone release into hypophyseal portal circulation. *Endocrinology*, **20**, 1083–8.

Petraglia, F., Vale, W. & Rivier, C. (1987b). Beta-endorphin and dynorphin participate in the stress-induced release of prolactin in the rat. *Neuroendocrinology*, **45**, 338–42.

Petraglia, F., Volpe, A., Genazzani, A.R., Rivier, J., Sawhenko, P.E. & Vale, W. (1990). Neuroendocrinology of the human placenta. *Frontiers in Neuroendocrinology*, **11**, 6–37.

Piercy, M. & Shin, S.H. (1980) Comparative studies of prolactin secretion in estradiol-primed and normal male rats induced by ether, stress, pimoxide and TRH. *Neuroendocrinology*, **31**, 270–5.

Pinkston, G. & Uphouse, L. (1988). Postovulatory reproduction of fertility in chlordecone treated female rats. *Reproductive Toxicology*, **2**, 105–9.

van der Poll, N.E., van Zanten, S. & de Jonge, F.H. (1986). Effects of testosterone, estrogen and dihydrotestosterone upon aggressive and sexual behaviour of female rats. *Hormones and Behaviour*, **20**, 418–31.

Powell, J.G. & Cochrane, R.L. (1982). The effects of a number of non-steroidal anti-inflammatory compounds on parturition in the rat. *Prostaglandins*, **23**, 469–88.

Prior, J.C. (1987). Physical exercise and the neuroendocrine control of reproduction. In *Clinical Endocrinology and Metabolism: Neuro-endocrinology of Stress*, ed. A. Grossman, pp. 299–318. London: Baillier Tindall.

Puri, J.C., Puri, V. & Anand Kumar, R.C. (1981). Serum levels of testosterone, cortisol, prolactin and bioactive luteinizing hormone in adult male rhesus monkeys following cage-restraint or anaesthetizing with ketamine hydrochloride. *Acta Endocrinologica*, **97**, 118–24.

Rabin, D., Gold, P.W., Margioris, A.N. & Chrousos, G.P. (1988). Stress and reproduction: Physiologic and pathophysiologic interaction between the stress and reproductive axes. *Advances in Experimental Medical Biology*, **245**, 377–87.

Racowsky, C., Hendricks, R.C. & Baldwin, R.V. (1989). Direct effects of nicotine on the meiotic maturation of hamster oocytes. *Reproductive Toxicology*, **3**, 13–22.

Ramahi-Ataya, A.J., Ataya, K.M., Subramanian, M.G. & Struck, R.F. (1988). The effect of 'activated' cyclophosphamide on rat granulosa cells *in vitro*. *Reproductive Toxicology*, **2**, 99–103.

Ramirez, R.V.D., Feder, H.H. & Sawyer, C.H. (1984). Role of brain catecholamines in the regulation of LH secretion: A critical inquiry. In *Frontiers in Neuroendocrinology* 8, ed. L. Martini & W.F. Ganong, pp. 27–83. New York: Raven Press.

Randall, C.L. (1987). Alcohol as a teratogen: A decade of research review. *Alcohol & Alcoholism*, Suppl. 1, pp. 125–32.

Rawitch, A.B., Schultz, K., Ebner, K. & Vardaris, R. (1977). Competition of delta-9-tetrahydro-cannabinol with estrogen in rat uterine estrogen receptor binding. *Science*, **197**, 1189–91.

Reel, J.R. & Lamb, J.C. (1985). Reproductive Toxicology of Chlordecone (Kepone). In *Reproductive Toxicology*, ed. R.L. Dixon, pp. 257–392. New York: Raven Press.

Reich, R., Miskin, R. & Tsafriri, A. (1986). Intrafollicular distribution of plasminogen activators and their hormonal regulation *in vitro*. *Endocrinology*, **119**, 1588–93.

Rettori, V., Skelley, C.W., McCann, S.M. & Dees, W.L. (1987). Detrimental effects of short-term ethanol exposure on reproductive function in the female rat. *Biology of Reproduction*, **37**, 1089–96.

Richards, C.D. & Hesketh, T.R. (1975). Implications for theories of anaesthesia of antagonism between anaesthetic and non-anaesthetic steroids. *Nature*, **256**, 179–82.

Richards, J.A. & Farookhi, R. (1978). Gonadotrophins and ovarian follicular growth. In *Clinics in Obstetrics & Gynaecology* 5, ed. J.E. Tysonje, pp. 363–74. London: W. B. Saunders Co. Ltd.

Richards, J.A., Schoch, P., Mohler, H. & Haefely, W. (1986). Mini-reviews. Benzodiazepine receptors resolved. *Experientia*, **42**, 121–6.

Richards, J.G. & Hedin, L. (1988). Molecular aspects of hormone action in ovarian follicular development, ovulation and luteinization. *Annual Review Physiology*, **50**, 441–63.

Rivier, C. & Vale, W. (1989). In the rat, interluekin-1α acts at the level of the brain and the gonads to interfere with gonadotropin and sex steroid secretion. *Endocrinology*, **124**, 2105–9.

Robson, J.M., Sullivan, F.M. & Wilson, C.A. (1971). The maintenance of pregnancy during the pre-implantation period in mice treated with phenelzine derivatives. *Journal of Endocrinology*, **49**, 635–48.

de Rosa, G., Corsello, S.M., de Rosa, E., Della Casa, S., Ruffilli, M.P., Grasso, P. & Pasargiklian, E. (1983). Endocrine study of anorexia nervosa. *Experimental Clinical Endocrinology*, **82**, 160–72.

Rosciszewska, D., Buntner, B., Guz, I. & Zawisza, L. (1986). Ovarian hormones, anticonvulsant drugs, and seizures during the menstrual cycle in women with epilepsy. *Journal of Neurology, Neurosurgery, and Psychiatry*, **49**, 47–51.

Rothschild, T.C., Calhoon, R.E. & Boylan, E.S. (1988). Genital tract abnormalities in female rats exposed to diethylstilbestrol in utero. *Reproductive Toxicology*, **1**, 193–202.

Roubenoff, R., Hoyt, J., Petri, M., Hochberg, M.C. & Hellmann, D.B. (1988). Effects of anti-inflammatory and immunosuppressive drugs on pregnancy and fertility. *Seminars in Arthritis and Rheumatism*, **18**, 88–110.

Roy, A.K. & Chatterjee, B. (1983). Sexual dimorphism in the liver. *Annual Review Physiology*, **45**, 37–50.

Rustin, G.J.S., Booth, M., Dent, J., Salt, S., Rustin, F. & Bagshawe, K.D. (1984). Pregnancy after cytotoxic chemotherapy for gestational trophoblastic tumours. *British Medical Journal*, **288**, 103–6.

Sakai, C.N. & Hodgen, G.D. (1988). Use of primate folliculogenesis models in understanding human reproductive biology and applicability to toxicology. *Reproductive Toxicology*, **1**, 207–21.

Sanchis, R., Esquifino, A. & Guerri, C. (1985). Chronic ethanol intake modifies estrous cyclicity and alters prolactin and LH levels. *Pharmacology, Biochemistry and Behaviour*, **23**, 221–4.

Sanders, J.E., Buckner, C.D., Leonard, J.M., Sullivan, K.M., Witherspoon, R.P., Deeg, H.J., Storb, R. & Thomas, E.D. (1983). Late effects on gonadal function of cyclophosphamide, total-body irradiation, and marrow transplantation. *Transplantation*, **36**, 252–5.

Sarker, D.P. & Yen, S.S.C. (1985). Hyperprolactinaemia decreases the luteinizing hormone-releasing hormone concentration in pituitary portal plasma: a possible role of β-endorphin as a mediator. *Endocrinology*, **116**, 2080–4.

Schade, R.R., Bonner, G., Gay, V.C. & van Thiel, D.H. (1983). Evidence for a direct inhibitory effect of ethanol upon gonadotropin secretion at the pituitary level. *Alcoholism: Clinical and Experimental Research*, **7**, 150–2.

Schaison, G. (1988). Pathophysiology of anovulation. *Human Reproduction*, **3**, 525–30.

Schildkraut, J.J. (1965). The catecholamine hypothesis of affective disorders: A review of supporting evidence. *American Journal of Physiology*, **122**, 509–22.

Schlesselmann, J.J. Oral contraceptives in relation to cancer of the breast and reproductive tract – an epidemiological review (1989). *British Journal of Family Planning*, **15**, 23–33.

Schmidt, G., Owman, Ch. & Sjoberg, N.-O. (1986). Histamine induces ovulation in the isolated perfused rat ovary. *Journal of Reproduction and Fertility*, **78**, 159–66.

Scialli, A.R. (1988). Is stress a developmental toxin? *Reproductive Toxicology*, **1**, 163–71.

Scott, J.R. (1977). Fetal growth retardation associated with maternal administration of immunosuppressive drugs. *American Journal of Obstetrics & Gynaecology*, **128**, 668–74.

Seeley, R.R. (1983). Effect of indomethacin on reproduction under laboratory and field conditions in deermice (*Peromyscus maniculatus*). *Biology of Reproduction*, **28**, 148–53.

Shamberger, R.C., Rosenberg, S.A., Seipp, C.A. & Sherins, R.J. (1981). Effects of high-dose methotrexate and vincristine on ovarian and testicular functions in patients undergoing postoperative adjuvant treatment of osteosarcoma. *Cancer Treatment Reports*, **65**, 739–46.

Shoental, R. (1977). Health hazards due to oestrogenic mycotoxins in certain foodstuffs. *International Journal of Environmental Studies*, **11**, 149–50.

Siever, L.J., Uhde, T.W. & Murphy, D.L. (1982). Possible subsensitization of alpha$_2$-adrenergic receptors by chronic monoamine oxidase inhibitor treatment in psychiatric patients. *Psychiatry Research*, **6**, 293–302.

Smith, C.G. & Asch, R.J. (1987). Drug abuse and reproduction. *Fertility and Sterility*, **48**, 355–73.

Smith, L.D. (1989). The induction of oocyte maturation: transmembrane signalling events and regulation of the cell cycle. *Development*, **107**, 685–99.

Solomon, J., Cocchia, M., Gray, R., Shattuck, D. & Vossmer, A. (1976). Uterotrophic effect of delta-9-tetrahydro cannabinol in ovariectomised rats. *Science*, **192**, 559–61.

Soules, M.R., Sutton, G.P., Hammond, C.B. & Haney, A.F. (1980). Endocrine changes at operation under general anaesthesia: reproductive hormone fluctuations in young women. *Fertility and Sterility*, **33**, 364–71.

Spangelo, B.L., MacLeod, R.M. & Isakson, P.C. (1990). Production of interleukin-6 by anterior pituitary cells *in vitro*. *Endocrinology*, **126**, 582–6.

Spicer, L.J. (1986). Catecholaminergic regulation of ovarian function in mammals: current concepts. *Life Sciences*, **39**, 1701–11.

Spitz, D.M., Tristram, S., Cohen, H., Anou, N. & di Rirth, D. (1979). Failure of metaclopramide to influence LH, FSH & TSH secretion or their response to releasing hormones. *Acta Endocrinologica*, **92**, 640–7.

Steger, R.W., Silverman, A.Y., Siler-Khodr, T.M. & Asch, R.H. (1980). The effect of $\Delta^9$-Tetrahydrocannabinol on the positive and negative feedback control of luteinizing hormone release. *Life Sciences*, **27**, 1911–16.

Steger, R.W., Silverman, A.Y., Johns, A. & Asch, R.H. (1981). Interactions of cocaine and Δ9 tetrahydrocannabinol with the hypothalamic-hypophyseal axis of the female rat. *Fertility and Sterility*, **35**, 567–72.

Stewart, J. & Cygan, D. (1980). Ovarian hormones act early in development to feminize adult open-field behavior in the rat. *Hormones and Behavior*, **14**, 20–32.

Stillman, R.J., Rosenberg, M.G. & Sachs, B.P. (1986). Smoking and Reproduction. *Fertility and Sterility*, **46**, 545–66.

Subramanian, M.G. & Gala, R.R. (1977). The effects of continuous chloroform and halothane anaesthesia on plasma prolactin levels in ovariectomised estrogen-treated rats. *Experientia*, **33**, 1245–6.

Subramanian, M.G. & Gala, R.R. (1978). The influence of adrenalectomy and of corticosterone administration on the ether-induced increase in plasma prolactin in ovariectomized estrogen-treated rats. *Proceedings of the Society for Experimental Biology and Medicine*, **157**, 415–17.

Suda, T., Tozawa, F., Ushiyama, T., Sumitomo, T., Yamada, M. & Demura, H. (1990). Interleukin-1 stimulates corticotropin-releasing factor gene expression in rat hypothalamus. *Endocrinology*, **126**, 1223–8.

Swartz, W.J. & Mall, G.M. (1989). Chlordecone-induced follicular toxicity in mouse ovaries. *Reproductive Toxicology*, **3**, 203–6.

Sylvester, P.W., van Vugt, D.A., Asylworth, C.F., Hanson, E.A. & Meites, J. (1982). Effects of morphine and naloxone on inhibition by ovarian hormones of pulsatile release of LH in ovariectomised rats. *Neuroendocrinology*, **34**, 269–73.

Taleisnik, S. & Sawyer, C.H. (1986). Activation of the CNS noradrenergic system may inhibit as well as facilitate pituitary luteinizing hormone release. *Neuroendocrinology*, **44**, 265–8.

Tallman, J.F. & Gallager, D.W. (1985). The gaba-ergic system: a locus of benzodiazepine action. *Annual Review Neuroscience*, **8**, 21–44.

Teoh, S.K., Mendelson, J.H., Mello, N.K. & Skupny, A. (1988). Alcohol effects on naltrexone-induced stimulation of pituitary, adrenal, and gonadal hormones during the early follicular phase of the menstrual cycle. *Journal of Clinical Endocrinology and Metabolism*, **66**, 1181–95.

Teschke, R. & Wiese, B. (1982). Sex-dependency of hepatic alcohol metabolizing enzymes. *Journal of Endocrinology Investigation*, **5**, 243–50.

van Thiel, D.H., Gavaler, J.S. & Lester, R. (1978). Alcohol-induced ovarian failure in the rat. *Journal of Clinical Investigation*, **61**, 624–32.

Thorner, M.O. & MacLeod, R.M. (1980). The lactotrope-regulation of its activity. In *Progress in Reproductive Biology* 6, ed. M. L'Hermite & S.J. Judd, pp. 1–23. Basel: Karger.

Tilders, F.J.H. & Berkenbosch, F. (1986). CRF and catecholamines; their place in the central and peripheral regulation of the stress response. *Acta Endocrinologica*, **112**, Suppl. 276, 63–75.

Tonetta, S.A. & diZerega, G. (1989). Intragonadal regulation of follicular maturation. *Endocrine Reviews*, **10**, 205–29.

Traurig, A.H., Papka, R.E. & Rush, M.E. (1988). Effects of capsaicin on reproductive function in the female rat: Role of peptide-containing primary afferent nerves innervating the uterine cervix in the neuroendocrine copulatory response. *Cell and Tissue Research*, **253**, 573–81.

Trounson, A., Rogers, P.A.W., Kola, I. & Saltrananthan, A.H. (1989). Fertilization, development and implantation. In *Obstetrics*, ed. A. Turnbull & G. Chamberlain, pp. 49–66. Edinburgh: Churchill Livingstone.

Tsafriri, A. (1988). Local nonsteroidal regulators of ovarian function. In *The Physiology of Reproduction* 1, ed. E. Knobil, J. D. Neill, pp. 527–66. New York: Raven Press.

Uphouse, L. & Williams, J. (1989). Sexual behaviour of intact female rats after treatment with o,p'-DDT or p,p'-DDT. *Reproductive Toxicology*, **3**, 33–41.

Vessey, M.P. (1989). Oral contraception and cancer. In *Contraception Science and Practice*, ed. M. Filshie & J. Guillebaud, pp. 52–68. Butterworths.

Walker, R.F. (1980). Serotonin circadian rhythm as a pacemaker for reproductive cycles in the female rat. In *Progress in Psychoneuroendocrinology*, ed. F. Brambilla, G. Racagni & D. de Wied, pp. 591–600. Elsevier/North Holland Biomedical Press.

Wardlaw, S.L., Wehrenberg, W.B., Ferin, M. & Frantz, A.G. (1980). Failure of β-endorphin to stimulate prolactin release in the pituitary stalk-sectioned monkey. *Endocrinology*, **107**, 1663–6.

Wathes, D.C., Swann, R.W. & Pickering, B.T. (1984). Variations in oxytocin, vasopressin and neurophysin concentrations in the bovine ovary during the oestrous cycle and pregnancy. *Journal of Reproduction & Fertility*, **71**, 551–7.

Watkins, J.C., Krogsgaard-Larson, P. & Honore, T. (1990). EEA. Pharmacology: structure-activity in the development of excitatory amino acid receptor agonists and competitive antagonists. *Trends in Pharmacological Sciences*, **11**, 25–33.

Weitlauf, H.M. (1988). Biology of implantation. In *The Physiology of Reproduction* 1, ed. E. Knobil & J.D. Neill, pp. 231–64. New York: Raven Press.

Whitehead, S.A. (1990). A gonadotrophin surge attenuating factor. *Journal of Endocrinology*, **126**, 1–4.

Wilcox, A., Weinberg, C. & Baird, D. (1988). Caffeinated beverages and decreased fertility. *The Lancet*, **2**, 1453–6.

Wilson, C.A. (1979). Hypothalamic neurotransmitters and gonadotrophin release. In *Oxford Reviews of Reproductive Biology* 1, ed. C.A. Finn, pp. 383–473. Oxford: Oxford Science Publications.

Wilson, C.A., Leigh, A.J. & Chapman, A.J. (1990). Gonadotrophin glycosylation and function. *Journal of Endocrinology*, **125**, 3–14.

Wilson, C.A. & Bonney, R.C. (1990). Phospholipase $A_2$ activity in the rat ovary during the oestrous cycle. *J. Endocrinological Investigations*, **13**, Suppl. 2, p. 303.

Yegnanarayan, R. & Joglekar, G.V. (1978). Anti-fertility effect of non-steroidal anti-inflammatory drugs. *Japanese Journal of Pharmacology*, **28**, 909–17.

Yen, S.S.C. (1986). The human menstrual cycle. In *Reproductive Endocrinology*, ed. S.S.C. Yen & R.B. Jaffe, pp. 200–36. Philadelphia: W.B. Saunders Co. Ltd.

Ying, S.-Y., Ling, N., Bohlen, P. & Guillemin, R. (1981). Gonadocrinins: Peptides in ovarian follicular fluid stimulating the secretion of pituitary gonadotropins. *Endocrinology*, **108**, 1206–15.

Yoshimura, Y., Maruyama, K., Shiraki, M., Kawakami, S., Fukushima, M. & Nakumura, Y. (1990). Prolactin inhibits plasminogen activator activity in the preovulatory follicles. *Endocrinology*, **126**, 631–6.

Yoshinaga, K., Rice, C., Krenn, J. & Pilot, R.L. (1979). Effects of nicotine on early pregnancy in the rat. *Biology of Reproduction*, **20**, 294–303.

# VI Other endocrine toxicological factors

MARY J. TUCKER

# 11    Dietary effects on endocrine tumours

## Introduction

Toxicologists have long been aware that the incidence of spontaneous tumours in rodents depends upon the species, strain and general environment in which the animals are maintained. Even the same inbred strain may show considerable differences in tumour patterns when maintained in different laboratories (Sabine, Horton & Wicks, 1973), indicating that environmental influences may override genetic characteristics. Although various factors such as caging, heating, lighting, and noise are all known to affect hormonal status in laboratory animals, dietary effects are the most widely studied and have the most marked influence on tumour development.

It was the actuarial records of an American insurance company that attracted the attention of Tannenbaum (1940a) when he observed that, in humans, individuals of average or less than average weight were not as likely to have cancer as those above average weight. This observation set in motion the first detailed studies of the relationship between diet and tumours in laboratory animals. Tannenbaum (1940b) described the effect of underfeeding mice and showed a reduction in the incidence of mammary and lung tumours in DBA mice and a delay in the onset of those which did develop. Once established, however, the tumours grew at a similar rate in the control and underfed mice. It is generally considered that diet may affect both initiation and promotion of tumours. It was several years before similar studies were undertaken in the rat but Saxton *et al.* (1948) also showed that restricting food intake significantly reduced tumour incidence. Food intake reduced to 46% of normal intake reduced tumours but did not affect skeletal growth or sexual maturity (Berg & Simms, 1960). Food restriction, even when started after the first few months of life, inhibits tumours (Nolen, 1972), but variable results have been reported for short periods of restriction followed by a return to *ad libitum* feeding. Nolen (1972) found no inhibiting effect but Ross & Bras

(1971) found that even a short period of seven weeks restriction followed by *ad libitum* feeding reduced tumour incidence. Increased longevity is the characteristic effect of food restriction in rats (Ross, 1961) and mice (Fernandez, Yunis & Good, 1976).

It has been suggested that the inhibitory effect of restricted food intake on tumours could be related to a reduced exposure to carcinogenic contaminants in the diet (Grasso, 1973). Synthetic and semi-synthetic diets, however, produce a significantly higher incidence of spontaneous tumours compared with 'natural' diets (Engel & Copeland, 1952) and promote higher incidences of tumours after induction with carcinogens or irradiation (Ershoff *et al.*, 1969).

Calorie restriction also has an inhibitory effect on tumours (Tannenbaum & Silverstone, 1949a; Yunis & Greenberg, 1974) and some strains of mice are more susceptible to calorie restriction than to restriction of total intake (Fernandez *et al.*, 1976). In the rat, tumours are exponentially related to calorie intake (Ross, Bras & Ragbeer, 1970).

Most of the experimental work on diet and hormonally dependent tumours in animals has been concerned with mammary tumours because breast cancer is an important disease of Western women and also because there are strains of rats and mice which develop high incidences of spontaneous mammary tumours and are also very susceptible to induction by various chemicals. In relation to those tumour type studies of the effects of individual components of the diet have been particularly fruitful. The level of fat in the diet has been implicated in mammary cancer in man and animals (Benson, Lear & Grand, 1956; Carroll & Khor, 1975). This is not simply a reflection of the high calorific value of high fat diets since Silverstone & Tannenbaum (1950) demonstrated increasing mammary tumours in animals fed isocaloric diets varying in fat from 1.6 to 24%. Fat content clearly affects specific tumour types and has a promoting rather than inhibiting effect (Carroll, Gammal & Plunkett, 1968; Carroll & Khor, 1975). In humans there is an established correlation between fat consumption and death rate from cancer of the breast and ovary (Lea, 1966), and hormone dependent cancers are claimed to be cancers of affluence and are related to a high fat intake in the populations where they are common (Berg, 1975). The effects of dietary protein levels are less clear; most standard laboratory diets contain 15–25% protein and restricting this level reduces the incidence of various tumours such as mammary tumours in C3H mice (White & Andervont, 1943) and liver tumours in the same strain (Tannenbaum & Silverstone, 1949b). Human epidemiology has shown that populations with a high protein intake have a high mortality from hormonally dependent cancers and lymphomas (Berg, 1975). It has been suggested that an excessive intake of protein may cause chronic immune stimulation and this may influence the development of lymphomas (Cunningham, 1976).

The importance of carbohydrate level in the diet appears to be related to its calorific value rather than to it having any direct effect upon tumours. The relevance of vitamins and trace elements has also to be established. It seems unlikely that they have any direct effect but may influence neoplasia through complex metabolic processes such as that suggested for vitamin C and its ability to prevent the nitrosation of amines and amides to carcinogenic nitrosamines and nitrosamides (Mirvish *et al.*, 1972). There has been no systematic study of the effects of diet on endocrine tumours of large laboratory animals (dog, monkey) since these species are rarely used for carcinogenicity studies. Most work has been done in the rat since this is the species which has a wide range and in many strains, a high incidence of spontaneous endocrine tumours. There is no evidence to suggest that pancreatic islet cell tumours in animals are affected by dietary factors.

All commonly used laboratory rat strains such as Sprague–Dawley, Fischer F344 and Wistar rats, as well as some inbred strains of mice, show high incidences of spontaneous tumours (adenomas) of the anterior lobe of the pituitary gland. The tumours are more common in females and although benign are a cause of high mortality because of their size and the elevated intra-cranial pressure and frequent cerebral haemorrhage produced by the expanding growth of the tumours. In females the adenomas are composed of prolactin producing cells and are associated with elevated levels of serum prolactin (Conybeare, 1988). As a consequence of this increased prolactin there is an associated high level of mammary tumours, mostly benign fibroadenomas. High levels of food intake, calorie intake, protein and fat have all been shown to be associated with high incidences of rat pituitary adenomas (Ross, 1961; Ross *et al.*, 1970; Moore & Tittle, 1973; Chan & Cohen, 1975). Spontaneous pituitary tumours in mice have been reviewed by Liebelt (1979) and are rare in most strains. A reduction in food intake by as little as 15–20% of *ad libitum* levels will significantly reduce pituitary tumours and the mammary tumours associated with them in the rat (Tucker, 1979).

The absence of sexual activity in experimental animals also appears to promote the development of pituitary tumours (Pickering & Pickering, 1984) and hormonal derangement of various kinds may produce tumours. Much of the understanding of the effects of hormonal imbalance has come from studies of the administration of exogenous hormones; oestrogens produce pituitary tumours in both rats (Furth, Nakane & Pasleels, 1976) and mice (Gardner, Pfeiffer & Trentin, 1959) albeit at high, 'non-physiological' doses. Nonetheless, there is the possibility that a diet could be contaminated by an unknown chemical or even contain a chemical constituent which has oestrogen-like activity. Blocking the hormone synthesis in other endocrine glands can produce pituitary tumours, for example antithyroid drugs will stimulate a feedback mechanism and will produce tumours which secrete thyroid stimulating hormone (TSH). Castration is another means of inducing pituitary tumours and the declining sexual function in old age may contribute to the spontaneous tumours. Dietary factors which affect sexual function, for example vitamin E in the rat, when deficient could produce tumours via this gonadal-pituitary axis.

Tumours of the thyroid gland can be readily induced by chemicals which have a direct effect on the gland or by hormonal imbalance produced by various mechanisms. There are a range of naturally occurring thyrostatic compounds such as brassica seeds which can produce follicular adenomas in the rat (Griesbach, Kennedy & Purves, 1945) as can diets which are deficient in iodine (daily intake 0–7 µg) which will produce varying incidences of follicular adenomas depending on strain and level of deficiency. In mice the pesticide, amitral, is goitrogenic and produced a high incidence of malignant thyroid tumours (Innes et al., 1969). Thyroid deficiency in the mouse will also eventually produce TSH secreting pituitary tumours and ultimately thyroid follicular adenomas. Spontaneous tumours of the adrenal gland are reported to be rare in mice but Frith (1983) reported incidences of 6.3% cortical adenomas and 1% cortical carcinomas in BALB/c female mice; in general incidences are less than 1% in most strains (Frith, 1983). The most common method of inducing cortical tumours in mice is by gonadectomy, although success depends upon the strain used; the numerous papers on this topic have been reviewed by Dunn (1970); it is thought that the induction of adrenocortical tumours by some chemical carcinogens is secondary to the castrating effect of the compound. Spontaneous medullary tumours are very rare in mice and no correlation with diet, or any other factor, can be defined. In contrast to the mouse adrenal tumours of the rat are common to some strains; a 90% incidence of cortical tumours has been recorded in Osborne Mendel female rats that are over 18 months of age and an 80% incidence of adrenal medullary tumours in M570 males over 18 months (Hollander and Snell, 1976). High oestrogen levels and gonadectomy induce cortical tumours in the rat (Heiman, 1944; Dunning, Curtis & Segaloff, 1953) and administration of growth hormone has been shown to induce medullary (phaeochromocytoma) tumours (Moon et al., 1956).

Proliferative (hyperplastic) lesions of the rat adrenal medulla are common in animals that are over 12 months of age in most strains of rat, either as a focal or diffuse condition, particularly in males. The pathogenesis of the lesion is not known but it can be induced by several stimuli including thiouracil, reserpine, growth hormone and nicotine. Phaeochromocytomas in the rat are similar, morphologically, to those observed in humans but there are few studies of the functional activity of the rat tumours and hyperplasias (Gilman, Gilbert & Spence, 1953). Cheng (1980) demonstrated some secretory activity in these tumours. Some workers consider that the hyperplastic medullary lesions progress to tumours with time (Hollander & Snell, 1976) but others consider that rat adrenal medullary tumours are not true phaeochromocytomas and do not resemble the human disease (Thompson *et al.*, 1981). Spontaneous tumours of the adrenal gland are likely to be a manifestation of hormonal imbalance as they often occur in association with tumours of other endocrine organs, such as the thyroid and pituitary. The link between hormonal imbalance, gonadectomy and adrenal cortical tumours suggests that any dietary factor which affects the hormonal environment has the ability, indirectly, to influence the development of adrenal tumours.

Spontaneous ovarian tumours are uncommon in laboratory rodents but they can be induced by various methods which generally depend on a direct disturbance of the pituitary/ovarian axis or perturbation of the hormonal environment. It is always difficult to study the factors which influence low incidence tumours but Saxton *et al.* (1948) were not able to demonstrate any effect on the incidence of ovarian tumours in rats due to variations in diet or nutrition. Spontaneous uterine tumours are rare in mice but not uncommon in many rat strains (Munoz, Dunn & Turusov, 1979; Marchant, 1982). Oestrogens will induce uterine tumours in mice and in rats produce proliferative lesions but few tumours. The induction of uterine tumours by chemicals and hormones has been reviewed by Baba & von Haan (1976). Deciduomas of the rat uterus have been recorded in animals fed vitamin E deficient diets (DeFeo, 1967).

Leydig cell tumours of the testis are very rare in mice but common in some strains of rat such as the F344 (Goodman *et al.*, 1979); all other histogenic types are uncommon in rodents. Leydig cell tumours can be induced in some mouse strains by oestrogenic compounds, reviewed by Mostofi & Bresler, 1979. In rats Leydig cell tumours have been induced by cadmium, a trace element in the diet (Roe *et al.*, 1964). Tumours of the prostate and seminal vesicle are exceedingly rare tumours, with the exception of a high incidence of prostate tumours in the rat strain ACI/segHAPBR, where genetic factors are of prime importance in the development of the tumours (Ward *et al.*, 1980).

## Dietary Effects

In discussing dietary effects in rodents it is important to state the species/ strain and diets used in experimental studies. In the following data the animals and diets included are those used at the ICI Laboratories at Alderley Park, Cheshire, UK. The Alderley Park (AP) rat strain is a specific pathogen free, closed colony of albino Wistar rats which have been continuously bred and used since 1957. The mice are from an inbred C57BL/10J strain originally obtained, as a breeding nucleus, from Bar Harbour, Maine, USA, and bred and used since 1975. The diets fed to both rats and mice were Powder 'O', which was used until the mid-seventies and was made to our own specification by a local miller, and, thereafter, PCD diet made by BP Nutrition. The specifications for these two diets are given in Table 11.1. It can be seen that in terms of the chief constituents the two diets are similar; the major difference between them is that wheat instead of barley is used in the PCD diet, and there is a high level of bran in the Powder 'O' diet (bran is not present in the PCD diet). The AP rat has a high spontaneous incidence of endocrine tumours but they are generally rare in the mouse strain. All of the histopathological examinations of the animals in the studies referred to hereafter were done by the author.

## Pituitary gland

Figure 11.1 shows the incidence of spontaneous tumours in the AP rat over a period of 25 years. At each five-year time point the data includes all of the tumours seen in control (untreated) animals in carcinogenicity studies completed in that year (minimum 100/sex). It can be seen that the incidence of pituitary tumours has increased significantly with time from about 10% in both sexes in 1960 to near 100% in females and 50% in males in 1985. The reason for this increase is considered to be an increase in size and food intake in the animals over the period of time. In the 1960s and early 1970s there were two serious outbreaks of infection in the colony, *Pasteurella pneumotropica* and *Sendai* virus; the bacterial infection caused pneumonia in large numbers of the animals while the virus infection, in the adult rat, tended to be subclinical producing a general malaise and failure to thrive. The general poor clinical condition of many of the experimental animals helped to maintain food intakes and body growth at a similar level for a long period of time. This smaller size also enabled the animals to be housed five to a cage. Over time, rederivation of the strain (within the closed colony) and vaccination of breeding stock irradicated the diseases, and during the next decade there was a marked increase in

Table 11.1. *Specifications for diets*

| Ingredient | Powder 'O' (%) | PCD (%) |
|---|---|---|
| Wheat | – | 20.0 |
| Wheat feed | – | 20.0 |
| Oats | 18.3 | 17.5 |
| Maize | 8.6 | 10.0 |
| Barley | 26.3 | 5.5 |
| Bran | 18.6 | – |
| Milk powder | 13.1 | 7.5 |
| Soyabean meal | – | 10.0 |
| White Fish meal | 4.4 | 5.0 |
| Meat and bone | 8.6 | – |
| Unextracted dried yeast | 1.3 | 2.5 |
| Vitamin/salt mix | 0.8 | 2.0 |
| | | |
| Total crude protein | 20.0 | 20.0 |
| Crude fat | 3.0 | 2.7 |
| Crude fibre | 4.8 | 4.0 |
| Vitamins/minerals | 0.8 | 2.0 |

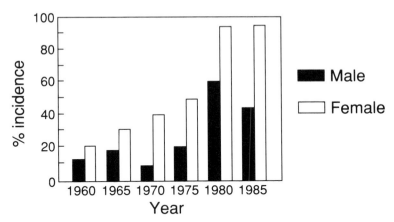

Fig. 11.1. Incidence of pituitary tumours in the AP rat.

body weight of the animals due to increased food intake. The increased size of the animals has necessitated the housing of males three/cage. The increasing body size seems to be a feature of specific pathogen-free animals and Nolen (1972) speculated that the control of infectious disease has allowed a fuller expression of the genes controlling growth. In the

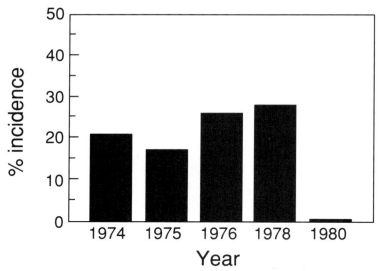

Fig. 11.2. Incidence of pituitary tumours in the C57BL/10S mice.

C57BL/10J mice pituitary tumours were a common tumour in the female when the strain was first bred and remained a feature for several years. Figure 11.2 shows the incidence over time. It can be seen that the incidence of pituitary tumours was around 28% in the first four studies (fed Powder 'O' diet) but in the fifth (fed PCD diet) this dropped to less than 1% and has remained at a low level in all subsequent studies. It is known that in untreated, *ad libitum*, fed rats serum prolactin levels increase as the animals age, reaching levels between 1000 and 2000 ng/ml in two-year-old females (Conybeare, 1988) and is followed by hyperplasia and then neoplasia of prolactin secreting cells in the pituitary. The increasing prolactin levels are related to a decrease in dopamine levels – dopamine inhibits prolactin release from the pituitary.

In a study by Atterwill *et al.* (1989) rats were fed on a restricted dietary regimen (6 hours/day) and compared with *ad libitum* fed animals; this demonstrated that serum prolactin concentrations were reduced in diet restricted females after 12 months, but not in males. There was no evidence that this was related to an increase in dopamine driven inhibition of prolactin secretion and the precise cause of the reduced prolactin levels is as yet unknown.

### Thyroid gland

Figure 11.3 shows the incidence of thyroid follicular tumours in the AP rat and reflects the marked variation in incidence of these tumours from

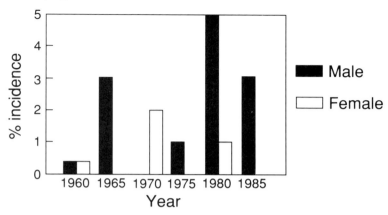

Fig. 11.3. Incidence of thyroid tumours in the AP rat.

one time-part to another. In general, they are not a common tumour (maximum incidence around 5%) and occur more frequently in males, but there is no pattern to the incidence with time as can be seen with pituitary tumours. It is impossible to draw an unequivocal conclusion about the causes of these tumours but the possibility of iodine deficiency, as a contributory factor, cannot be excluded since this element is not measured in the standard vitamin/salt mix which is a constituent of the diet. There is always a possibility that batches of diet vary in iodine levels. In toxicology studies a reduction of body weight in the treatment groups is a common side-effect and the reduced food intake could change a marginal adequacy in iodine into a deficiency sufficient to produce a small increase in thyroid tumours. In addition protein levels significantly affect liver enzyme activity (Butler & Dauterman, 1988) so lowered protein intake may influence thyroxine metabolism and cause a feedback to the pituitary to increase TSH production with a subsequent increase in follicular tumours.

## Adrenal gland

Figure 11.4 shows the incidence of adrenocortical tumours in the AP rat and shows that there has been a decline in this type of tumour with time and the sex difference apparent in the earlier studies (more frequent in males) has disappeared. As for thyroid tumours it is impossible to pinpoint the cause of such variation. It is known that any type of stress, such as overcrowding, ill health, experimental procedures, increase the output of pituitary adrenocorticotrophic hormone (ACTH); exogenous administration of this hormone can produce cortical tumours so in the

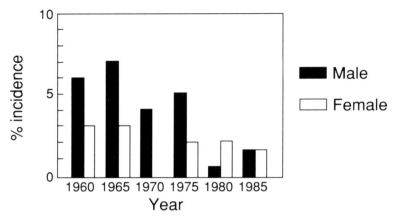

Fig. 11.4. Incidence of adrenocortical tumours in the AP rat.

early studies 'stress' levels may have been high due to intercurrent infections and gang housing; the improved health and caging density of the animals in later studies may have reduced stress and ACTH production with a consequent fall in the incidence of cortical tumours. Gonadectomy is a standard method of inducing cortical tumours so that declining sexual function with age or any dietary factor which affects the gonad-pituitary axis could also affect tumour incidence.

## Discussion

Laboratory diets for rodents, are, in general, designed for breeding purposes, and aim to produce animals of a reasonable size and sexual maturity as quickly as possible. The use of such diets in long term studies is inappropriate and in combination with lack of exercise and sexual activity results in obese animals with high levels of spontaneous tumours.

Long term monitoring of spontaneous tumour incidence in rodents is not common since most laboratories obtain these animals from commercial sources. In the AP rodents such monitoring shows that there are significant changes in tumour patterns, in rats and mice, in closed colonies and inbred strains, and that environmental factors particularly the diet, must be affecting these patterns. The evidence that overnutrition produces high spontaneous tumour levels is overwhelming but the aetiology of almost all individual types remains unknown. It is possible that minor changes in the diet can produce major effects in the animal.

Most 'natural' diets are based on cereals and in most, the level of the major components, such as protein, is an assumption calculated from the type and amount of the constituents but there can be wide differences in protein yield in cereals from different sources and pesticide residues will also vary from one country to another. In the ICI diets the high level of bran in Powder 'O' diet may have produced a shorter intestinal transit time and helped to maintain a low body weight compared with PCD which contains no bran. Transitory deficiencies in trace elements or vitamins could affect the function of various systems in susceptible individuals.

The extensive literature on the subject of diet and tumour incidence would suggest that there is a great diversity in the types of tumour which are inhibited by food restriction – hepatic, pulmonary, endocrine and lymphoreticular tumours – the effect varies with the strain and species and this might suggest a common mechanism for the effect; the literature shows that in all studies the inhibitory effect occurs in the tumour most common in the strain used. This is more a reflection of the difficulties in detecting effects in tumour types of low and variable incidence than a genuine lack of effect on less common tumours. In standard carcinogenic studies a group size of 50–100 animals/sex is usual; it is relatively simple to demonstrate a statistically significant inhibition in a tumour type which constantly occurs at a level of 30% or more and virtually impossible to show an effect on a spontaneous tumour with an incidence which varies from 0–10% (0–5 animals in a group of 50). It is a feature of diet restriction experiments (Tucker, 1979) that the majority of tumour types are numerically reduced but statistical methods can only establish significance for the common types.

The other question to be addressed is the relevance to humans of the endocrine tumours seen in other animals. It would be simplistic to conclude that they must be similar since they relate to 'hormone imbalance', when the nature and cause of the imbalance may be very different. Pituitary and mammary tumours in the rat are related to the elevated levels of prolactin and tumours in these organs can be significantly reduced by control of food or protein intake. In women, breast cancer is not related to elevated prolactin or pituitary tumours – oestrogens and dietary fat are two of the factors implicated in the development of the disease. Thyroid tumours in humans are uncommon except for populations exposed to low levels of iodine or ionizing radiation; the factors causing spontaneous thyroid tumours in rodents are not known but could include iodine deficiency. Adrenal tumours are rare in humans and rodents, except for a few strains of rat; the ease of induction of cortical tumours in rodents following gonadectomy suggests a causal hormonal factor as yet undefined. In humans adrenocortical tumours may be associated with Cushing's syndrome and in this disease, pituitary tumours which secrete ACTH have been identified. Tumours of the reproductive system show considerable differences between the species; testicular tumours are rare in most rodents, with the exception of the F344 rat, and also in men; in rodents they tend to occur in old animals where testicular function has declined; in men they usually occur between the ages of 20 and 50, when testicular function is likely to be normal. Prostate disease of men, however, occurs in an older age group and may be related to changing androgen levels; it is a rare disease in the rodent. Similarly tumours of the female genital tract show differences in type and functional activity such as cervical tumours which are rare in rodents but not uncommon in women.

There can be no doubt that the interrelationship between the endocrine glands is as complex in rodents as in humans but is much less well defined. In most laboratory rodents normal hormonal status and serum hormone levels at different ages remain to be established; there is some evidence to suggest differences exist between strains, for example thyroid hormone levels in SD and Fischer F344 rats (Chen & Walfish, 1979; Waner & Nyska, 1988). Now that appropriate techniques are available it is to be hoped that more data will be published and all toxicologists will consider the value of acquiring reference ranges for hormones in their laboratory animals in a similar way to the data on clinical chemistry and haematology parameters. It is through this means that we shall be able to study and understand the factors which influence the spontaneous and induced tumours of the endocrine system, and to predict, more accurately, the relevance of such tumours to humans.

## References

Atterwill, C.K., Brown, C.G., Conybeare, G., Holland, C.W. & Jones, C.A. (1989). Relation between dopaminergic control of pituitary lactotrophic function and deceleration of age related changes in serum prolactin of diet restricted rats. *Fd. Chem. Toxic.*, **27**, 97–103.

Baba, N. & von Haan, E. (1976). Tumours of the vagina, uterus, placenta and oviducts. In *Pathology of Tumours in Laboratory Animals. Tumours of the Rat*, part 2, ed. V.S. Turusov, pp. 161–88. IARC Scientific Publication No. 6, Lyon.

Benson, J., Lear, M. & Grand, C.G. (1956). Enhancement of mammary fibrodenomas in the female rat by a high fat diet. *Cancer Res.*, **16**, 135–7.

Berg, B.N. & Simms, H.S. (1960). Nutrition and longevity in the rat. II. Longevity and onset of disease with different levels of food intake. *J. Nutr.*, **71**, 255–63.

Berg, J.W. (1975). Can nutrition explain the pattern of international epidemiology of hormone dependant cancers. *Cancer Res.*, **35**, (II Pt 2), 3345–50.

Butler, L.E. & Dauterman, W.C. (1988). The effect of dietary protein levels on xenobiotic biotransformation on F344 male rats. *Toxicol. Appl. Pharmacol.*, **95**, 301–10.

Carroll, K., Gammal, E.B. & Plunkett, E.R. (1968). Dietary fat and mammary cancer. *Can. Med. Assoc. J.*, **98**, 590–4.

Carroll, K. & Khor, J.J. (1975). Dietary fat in relation to tumorigenesis. *Prog. Biochem. Pharmacol.*, **10**, 338–53.

Chan, P. & Cohen, L.A. (1975). Effect of diet, antioestrogen and anti-prolactin on the development of mammary tumours in rats. *J. Natl. Cancer Inst.*, **52**, 25–30.

Chen, H.J. & Walfish, P.G. (1979). Effects of age and testicular function on the pituitary/thyroid system in male rats. *J. Endocrin.*, **22**, 276–80.

Cheng, L. (1980). Phaeochromocytoma in rats. Incidence, etiology, morphology and functional activity. *J. Environ. Pathol. Microbiol.*, **4**, 219–28.

Conybeare, G. (1988). Modulating factors: challenges to experimental design. In *Carcinogenicity: The Design, Analysis and Interpretation of Long-term Animal Studies*, ed. H. Grice & J.L. Ciminera, chapter 18, pp. 150–72. ILSI Monographs. Berlin: Springer-Verlag.

Cunningham, A.S. (1976). Lymphomas and animal protein consumption. *Lancet*, **11**, 1184–6.

DeFeo, V.J. (1967). Decidualization. In *Cellular Biology of the Uterus*, ed. R.M. Wynn, pp. 190–290. New York: Meredith.

Dunn, T.B. (1970). Normal and pathologic anatomy of the adrenal gland of the mouse, including neoplasms. *J. Natl. Cancer Inst.*, **44**, 1323–89.

Dunning, W.F., Curtis, M.R. & Segaloff, A. (1953). Strain differences in response to estrone and the induction of mammary gland, adrenal and bladder cancer in rats. *Cancer Res.*, **13**, 430–2.

Engel, R.W. & Copeland, D.M. (1952). Protective action of stock diets against the cancer inducing action of 2-acetylamino fluorene in rats. *Cancer Res.*, **29**, 780–8.

Ershoff, B.M., Bajua, G.S., Field, J.B. & Boretta, L.A. (1969). Comparative effects of purified diets and a natural stock ration on the tumour incidence of mice exposed to sublethal doses of x-irradiation. *Cancer Res.*, **29**, 780–8.

Fernandez, G., Yunis, E.J. & Good, R.A. (1976). Influence of diet on survival of mice. *Proc. Natl. Acad. Sci.*, **73**(4), 1279–84.

Frith, C.H., Littlefield, N.A. & Umholtz, R. (1981). Incidence of pulmonary metastases for various neoplasms in BALB/cStCrlFC3H/ Nctr female mice fed N-Z-fluoroenylacetamide. *J. Natl. Cancer Inst.*, **66**, 703–12.

Frith, C.H. (1983). Adenoma and carcinoma, adrenal cortex, mice. In *Endocrine System. Monographs on Pathology of Laboratory Animals*, ed. T.C. Jones, U. Mohr & R.D. Hunter, pp. 49–56. Berlin: Springer.

Furth, J., Nakane, P.K. & Pasleels, J.L. (1976). Tumours of the pituitary gland. In *Pathology of Tumours of Laboratory Animals*, vol. 1. *Tumours of the rat*, part 2, ed. V.S. Turusov, pp. 201–38. IARC Scientific Publications No 6, Lyon.

Gardner, W.U., Pfeiffer, C.A. & Trentin, J.J. (1959). Hormonal factors in experimental carcinogenesis. In *The Physiopathology of Cancer*, ed. F. Homburger, pp. 152–237. New York: Hoeber.

Gilman, J., Gilbert, C. & Spence, I. (1953). Phaeochromocytoma in the rat. Pathogenesis and collateral reactions and its relation to comparable tumours in man. *Cancer*, **6**, 494–511.

Goodman, D.G., Ward, J.M., Sqire, R.A., Chu, K.C. & Linhart, M.S. (1979). Neoplastic and non-neoplastic lesions in aging F344 rats. *Toxicol. Appl. Pharmacol.*, **48**, 237–48.

Grasso, P. (1973). The range of carcinogenic substances in human foods and the problems of testing for them. *Proc. Roy. Soc. Med.*, **66**, 20–7.

Griesbach, W.E., Kennedy, T.H. & Purves, H.D. (1945). Studies on experimental goitre. IV Thyroid adenomata in rats on Bassica seed diet. *Brit. J. exp. Path.*, **26**, 18–24.

Hollander, C.F. & Snell, C.K. (1976). Tumours of the adrenal gland. In *Pathology of the Tumours of Laboratory Animals. Tumours of the rat*, vol. 1, ed. V.S. Turusov, pp. 273–93, IARC Scientific Publication No. 6, Lyon.

Heiman, J. (1944). Spontaneous tumours of the adrenal cortex in a castrated male rat. *Cancer Res.*, **4**, 430–2.

Innes, J.R.M., Ulland, B.M., Vallerio, M.G., Petrucelli, L., Fishbein, L., Hart, E.R., Pallota, A.J., Bates, R.R., Falk, M.L., Gort, J.J., Klein, M., Mitchell, I. & Peters, J. (1969). Bioassay of pesticides and industrial chemicals for tumorgenisis in mice: a preliminary note. *J. Natl. Cancer Inst.*, **42**, 1101–14.

Lea, A.J. (1966). Dietary effects associated with death rates from certain neoplasms in man. *Lancet*, **2**, 332–3.

Liebelt, A.G. (1979). Tumours of the pituitary gland. In *Pathology of Tumours in Laboratory Animals. II Tumours of the Mouse*, ed. V.S. Turusov, pp. 411–50. IARC Scientific Publications, Lyon.

Marchant, J. (1982). Animal models for tumours of the female genital tract. In *Pathology of the Female Genital Tract*, 2nd edn, ed. A. Blaustein, pp. 452–64. Berlin: Springer-Verlag.

Mirvish, S.S., Wallcare, L., Eagen, M. & Shubik, P. (1972). Ascorbate-nitrite reaction – Possible means of blocking the formation of carcinogenic N-nitrosa-compounds. *Science*, **177**, 65–8.

Moon, H.D., Koneff, A.A., Li, C.H. & Simpson, M.E. (1956). Phaeochromocytomas of the adrenals in male rats chronically injected with pituitary growth hormone. *Proc. Soc. exp. Biol. (N.Y.)*, **93**, 74–7.

Moore, C. & Tittle, P.W. (1973). Muscle activity, body fat and induced rat mammary tumours. *Surgery*, **73**, 329–32.

Mostofi, F.K. & Bresler, V.M. (1979). Tumours of the testis. In *Pathology of the Tumours of Laboratory Animals*, vol. 2, *Tumours of the Mouse*, ed. V.S. Turusov, pp. 325–50. IARC Scientific Publication No. 23, Lyon.

Munoz, N., Dunn, T.B. & Turusov, V.S. (1979). Tumours of the vagina and uterus. In *Pathology of Tumours in Laboratory Animals*, vol. 2, *Tumours of the Mouse*, ed. V.S. Turusov, pp. 359–84. IARC Scientific Publication No. 23, Lyon.

Nolen, G.A. (1972). Lasting influence of early caloric restriction on prevalence of neoplasms in the rat. *J. Nutr.*, **75**, 197–210.

Pickering, C.E. & Pickering, R.G. (1984). The effect of repeated reproduction on the incidence of pituitary tumours in Wistar rats. *Lab. Anim.*, **18**, 371–8.

Roe, F.J.C., Dukes, C.E., Cameron, K.M., Pugh, R.C.B. & Mitchley, B.C.V. (1964). Cadmium neoplasia. Testicular atrophy and Leydig cell hyperplasia and neoplasia in rats and mice following subcutaneous injection of cadmium salts. *Brit. J. Cancer*, **18**, 674–81.

Ross, M.H. (1961). Length of life and nutrition in the rat. *J. Nutr.*, **75**, 197–210.

Ross, M.H., Bras, G. & Ragbeer, M.S. (1970). Influence of protein and calorie intake upon spontaneous tumour incidence of the anterior pituitary gland in the rat. *J. Nutr.*, **100**, 177–89.

Ross, M.H. & Bras, G. (1971). Lasting influence of early calorie restriction on prevalence of neoplasms in the rat. *J. Natl. Cancer Inst.*, **47**(5), 1095–113.

Sabine, J.R., Horton, B.J. & Wicks, H.B. (1973). Spontaneous tumours in C3H-A$^{vy}$ and C3H-A$^{vy}$FB mice. High incidence in the United States and low incidence in Australia. *J. Natl. Cancer Inst.*, **50**, 1237–42.

Saxton, J.A., Sperling, G.A., Barnes, L.L. & McKay, C.M. (1948). The influence of nutrition upon the incidence of spontaneous tumours on the rat in longevity and onset of disease with different levels of food intake. Acta Unio. *Int. Contra Cancrum*, **6**, 423–31.

Silverstone, H. & Tannenbaum, A. (1950). The effect of the proportion of dietary fat on the rate of mammary carcinoma in mice. *Cancer Res.*, **10**, 448–53.

Tannenbaum, A. (1940a). Relationship of body weight to cancer incidence. *Arch. Path.*, **30**, 504–17.

Tannenbaum, A. (1940b). Initiation and growth of tumours, effects of underfeeding. *Am. J. Cancer*, **38**, 335–50.

Tannenbaum, A. & Silverstone, H. (1949a). The influence of the degree of calorie restriction on the formation of skin tumours and hepatomas in mice. *Cancer Res.*, **9**, 724–7.

Tannenbaum, A. & Silverstone, H. (1949b). The genesis and growth of tumours. IV Effects of varying the proportion of protein (casein) in the diet. *Cancer Res.*, **9**, 162–73.

Thompson, S.W., Rac, V.S., Semonick, D.E., Antonchak, B., Spaet, R.H. & Schellhammer, L.E. (1981). *The Adrenal Medulla of Rats.* Springfield, Ill: Thomas.

Tucker, M.J. (1979). Effects of long term diet restriction on tumours in rodents. *Int. J. Cancer*, **23**, 803–7.

Waner, T. & Nyska, A. (1988). Thyroxine (T4) and triiodothyronine (T3) levels in Fischer F344 inbred rats. *Lab. Anim.*, **22**, 276–80.

Ward, J.M., Renzil, G., Stinson, S.F., Lattuada, C.P., Longfellow, D.G. & Cameron, T.P. (1980). Histogenesis and morphology of naturally occurring prostate carcinoma in the ACI/segHAPBR rat. *Lab. Invest.*, **43**, 517–22.

White, J. & Andervont, H.B. (1943). Effects of a diet relatively low in cystine on the production of spontaneous mammary gland tumours in the strain C3H female mice. *J. Natl. Cancer Inst.*, **3**, 449–87.

Yunis, E.J. & Greenberg, L.J. (1974). Immunopathology of ageing. *Fed. Proc.*, **33**, 2017–19.

G.R. BETTON

# 12 Toxicology of the diffuse neuroendocrine system

## Introduction

The diffuse neuroendocrine system (DNES) represents the largest population of endocrine cells in the body and is distributed in a wide range of organs outside the central nervous system. This population is heterogeneous in its composition and distribution. Initial theories of a neural crest origin have been disproved but the stem cell differentiation from embryonic endodermal or ectodermal elements into neuro-endocrine or epithelial elements at an early stage holds true in most cases. Neuroendocrine cells are characterized by silver staining reactions with or without reducing agents (argentaffin and argyrophil cells, Grimelius & Wilander, 1980) related to amine content of secretory granules. The term APUD system (amine precursor uptake and decarboxylase) coined by Pearse (1968) has been alternatively used to describe the DNES but not all cells of the system have APUD activity. Some common markers of neuroendocrine cells are listed in Table 12.1.

## Anatomy and physiology

The diffuse distribution of cells of the DNES is intimately related to the regulatory function of neuroendocrine cells in monitoring the local milieu and signalling target cells locally or at a distance through a peptide or amine mediator. Thus factors such as $P_{CO_2}$ or $P_{O_2}$ in the lung, pH of gastric juice, or nutrients in the small intestine are monitored by apical membranes of neuroendocrine cells in contact with body interfaces. Implicit in their name is the close inter-relationship between endocrine cells and the local (autonomic) innervation by the sympathetic and parasympathetic nervous systems. Microanatomical groupings of cells with stimulatory and inhibitory neuroendocrine cells functioning in a (local) paracrine fashion allows for the integration of positive and negative inputs at a given site, for example the antral mucosa of the stomach. Release of a peptide hormone mediator, active at a receptor distant from

Table 12.1. *Common (shared) markers of neuroendocrine cells*

| Components | Markers |
|---|---|
| Aromatic amines | – formaldehyde-induced fluorescence amine precursor uptake amino acid decarboxylalse |
| Acidic secretory vacuoles | – $Mg^{++}$-dependant $H^+/K^+$ ATPase<br>ATP |
| Neurosecretory granules | – Specific peptide hormone for cell type<br>Chromogranins (Cohn *et al.*, 1963; Angeletti, 1986; Hagn *et al.*, 1986)<br>Neuron-specific enolase (Bishop *et al.*, 1982)<br>Synaptophysian (Gould *et al.*, 1987)<br>Specific proteases<br>Non-specific esterase |

the secreting cell can, therefore, be appropriate to a multifactorial environment.

Some hormone mediators secreted by neuroendocrine cells have also been shown to stimulate receptors on the secreting cell (autocrine effect), for example the secretion of gastrin releasing peptide (GRP), the mammalian analogue to bombesin of amphibians, is secreted by lungs in oat cell carcinoma (bronchial neuroendocrine cell in origin).

Expression of neuroendocrine secretory function of neoplastic cells has also been reported in tumours of a wide range of epithelial cell types but not primarily of neuroendocrine cell origin, for example in hepatocellular carcinogenesis in the rat (Seglen *et al.*, 1989).

Physiological regulation of the DNES is highly specific for each of the cell types involved, some of which are listed in Table 12.2. With such a plethora of cell types (Solcia *et al.*, 1980), peptide hormone products, and control mechanisms (some of which show interspecies variation in their relative importance), this review will address only selected examples within the DNES for discussion. In general, stimulation of cells of the DNES to secrete peptide hormones over a prolonged period can result in a resetting of the feedback control to a new (compensated) steady state with no hypertrophy of hyperplasia of the neuroendocrine cell concerned. However, in other cases a condition of prolonged marked hyperplasia and hypertrophy with ultimate elevation in the frequency of benign or malignant tumours of neuroendocrine origin ('carcinoids') may result. In general, laboratory animals show an extremely low or zero incidence of spontaneous tumours of this type and therefore a toxicological mechanism for tumour induction may be readily identifiable. This is in contrast to

Table 12.2. *Neuroendocrine cell types (diffuse system)*

| Cell | Organ | Polypeptide hormone |
|------|-------|---------------------|
| | Thymus | ACTH |
| | Thymus | Calcitonin |
| | Thymus | CGRP |
| | Thymus | CCK |
| | Thymus | Gastrin |
| | Thymus | Neurotensin |
| | Thymus | Somatostatin |
| | Thymus | Substance P |
| NEBs ($P_2$) | Lung | Bombesin |
| NEBs ($P_2$) | Lung | ACTH (in hamsters on nitrosamines) |
| NEBs ($P_2$) | Lung | VIP (in man) |
| NEBs ($P_2$) | Lung | Calcitonin |
| NEBs ($P_2$) | Lung | CGRP |
| Solid NE cells | Lung | Leu-encephalin |
| Merkel | Skin | Enkephalin (rodents) |
| ECL | Stomach fundus | (histamine) |
| A | Stomach fundus | Glucagon |
| D | Stomach antrum | Somatostatin |
| G | Stomach antrum | Gastrin |
| EC1 | Intestine | Substance P |
| EC2 | Intestine | Motilin |
| D | Intestine | Somatostatin |
| S | Intestine | Secretin |
| I | Intestine | Cholecystokinin |
| K | Intestine | Gastric inhibitory peptide |
| N | Intestine | Neurotensin |
| L | Intestine | Glicentin |
| PP | Pancreas Ducts | Pancreatic polypeptide, GRF |
| A | Pancreas Islets | Glucagon, CRF |
| B | Pancreas | Insulin, TRH |

ACTH = adrenocorticotropin; CCK = cholecystokinin; CGRP = calcitonin gene related peptide; CRF = corticotropin releasing factor; GRF = growth hormone releasing factor; TRH = thyrotropin-releasing hormone; VIP = vasoactive intestinal peptide; NEB = neuroepithelial bodies.

other discrete endocrine organs where spontaneous incidence and sensitivity to variation in non-specific factors such as nutrition may confound interpretation.

A second sequela to perturbation of the DNES by xenobiotics is the hypersecretion of peptide hormones which, if trophic in action, causes proliferation of cells of the target organ and, may result in hyperplasia and neoplasia of exocrine or other tissues, for example the action of cholecystokinin (CCK) on exocrine pancreatic cells.

## Pathophysiology and toxicology

Exposure of humans or other animals to xenobiotics may result in a pathophysiological disturbance ranging from a minor fully compensated resetting of endocrine feedback loops to a deregulated hypersecretion and degeneration or neoplastic progression in specific cell population of the DNES.

Categories of xenobiotic action are listed in Table 12.3.

Specific examples of the effects of xenobiotics of the DNES of toxicological significance are listed according to organ systems as follows:

### Thymic neuroendocrine cells

The thymus develops from a migration of branchial pouch epithelium into the cranial thorax where the thymic epithelial cells differentiate into the well-recognized Hassal's corpuscles. These are comprised of thymosin-secreting epithelial cells which serve to organize and regulate bone-marrow derived lymphocytes to differentiate into T-lymphocytes depleted of auto-reactive clones. In addition, nests of neuroendocrine cells of uncertain (neural crest or foregut) origin are identifiable and are more prominent in the aged rat following thymic atrophy. The function of these cells is unclear but recent focus on neuroendocrine and immune system interactions may soon resolve these questions. Neuroendocrine 'carcinoid' tumours of the thymus in man have been reported to be derived from a range of cell types (Herbst et al., 1987) and have clinically been shown to be a source of ectopic adrenocorticotrophin (ACTH) production in Cushing's syndrome (Salyer, Salyer & Eggleston, 1976; Wick & Scheithauer, 1984). Thymic carcinoids have been reported in control rats only rarely (Naylor, Krinke & Ruefenacht, 1988) and have not been described as a target organ effect of xenobiotic exposure.

### Respiratory neuroendocrine cells

The bronchopulmonary tract contains solitary or groups (neuroepithelial bodies, NEBs) of neuroendocrine cells within the major and minor airway epithelial lining (Lauweryns, Cokelaere & Theunynck, 1972; Sorokin, Hoyt & Pearsall, 1983). A range of peptide hormones has been identified within these cells and within bronchopulmonary carcinoids and

Table 12.3. *Categories of neuroendocrine effects of xenobiotics*

| Type | Mechanisms | Example |
|------|-----------|---------|
| CNS | Changes in automatic nervous system | 'Stress' and ACTH |
| Receptor mediated | Agonists or antagonists of DNES cells | Somatostatin analogues |
| Metabolic | Enzyme induction or inhibition | Phenbarbitone |
| Target organ toxicity | Bystander tissue injury altering local milieu | Pneumocyte injury/ alveolar macrophage increase |
| Pharmacological action | Modification of cellular function | Gastric antisecretory agents |

ACTH = adrenocorticotrophin; DNES = diffuse neuroendocrine system

neuroendocrine carcinomas derived from them (Gould *et al.*, 1983). Bombesin/GRP and ACTH are the most frequently expressed hormones in 'oat cell' carcinoma in human clinical practice.

Some tumours show mixed neuroendocrine and epithelial cell markers (Blobel *et al.*. 1985), indicative of dedifferentiation. Bronchial neuroendocrine cells in rodents have demonstrated changes in granule content under conditions of hypobaric hypoxia (Moosavi, Smith & Heath, 1973) and, in hamsters, after exposure to cigarette smoke when calcitonin and bombesin/GRP secretion was increased (Tabassian *et al.*, 1989). In association with pneumocyte injury, rats exposed to diethylnitrosamine (Linnoila, 1982), nitrogen dioxide (Kleinerman, Marchevsky & Thornton, 1981), or chysotile or crocidolite (Johnson, Wagner & Wills, 1980), and hamsters injected with 4-nitroquinoline-1-oxide (Ito *et al.*, 1988) showed proliferation of pulmonary neuroendocrine cells (NEBs) in addition to other target organ effects. Whether these changes were direct effects or indirect secondary actions of lung injury and hypoxia has not been determined.

Of comparative interest is the neuroendocrine chief cell hyperplasia within carotid bodies of patients with cardiopulmonary disease (Heath, Smith & Jago, 1984) and in rats with a variety of pathologies causing hypoxia (Van Zwieten *et al.*, 1979).

## Intestinal neuroendocrine cells and the pancreas

The development of endocrine cells in the gastrointestinal tract and its embryological derivatives (pancreas, liver) has been the subject of scientific investigation for decades. The wide range of cell types and their associated specific peptide hormone products has been reviewed by Solcia *et al.* (1980) and Buchan & Polak (1980). The identification of associated peptidergic neuronal regulation of gastrointestinal motility, secretion and hormonal secretion opens the way for resolution of the underlying mechanisms in many areas of gastrointestinal (GI) toxicology. Applications of molecular biology techniques to localize early events in DNES function have revealed that related peptide hormones such as enteroglucagon and glicentin (Holst, 1983) are in fact coded for by large genes for hormone precursors ('pre-pro-peptides') which can liberate different peptides according to the cleavage site of translated proteins. Small 'flanking' peptides may play an important yet presently poorly understood means of feedback regulation.

Many GI peptide hormones serve to regulate exocrine secretory function, water and electrolyte balance and/or smooth muscle contraction during the digestive process. Significant central nervous system (CNS) and autonomic neuronal inputs and local and distant endocrine signals serve to regulate the process. Synergistic effects are also important (Mori *et al.*, 1986; Damge *et al.*, 1988).

Cholecystokinin (CCK) secreted by I cells of the small intestine acts at specific receptors on pancreatic acinar cells causing secretion *in vitro* and *in vivo* (Jensen, Lemp & Gardner, 1982). In addition to its secretagogue actions, CCK also has a trophic (proliferative) action on pancreatic exocrine tissue. These trophic actions can serve to promote the carcinogenic action of genotoxic chemicals. The essential fatty acid unsaturated linoleic acid increased the asaserine-induced pancreatic hyperplasias and tumours (Roebuck *et al.*, 1985) in the rat. CCK promoted pancreatic carcinogenesis in the hamster N-nitro-bis (2-oxypropyl) amine (BOP) model (Howatson & Carter, 1985) although other workers found no effect if administered 0–3 h post-BOP administration (Pour *et al.*, 1988). A high fat diet was, however, found to enhance BOP pancreatic carcinogenesis in the hamster (Birt *et al.*, 1989).

In the absence of exogenous genotoxic carcinogens, corn oil, often used as a vehicle, was found to cause a five-fold rise in pancreatic exocrine focal hyperplasias and adenoma (Eustis & Boorman, 1985). Raw soya flour (RSF) containing a heat labile trypsin inhibitor has been shown to induce raised plasma CCK (Loser *et al.*, 1988) and pancreatic acinar cell hyperplasia (Fig. 12.1) and neoplasia (Fig. 12.2) in the rat (McGuiness, Morgan & Wormsley, 1984). This effect is absent after heat inactivation of soya flour trypsin inhibitor. The early hypertrophy and hyperplasia seen after four days on RSF diets could be specifically inhibited by the specific CCK antagonist L364, 718 (Sundaram & Dayan,

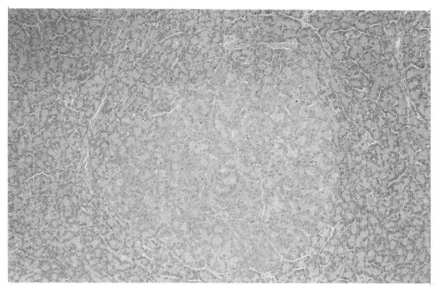

Fig. 12.1. Focal hyperplasia of pancreatic acinar cells. Note change in staining characteristics and lobular organisation. H/E

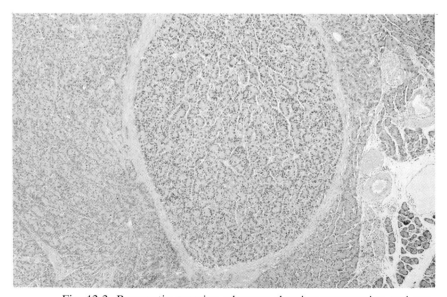

Fig. 12.2. Pancreatic exocrine adenoma showing compression and capsule formation in a 2-year-old rat fed on diet containing raw soya flour. H/E

1989). Similarly, the trypsin inhibitor, camostate, which has a potent trophic action on the rat exocrine pancreas, produced no effect if co-administered with L-364,718 (Wisner *et al.*, 1988). Induction or promotion of pancreatic exocrine neoplasia, therefore, was related to elevations in CCK from intestinal CCK-secreting I cells responding to dietary effect, probably related to an inhibitory luminal signal peptide regulating protease activity in the small intestine. Despite chronic hypersecretion of CCK by I cells, these cells *per se* do not proliferate to form neuro-endocrine tumours themselves.

### Gastric neuroendocrine cells

#### Anatomy and physiology

The stomach shows considerable anatomical variation during mammalian evolution with considerable specialization of the squamous epithelial-lined forestomach or non-glandular stomach, reaching a peak in the ruminants. The squamous epithelium of the forestomach is sharply demarcated from the acid-secreting oxyntic glandular mucosa by a limiting ridge and narrow band of mucus-secreting cardiac glands. The thinner antral mucosa extends from the pylorus almost to the limiting ridge along the lesser curvature but only about one quarter of the way along the greater curvature. The boundary is visible on naked eye examination of the stomach after opening along the greater curvature, removal of food, and pinning out. Omnivores and carnivores such as humans and the dog lack a forestomach and have a simple glandular stomach lined by cardiac, oxyntic (fundic) and antral mucosae.

The gastric mucosal reactions to dietary, neuronal, and endocrine factors are complex and for details the reader is referred to reviews of gastric physiology (Johnson, 1988). The principal functions are to serve as a food reservoir bathed in gastric acid and associated acid-activated enzymes. These functions are regulated primarily by direct vagal innervation, activated by higher CNS centres in response to the stimulus of eating, and by the potent secretagogue gastrin secreted by antral G cells. Antral G cells and D cells are juxtaposed in the antral mucosa, and D cell processes deliver somatostatin directly to receptors on G cells, shutting off gastrin secretion when local pH falls. This negative paracrine effect also regulates gastrin secretion via antral D cells in response to cholinergic (vagal) inputs and other factors. Regions within the stomach, therefore, interplay on the regulation of gastric acid secretion both by autonomic, neuronal, paracrine, and circulatory endocrine factors.

The normal histology of an oxyntic gland from the gastric body or fundus of many species has a typical architecture with specialized cell

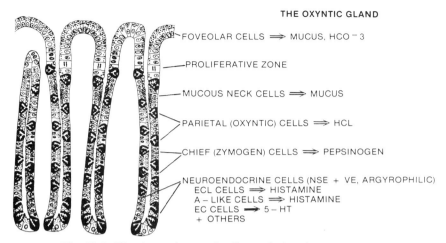

THE OXYNTIC GLAND

FOVEOLAR CELLS ⟹ MUCUS, HCO⁻3

PROLIFERATIVE ZONE

MUCOUS NECK CELLS ⟹ MUCUS

PARIETAL (OXYNTIC) CELLS ⟹ HCL

CHIEF (ZYMOGEN) CELLS ⟹ PEPSINOGEN

NEUROENDOCRINE CELLS (NSE + VE, ARGYROPHILIC)
ECL CELLS ⟹ HISTAMINE
A – LIKE CELLS ⟹ HISTAMINE
EC CELLS ⟹ 5 – HT
+ OTHERS

Fig. 12.3. Histology of normal cell populations in rat oxyntic mucosa.

functions (Fig. 12.3). It is essential to appreciate the presence of the proliferative zone at the base of the gastric pits (foveolae) from which (i) mucous foveolar cells with bicarbonate secreting capacity are produced by upward migration (life span 3–6 days), and (ii) gastric gland cells (parietal cells, chief cells, mucous neck cells, and neuroendocrine cells) are produced by local mitosis, and by downward migration, with pro-longed lifespans (up to 120 days for parietal cells) (Willems *et al.*, 1972; Fujita & Hattori, 1977; Helander, 1981).

It is for this reason that although normal gastric mucosa shows a higher fraction of gastric gland cells versus foveolar cells under conditions of higher cell production, the proportion of foveolar cells in a hyperplastic mucosa appears to increase disproportionately. In addition, superficial injury to the surface epithelial cells can be rapidly repaired by migration and flattening out of mucous cells from gastric pits to cover damaged basement membrane (Lacy & Ito, 1984).

In contrast, the antral mucosa is divided into surface mucous cells of the pits with a lifespan of 1–1.5 days in rodents and gland cells with a lifespan of 2–8 days. The neuroendocrine G cell component, however, has a lifespan of 2–4 months in the mouse. Circadian rhythms in cell proliferation have been observed in antral mucosa.

Acid secretion by the gastric mucosa is a specialized function of parietal (oxyntic) cells located in the body and fundus of the stomach. Parietal cells are absent from the antral mucosa, therefore gastrin-secreting G cells confined to the antrum are exposed only to luminal and not to locally produced gastric acid.

424     G.R. BETTON

## STRUCTURE OF RAT LITTLE GASTRIN

| | 1 | 2 | 3 | 4 | 5 | 6 | 7 | 8 | 9 | 10 | 11 | 12 | 13 | 14 | 15 | 16 | 17 |
|---|---|---|---|---|---|---|---|---|---|---|---|---|---|---|---|---|---|
| Rat | Glp-Arg-Pro-Pro-Met-Glu-Glu-Glu-Glu-Ala-Tyr-Gly-Trp-Met-Asp-Phe-NH₂ |
| Hog | | | -Gly- | -Trp- |
| Dog | | | -Gly- | -Trp- | | | -Ala- |
| Cat | | | -Gly- | -Trp- | | | | -Ala- |
| Man | | | -Gly- | -Trp-Leu- |
| Cow and sheep | | | -Gly- | -Trp-Val- | | | | -Ala- |

Comparison of the sequence of rat gastrin with that of heptadecapetide gastrins from other species.

Fig. 12.4. Amino acid sequence of gastrin G-17 in various species.

Gastrin was one of the earliest peptide hormones to be isolated and was characterized as a potent gastric secretagogue. Its amino-acid sequence (Fig. 12.4) is highly conserved (Reeve et al., 1981) with the C-terminal 5-amino acid sequence (pentagastrin) having potent secretory actions in a wide range of species. There is homology with CCK at the 4 C-terminal amino acids. Gastrin receptors have been demonstrated on the parietal cell and operate via a c′-AMP second messenger. The tyrosine near the C-terminus can also be phosphorylated via a protein kinase mechanism linked to the epidermal growth factor (EGF) receptor. EGF is known to be a trophic hormone for the oxyntic mucosa with ornithine decarboxylase expression and DNA and RNA synthesis being induced. The molecular form in which gastrin is secreted by the antral G cells (G-17, G-34 and other forms) is subject to considerable modification by serum proteases and molecular forms have been shown to vary in their biological activity and half-life in the circulation. Gastrin receptors on glandular cells in the fundic mucosa other than the parietal cell have not been fully characterized, but are presumed to be present on enterochromaffin-like (ECL) cells as well as the cells of the proliferative zone in which trophic effects are expressed (Johnson, 1988).

Inhibition of acid secretion

The identification of the histamine H₂-receptor in the gastric mucosa and the recognition that antagonists at this receptor were potent inhibitors of both histamine and gastrin-stimulated acid secretion as well as being active in some neuronally-mediated hypersecretory states, revolutionized the therapy of peptic ulcer disease, both gastric and duodenal. First

Table 12.4. *Antisecretory agents and ECL cell changes in rodent toxicity studies*

| | H$_2$-receptor antagonists: short-acting | | | | |
| | Cimetidine | Ranitidine | Oxmetidine | Famotidine | Nizatidine |
|---|---|---|---|---|---|
| Hypergastrinaemia | + | + | + | + | ? |
| Diffuse ECL cell hyperplasia | + | + | + | ? | + + |
| Focal ECL cell hyperplasia | – | – | – | – | – |
| Neuroendocrine tumours | | | | | |
| rat | – | – | – | – | – |
| mouse | – | – | – | – | – |

generation histamine H$_2$-receptor antagonists (H$_2$RAs, cimetidine, ranitidine, nizatidine and famotidine), were all free of gastric carcinogenic effects in rodents (Leslie *et al.*, 1981; Poynter *et al.*, 1982; Morton, 1987; Burek, Majka & Bokelman, 1985, see Table 12.4). These agents are characteristically short acting and generally of low pharmacological potency requiring twice daily or more frequent dosing unless large (over) doses are administered. Although these agents have been effective in the acute therapy and maintenance of peptic ulcers in 90–95% of subjects, a resistant group of ulcer patients, such as cigarette smokers, can be identified. First generation agents have also been relatively ineffective in gastrinoma (Zollinger–Ellison, Z–E) patients and in gastroesophageal reflux disease (GERD).

In the search for more potent longer acting agents, a second generation of H$_2$RAs has emerged – SK&F93479, loxtidine, BL6341, ICI162846. Whilst demonstrating improved therapeutic potential where tested, these agents have been uniformly distinguished by their ability to produce neuroendocrine carcinoid tumours in the stomach of rodents (Poynter *et al.*, 1985, 1986; Betton *et al.*, 1988; Hirth *et al.*, 1988; Streett, Robertson & Crissman, 1988, see Table 12.5). Although all were shown to be potent antagonists at the histamine H$_2$-receptor, sometimes with slowly reversible or 'unsurmountable' dissociation from the receptor, these second generation agents showed considerable chemical diversity.

Omeprazole, a substituted benzimidazole, enters the parietal cell acidic compartment where it is activated to a reactive species capable of covalently linking to and inhibiting the H$^+$/K$^+$ ATPase enzyme. Omeprazole, therefore, acts at the final common (H$^+$ secreting) pathway in the parietal cell, which is still stimulated by agonist mediators. Results of animal and human pharmacology, and therapeutic studies indicate a

Table 12.5. *Antisecretory agents and ECL cell changes in rodent toxicity studies*

| | H$_2$-receptor antagonists, potent long-acting, and omeprazole | | | | |
| | SK&F 93479 | Loxitidine | BL 6431 | ICI 162846 | Omeprazole |
|---|---|---|---|---|---|
| Hypergastrinaemia | +++ | ? | +++ | ? | ++++ |
| Diffuse ECL cell hyperplasia | +++ | ? | +++ | +++ | ++++ |
| Focal ECL cell hyperplasia | +++ | +++ | ++ | +++ | ++++ |
| Percentage oxyntic neuroendocrine (ECL) tumours (carcinoids) | | | | | |
|   rat (m/f) | 17/22 | 2/16 | 6/4 | +++ | 10/40 |
|   mouse | – | ++ | ND | ++ | –* |
| Sex difference | m=f | m<f | m>f | ? | m<f |
| No effect dose (rat) | 200mg/kg | <50mg/kg | 55mg/kg | ? | <1mg/kg |

*–mouse study only 18 months duration

high level of efficacy, even in those subjects showing poor responses to first generation H$_2$-receptor antagonists, and omeprazole was shown to induce gastric carcinoid tumours in the rat (Ekman *et al.*, 1985; Carlsson *et al.*, 1986; Table 12.5).

### Short-term effects of antisecretory agents in animals
Indirect effects of antisecretory agents are thought to share a common pathophysiology through the compensatory secretion of gastrin in response to raised intragastric pH. This example of endocrine feedback, attempting to restore homeostasis after pharmacological intervention, is the basis of the so called 'gastrin hypothesis' for ECL cell hyperplasia and carcinoid tumour induction, as depicted in Fig. 12.5.

The gastrin-producing G cells of the antral mucosa synthesize and secrete gastrin in its various molecular forms in response to a range of factors, the most important of which is considered to be elevation of the pH gastric juice in the antrum. Surgical models for Bilroth II resections such as antral transplantation to the colon or Roux-en-Y reconstructions result in diversion of gastric acid secretion from the antrum with resultant hypergastrinaemia and antral G cell hyperplasia in both humans and rat. The local control of gastrin secretions within the antral mucosa is however complex, with vagal innervation and paracrine inputs by inhibitory somatostatin secreting D cells, playing a modulatory role.

Short-term therapy with antisecretory agents (Decktor *et al.*, 1988) or the administration of antacids can be shown to increase circulating gastrin but antral G and D cell populations are generally changed only on chronic

## PHYSIOLOGY OF CHRONIC ACID SUPPRESSION

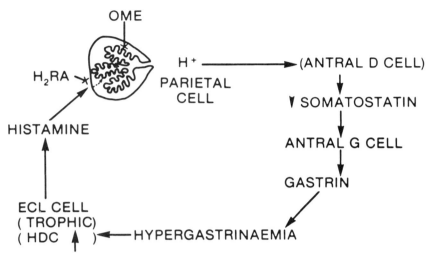

H$_2$RA = POTENT H$_2$-RECEPTOR ANTAGONIST, EG SK&F 93479

OME = H$^+$/K$^+$ ATPase INHIBITOR, EG OMEPRAZOLE

HDC = HISTIDINE DECARBOXYLASE

Fig. 12.5. Physiology of chronic acid suppression with hypergastrinaemia leading to proliferation of ECL cells.

treatment. It is particularly significant that G cell hyperplasia has never been reported to progress to gastrinoma in either humans or experimental animals.

The oxyntic mucosa, however, shows a close dependency on circulating gastrin for its proliferative activity. Antrectomy (removing G cells) results in atrophy of the oxyntic mucosa and reduction in ECL cell numbers (Hakanson *et al.*, 1976), whereas sustained hypergastrinaemia is invariably associated with increased proliferative zone activity of the oxyntic mucosa. The 'atrophic gastritis' of the oxyntic mucosa of humans (Type A) shows a loss of secretory glandular elements but the foveolar cells and subsequent intestinal metaplasias are certainly not 'atrophic'.

Under conditions of sustained hypergastrinaemia, the oxyntic mucosa shows a specific classic trophic response with increased thymidine uptake and mitotic activity in the proliferative zone, with a subsequent overall increase in mucosal height and stomach weight in a range of species (Hakanson *et al.*, 1988). The chronic stimulation of proliferative activity results in an increased mass of cells of all types. Increased parietal cell mass, for example, can be seen in rats treated with antacids for 60 days (Mazzacca *et al.*, 1978) and in patients treated with cimetidine (Svendson *et al.*, 1986) and this increased parietal cell mass may explain the reduction in sustained achlorhydria on chronic versus acute administration of potent long-acting anti-secretory agents.

Enterochromaffin-like (ECL) cells have been the subject of particular interest since, unlike the antral G cells, they have exhibited a full spectrum of progression from diffuse hyperplasia to focal hyperplasia to neuroendocrine (carcinoid) tumour formation in the rat, mouse, and humans under conditions causing sustained marked hypergastrinaemia.

ECL-cells show differences in term of both their frequency and functions between species, with mucosal histamine production being primarily of ECL-cell origin in rodents but is of mast cell origin in humans and the dog. ECL cells are also most numerous in the rodent compared to the dog and humans. Gastrin receptors are presumed to be present on the ECL cell surface since gastrin rapidly activates the enzyme histidine decarboxylase in these cells (Hakanson *et al.*, 1976). Full characterization of the ECL-cell gastrin receptor and its homology with the parietal cell gastrin receptor is awaited. Gastrin shows considerable sequence homology with the middle T-antigen/oncogene of polyoma virus (Baldwin, 1982).

The trophic action of gastrin on the ECL cell would appear to be a direct one based on labelling studies (Willems *et al.*, 1972), rather than being a consequence of trophic effects on the pleuripotential stem cell of the proliferative zone. This supposition is supported by the fact that expansion of the oxyntic mucosal ECL cell population appears to take place from the basal third of the gastric gland, where they are normally situated, upwards towards the proliferative zone at the top of the gland, rather than downwards. Altered maturation rates of cells destined to express neuroendocrine cell differentiation would, however, also explain this distribution pattern in conditions of hypergastrinaemia. Hypertrophy of ECL cells following four weeks exposure to synthetic gastrin or 2–10 weeks oral omeprazole treatment were ultrastructurally identified in a number of rodent species (Bottcher *et al.*, 1989).

### Long-term actions of antisecretory agents

During the course of animal studies of antisecretory agents of the short acting $H_2$-RA type, few target organ effects were reported in the gastric mucosa of rats (Table 12.4), dogs and mice even after long term (1–2 year) treatment at high toxicological doses (Leslie *et al.*, 1981; Poynter *et al.*, 1982; Burek, Majka & Bokelman, 1985; Morton, 1987). Some general trophic effects on the oxyntic mucosa and diffuse changes in ECL cell populations were, however, subsequently demonstrable on more detailed evaluation of these compounds. Nevertheless, these agents were insufficiently potent or too short-acting to progress the ECL cell diffuse hyperplasia stage through to focal hyperplasia, or neuroendocrine (carcinoid) tumour formation.

In contrast, a series of potent long-acting $H_2RAs$ (Table 12.5) and the proton pump inhibitor (PPI) omeprazole (Table 12.5) were shown in rapid succession to be capable of inducing diffuse and focal ECL cell hyperplasia and neuroendocrine tumours (Figs 12.6 and 12.7) of the oxyntic mucosa of the rat and, in some cases, the mouse. This tumour type, with the exception of one reported spontaneous case in the rat (Majke & Sher, 1989), has been uniquely associated with compounds having antisecretory activity and has not been observed following treatment with genotoxic gastric carcinogens such as N-methyl-N'-nitro-N'-nitrosoguanidine (MNNG) causing gastric exocrine adenocarcinomas, with the exception of one report (Tahara *et al.*, 1981). These observations lead to the simultaneous conclusion by a number of workers that the mechanism of gastric neuroendocrine tumour formation in the rat was an indirect non-genotoxic one linked to the homeostatic perturbation by antisecretory agents and the subsequent trophic effects of hypergastrinaemia (Fig. 12.5).

Thus, the potent long acting $H_2RAs$ SK&F 93479 (Betton *et al.*, 1988), loxtidine (Poynter *et al.*, 1985), ICI 162846 (Streett *et al.*, 1988), and BL 6341 (Hirth *et al.*, 1988) and the PPI omeprazole (Ekman *et al.*, 1985) presented compelling evidence for a correlation with potency and duration of antisecretory action as being critical elements for ECL cell hyperplasia of sufficient degree to progress to neoplasia. The ultimate transformation event from hyperplasia to neoplasia, nevertheless, remains unknown since the long latent period for carcinoid tumour expression ($>80$ weeks) and the absence of studies on the effects of cessation of drug treatment at various timepoints beyond 52 weeks during a lifespan oncogenicity study make this aspect of the progression from hyperplasia to neoplasia sequence technically difficult to study.

Studies of the effects of surgical excision of 75% of the oxyntic mucosa by 75% fundectomy resulted in the lifetime suppression of gastric acid secretion and subsequent hypergastrinaemia in rats without the administration of xenobiotics. Using this procedure, the residual 25% of the oxyntic mucosa was shown to develop ECL cell hyperplasia and neuroendocrine carcinoid tumour formation by two years.

Lifetime exposure of mice to potent long-acting antisecretory agents

A

B

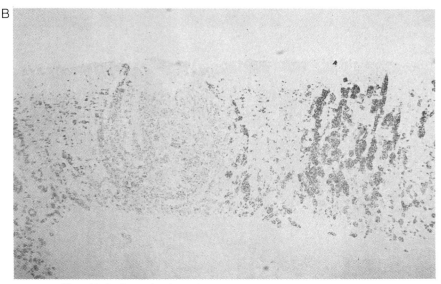

Fig. 12.6. Oxyntic gland histology in rat treated for two years with a potent long-acting histamine H-2 receptor antagonist, SK&F 93479. Diffuse and focal hyperplasia of neuroendocrine ECL cells and an intramucosal carcinoid tumour. (A) H/E ×15.7. (B) Anti-chromogranin A PAP stained section showing positive staining of neuroendocrine cells in hyperplastic regions and partial loss of staining of neuroendocrine tumour cells.

has produced a somewhat different pattern of gastric mucosal pathology from that seen in the rat.

Whereas in the rat the general trophic effect on the mucosa is expressed as an increase in mucosal height with little change in normal architecture, the long-acting $H_2$-receptors loxtidine, ICI 162846, and SK&F 93479 produced a multifocal glandular hyperplasia of the oxyntic glands with associated cyst formation and, in some mice, penetration of the exocrine glandular elements into the submucosa (Streett *et al.*, 1988; Betton *et al*, 1988; Poynter *et al.*, 1986). This pattern of glandular hyperplasia with increased foveolar/parietal-chief cell ratio is also seen as a spontaneous lesion with genetic (Stewart & Andervont, 1938), nutritional (Rehm, Sommer & Deerberg, 1987), environmental (Greaves & Boiziau, 1984) and autoimmune factors (Kishimoti *et al.*, 1984) implicated in its pathogenesis. The role of hypergastrinaemia as mediator of this change remains to be a proven factor. Submucosal penetration and cyst formation seen in treated mice shows some similarities to gastritis cystica pro-

A

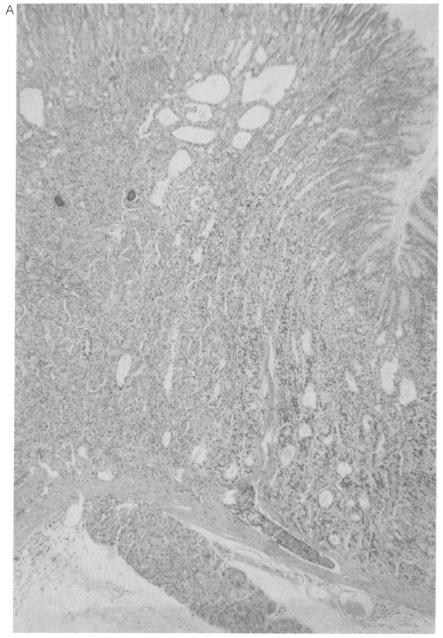

Fig. 12.7. Intramucosal neuroendocrine (carcinoid) tumour in 2-year-old
SK&F 93479 treated rat. Note poorly demarcated form of tumour with

B

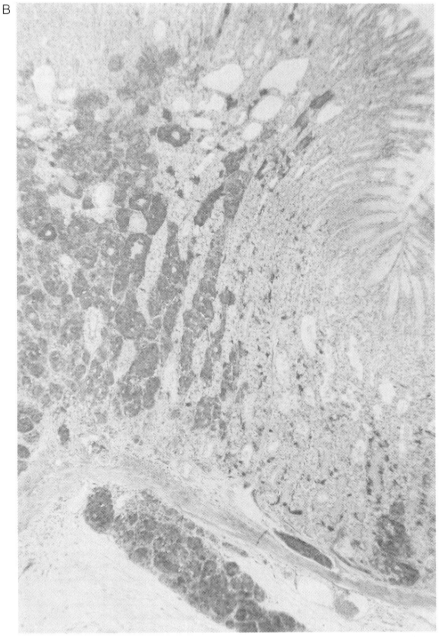

invasion of submucosa. (A) H/E. (B) Anti-neuron-specific enolase PAP stained.

funda of macaques (Scotti, 1973) and of humans (Franzin & Novelli, 1981). Morphologically comparable glandular hypertrophy and hyperplasia have been observed in dogs treated for one year with the PPI omeprazole (Ekman *et al.*, 1985). Simoens, Woudden-Colle & Graef (1989) induced hypergastrinaemia in dogs by omeprazole treatment.

In addition to non-neoplastic effects on the exocrine glandular elements in mice, some potent long-acting antisecretory agents have been reported to induce diffuse neuroendocrine cell hyperplasia alone (Betton *et al.*, 1988) or complete progression to focal hyperplasia and carcinoid tumour formation in mice (Streett *et al.*, 1988; Poynter *et al.*, 1986). It should be noted that all agents causing carcinoids in mice also caused carcinoids in rats but not *vice versa*. It may be that the shorter length (18 months) of the mouse carcinogenicity study for omeprazole contributed to this observation. Because of the known trophic effects of gastrin on the gastric mucosa, the interaction of gastrin on exocrine gastric adenocarcinoma by MNNG and other agents has been studied with rather variable results. Some workers have found exogenously administered gastrin (Yasui & Tahara, 1985) and hypergastrinaemia secondary to autoimmune or chemically induced atrophic gastric (Kishimoto *et al.*, 1984) potentiated MNNG carcinogenesis to produce adenocarcinomas, mainly in the antral mucosa. Other workers (Tatsuta *et al.*, 1980, 1982) however, have shown a reduction in MNNG-induced adenocarcinoma incidence after the administration of exogenous tetragastrin. Until such findings can be reconciled, the ability of gastrin to function as a promoter remains speculative. Interestingly, some MNNG plus gastrin treated groups also showed induction of neuroendocrine tumours but the absence of a gastrin-alone control group precludes a conclusion that these tumours were induced by gastrin *per se*. In clinically normal human subjects, an age related increase in plasma gastrin and fundic ECL-cell counts in females but not males has been reported (Green *et al.*, 1989).

### Comparative pathology of gastric neuroendocrine tumours

The spontaneous occurrence of gastric neuroendocrine tumours in animals is extremely rare. With the exception of one spontaneous gastric carcinoid in a rat (Majke & Sher, 1989), no naturally occurring cases of neuroendocrine tumours of the oxyntic mucosa of rodents (apart from *Mastomys* mouse, *vide infra*) have been reported. Similarly, gastric neuroendocrine tumours of other mammalian species are rare. The unique animal model represented by *Mastomys natalensis*, in which certain strains of this multimammate mouse have a high incidence of gastric ECL-cell carcinoid tumours formation (Soga *et al.*, 1975; Solleveld, 1981) is, however, somewhat atypical in that hypergastrinaemia does not precede ECL-cell hyperplasia and subsequent tumour formation. There is also a range of other neoplasms and auto-immune conditions in this species. The natural history of gastrointestinal neuroendocrine tumour formation in humans is interesting because of the association between gastric carcinoids and Type A chronic atrophic gastritis (CAG). Gastric carcinoids represent only about 2% of all gastrointestinal carcinoid tumours and, being of foregut origin, are rarely associated with a carcinoid syndrome. On this basis, a nomenclature of neuroendocrine tumour is preferable. Gastric neuroendocrine tumours of the oxyntic mucosa (non-antral) have been observed on electron microscopy to have the morphology of ECL cells (Bordi *et al.*, 1978) and were associated with multifocal areas of hyperplastic neuroendocrine cells (Rubin, 1969; Moses *et al.*, 1986). Areas of intestinal metaplasia in CAG patients also showed a variety hyperplastic neuroendocrine cell types (Rode *et al.*, 1986), but include typical ECL-cell carcinoid tumours (Hodges *et al.*, 1981). The key association between CAG and the risk of carcinoid tumour development would appear to be the presence of hypergastrinaemia. The association of type A (fundic or oxyntic) but not type B (antral) CAG with carcinoid tumours would add further support for this hypothesis. Indeed, stratification of patients with fundic CAG according to degree of hypergastrinaemia shows a strong correlation between gastrin and degree of oxyntic neuroendocrine cell hyperplasia and presence of carcinoid tumour (Borch *et al.*, 1986). The latter patient population had mean plasma gastrin of 1659 pmol/L compared to 304 pmol/L in patients having only diffuse hyperplasia.

The association of gastric endocrine cell hyperplasia with Zollinger–Ellison syndrome (Z–E) patients (Bordi *et al.*, 1974, 1978; Mignon *et al.*, 1987) is more tenuous but would again point to the role of gastrin as a trophic tumourigenic factor. No further increase in fundic carcinoids occurred in Z–E patients on omeprazole therapy for up to 51 months (Maton *et al.*, 1989). Since Z–E patients typically have functional gastrinomas of the pancreas and are hypersecretors (as opposed to type A CAG patients who are achlorhydric), this also points to achlorhydria *not* being the primary aetiological factor in CAG patients since only hypergastrinaemia is a common factor in these two conditions.

## Conclusions and future directions

Laboratory animal models of pancreatic exocrine neoplasia show important differences in their histogenetic origin, that is, acinar cell types in the rat versus ductal cell origin in the hamster. Nevertheless, in both species, the role of cholecystokinin in enhancing or promoting the action of genotoxic carcinogens or the spontaneous background incidence, either directly or subsequent to dietary factors, is relevant to humans where dietary fat intake is one risk factor for pancreatic exocrine adenocarcinoma.

Laboratory rodents, that is the rat, and to a lesser degree, the mouse, are uniquely susceptible to ECL-cell carcinoid tumour induction following lifespan administration of high doses of potent long-acting antisecretory agents. Although carcinoid tumour induction has a latent period of >80 weeks, early changes of sustained hypergastrinaemia and ECL-cell hyperplasia in the oxyntic mucosa can be observed within weeks of treatment. Short-acting or less potent antisecretory H$_2$RAs cause only low grade hypergastrinaemia of short duration and lesser degrees of ECL-cell hyperplasia which does not progress to carcinoid tumour formation.

Although hypergastrinaemia in humans is considered to be a factor in the induction of gastric carcinoids of CAG patients (Bordi et al., 1974; Moses et al., 1986; Rode et al., 1986; Hodges et al., 1981; Borch et al., 1986; Capella et al., 1980), the degree of hypergastrinaemia present over the long history of CAG far exceeds the degree of hypergastrinaemia produced by therapy of duodenal ulcer patients with either the short acting H$_2$RA ranitidine or the potent long acting PPI omeprazole (Lanzon Miller et al., 1987). On this basis, it is considered that the clinical use of H$_2$RAs or PPIs in the therapy of peptic ulcer disease in humans will not result in a degree and duration of hypergastrinaemia to place patients at risk of developing gastric carcinoid tumours. To date, the clinical use of such agents in long-term maintenance therapy has also failed to produce focal hyperplasia or neuroendocrine tumours. The induction of carcinoid tumours in rodent oncogenicity studies is, therefore, considered to be a pharmacology-related non-genotoxic gastrin-mediated process resulting from a degree of hypergastrinaemia far in excess of that induced by peptic ulcer therapy. Although some authors (Elder, 1985; Penston & Wormsley, 1987) have claimed that any degree of hypergastrinaemia or even achlorhydria represents a risk factor for gastric carcinogenesis, there is no evidence that therapy with antisecretory agents leads even to a diffuse ECL cell hyperplasia (Bordi et al., 1987). The comparative pathology of the rare event of carcinoid tumour induction in CAG patients indicated that therapeutic doses of even potent long-acting antisecretory agents produce insufficient hypergastrinaemia to result in ECL hyperplasia or neoplasia.

## Acknowledgements

The author wishes to thank Dr Carolyn Price, Charles Dormer, Pauline Pert, and Terry Wells formerly of Smith Kline and French Ltd for their scientific collaboration and Professor Julia Polak for inspiration. Thanks are also due to Ann Powell for typing the manuscript and Andrew Shaw for the photography.

## References

Angeletti, R.H. (1986). Chromatogranins and neuroendocrine secretion. *Laboratory Investigation*, **55**, 387–90.

Baldwin, G.S. (1982). Gastrin and the transforming protein of polyoma virus have evolved from a common ancestor. *FEBS Letters*, **137**, 1–5.

Betton, G.R., Dormer, C.S., Wells, T., Pert, P., Price, C.A. & Buckley, P. (1988). Gastric ECL-cell hyperplasia and carcinoids in rodents following chronic administration of H$_2$-antagonists SK&F 93479 and oxmetidine and omeprazole. *Toxicologic Pathology*, **16**, 288–98.

Birt, D.F., Julius, A.D., White, L.T. & Pour, P.M. (1989). Enhancement of pancreatic carcinogenesis in hamsters fed a high-fat diet ad libitum and at a controlled caloric intake. *Cancer Res.*, **49**, 5848–51.

Bishop, A.E., Polak, J.M., Facer, P., Ferri, G.L., Marangos, P.J. & Pearse, A.G.E. (1982). Neuron specific enolase: a common marker for the endocrine cells and innervation of the gut and pancrease. *Gastroenterology*, **83**, 902–15.

Blobel, G.A., Gould, V.E., Moll, R., Lee, I., Huszar, M., Geiger, B. & Franke, W.W. (1985). Coexpression of neuroendocrine markers and epithelial cytoskeletal proteins in bronchopulmonary neuroendocrine neoplasms. *Laboratory Investigation*, **52**, 39–51.

Borch, K., Renvall, H., Liedberg, G. & Andersen, B.N. (1986). Relations between circulating gastrin and endocrine cell proliferation in the atrophic gastric fundic mucosa. *Scandinavian Journal Gastroenterology*, **21**, 357–63.

Bordi, C., Cocconi, G., Togni, R., Vezzadini, P. & Missale, G. (1974). Gastric endocrine cell proliferation. *Archives Pathology*, **98**, 274–8.

Bordi, C., Gabrielli, M. & Missale, G. (1978). Pathological changes of endocrine cells in chronic atrophic gastritis. *Archives of Pathology and Laboratory Medicine*, **102**, 129–35.

Bordi, C., Creutzfeldt, W., Hakanson, R., Solcia, E. & Sundler, F. (1987). Achlorhydria:hypergastrinaemia:carcinoids – a flawed hypothesis. *Gut*, **28**, 1189–91.

Bottcher, C., Hakanson, R., Nilsson, G., Seensalu, R. & Sundler, F. (1989). Effects of long-term hypergastrinaemia on the ultrastructure of enterochromaffin-like cells in the stomach of the rat, hamster and guinea pig. *Cell Tissue Research*, **256**, 247–57.

Buchan, A.M.J. & Polak, J.M. (1980). The classification of the human gastroenteropancreatic endocrine cells. *Investigative Cellular Pathology*, **3**, 51–71.

Burek, J.D., Majka, J.A. & Bokelman, D.L. (1985). Famotidine: summary of preclinical safety assessment. *Digestion*, **32** (Suppl 1), 7–14.

Capella, C., Polak, J.M., Timson, C.M., Frigerio, B. & Solcia, E. (1980). Gastric carcinoids of argyrophil ECL cells. *Ultrastructural Pathology*, **1**, 411–18.

Carlsson, E., Larsson, H., Mattsson, H., Ryberg, B. & Sundell, G. (1986). Pharmacology and toxicology of omeprazole – with special reference to the effects on the gastric mucosa. *Scandinavian Journal of Gastroenterology*, **118** (Suppl.), 31–8.

Cohn, D.V., Elting, J.J., Frick, M. & Elde, R. (1963). Selective localizaton of the parathyroid secretory protein-I adrenal medulla chromatogranin A protein family in a wide variety of endocrine cells of the rat. *Endocrinology*, **114**, 1963–74.

Damge, C., Hajri, A., Lhoste, E. & Aprahamian, M. (1988). Comparative effect of chronic bombesin, gastrin-releasing peptide and caerulein on the rat pancreas. *Regulatory Peptides*, **20**, 141–50.

Decktor, D.L., Pendleton, R.G., Kellner, A.T. & Davis, M.A. (1988). Acute effects of ranitidine, famotidine and omeprazole on plasma gastrin in the rat. *Journal of Pharmacology and Experimental Therapeutics*, **249**, 1–5.

Ekman, L., Hansson, E., Havu, N., Carlsson, E. & Lundberg, C. (1985). Toxicological studies on omeprazole. *Scandinavian Journal of Gastroenterology*, **20** (Suppl 108), 53–69.

Elder, J.B. (1985). Inhibition of acid and gastric carcinoids. *Gut*, **26**, 1279–83.

Eustis, S.L. & Boorman, G.A. (1985). Proliferative lesions of the exocrine pancreas relationship to corn oil gavage in the National Toxicology Program. *Journal of the National Cancer Institute*, **75**, 1067–73.

Franzin, G. & Novelli, P. (1981). Gastritis cystica profunda. *Histopathology*, **5**, 535–47.

Fujita, S. & Hattori, T. (1977). Cell proliferation, differentiation, and migration in the gastric mucosa: a study on the background of carcinogenesis. In *Pathophysiology of Carcinogenesis in Digestive Organs*, ed. E. Farber et al., pp. 21–36. Baltimore: University Park Press.

Gould, V.E., Linnoila, R.I., Memoli, V.A. & Warren, W.H. (1983). Biology of disease. Neuroendocrine components of the bronchopulmonary bract: hyperplasias, dysplasias, and neoplasms. *Laboratory Investigation*, **49**, 519–37.

Gould, V.E., Wiedenmann, B., Lee, I., Schwechheimer, K., Dockhorn-Dworniczak, B., Radosevich, J.A., Moll, R. & Franke, W.W. (1987). Synaptophysin expression in neuroendocrine neoplasms as determined by immunocytochemistry. *American Journal of Pathology*, **126**, 243–57.

Greaves, P. & Boiziau, J.-L. (1984). Altered patterns of mucin secretion in gastric hyperplasia in mice. *Veterinary Pathology*, **21**, 224–8.

Green, D.M., Bishop, A.E., Rindi, G., Lee, F.I., Daly, M.J., Domin, J., Bloom, S.R. & Polak, J.M. (1989). Enterochromaffin-like cell populations in human fundic mucosa: quantitative studies of their variants with age, sex, and plasma gastrin levels. *Journal of Pathology*, **157**, 235–41.

Grimelius, L. & Wilander, E. (1980). Silver stains in the study of endocrine cells of the gut and pancreas. *Investigative Cellular Pathology*, **3**, 3–12.

Hagn, C., Schmid, K.W., Fischer-Colbrie, R. & Winkler, H. (1986). Chromogranin A, B, and C in human adrenal medulla and endocrine tissues. *Laboratory Investigation*, **55**, 405–11.

Hakanson, R., Larsson, L.-I., Leidberg, G. & Sundler, F. (1976). The histamine-storing enterochromaffin-like cells of the rat stomach. In *Chromaffin, Enterochromaffin and Related Cells*, ed. R.E. Coupland & T. Fujita, pp. 243–63. Amsterdam: Elsevier.

Hakanson, R., Axelson, J., Ekman, R. & Sundler, F. (1988). Hypergastrinaemia evoked by omeprazole stimulates growth of gastric mucosa but not of pancreas or intestines in hamster, guinea pig and chicken. *Regulatory Peptides*, **23**, 105–15.

Heath, D., Smith, P. & Jago, R. (1984). Dark cell proliferation in carotid body hyperplasia. *Journal of Pathology*, **142**, 39–49.

Helander, H.F. (1981). The cells of the gastric mucosa. *International Review of Cytology*, **70**, 217–89.

Herbst, W.M., Kummer, W., Hofman, W., Otto, H. & Heym, C. (1987). Carcinoid tumours of the thymus. An immunohistochemical study. *Cancer*, **60**, 2465–70.

Hirth, R.S., Evans, L.D., Buroker, R.A. & Oleson, F. (1988). Gastric enterochromaffin-like cell hyperplasia and neoplasia in the rat: an indirect effect of the histamine $H_2$-receptor antagonist, BL-6341. *Toxicologic Pathology*, **16**, 273–87.

Hodges, J.R., Isaacson, P. & Wright, R. (1981). Diffuse enterochromaffin-like (ECL) cell hyperplasia and multiple gastric carcinoids: a complication of pernicious anaemia. *Gut*, **22**, 237–41.

Holst, J.J. (1983). Gut glucagon, enteroglucagon, gut glucagonlike immunoreactivity, glicentin – current status. *Gastroenterology*, **84**, 1602–13.

Howatson, A.G. & Carter, D.C. (1985). Pancreatic carcinogenesis-enhancement by cholecystokinin in the hamster-nitrosamine model. *British Journal of Cancer*, **51**, 107–14.

Ito, T., Kitamura, H., Inayama, Y. & Kanisawa, M. (1988). Pulmonary adenoma and endocrine cell hyperplasia in Syrian golden hamster treated with 4-nitroquinoline 1-oxide. *Acta Pathologia Japonica*, **38**, 1097–104.

Ito, S. (1981). Functional gastric morphology. In *Physiology of the*

*Gastrointestinal Tract*, ed. L.R. Johnson, pp. 517–50. New York: Raven Press.

Jensen, R.T., Lemp, G.F. & Gardner, J.D. (1982). Interactions of COOH-terminal fragments of cholecystokinin with receptors on dispersed acini from guinea pig pancreas. *The Journal of Biological Chemistry*, **257**, 5554–9.

Johnson, N.F., Wagner, J.C. & Wills, H.A. (1980). Endocrine cell proliferation in the rat lung following asbestos inhalation. *Lung*, **158**, 221–8.

Johnson, L.R. (1988). Regulation of gastrointestinal mucosal growth. *Physiological Reviews*, **68**, 456–502.

Kishimoto, S., Konemori, R., Mukai, T., Kambara, A., Okamoto, K., Shimizu, S., Iwasaki, Y., Daitoku, K., Kajiyama, G. & Miyoski, A. (1984). Distribution of GEP endocrine cells in the gastric mucosa of mice with experimental gastritis. *Hiroshima Journal of Medical Sciences*, **33**, 469–657.

Kleinerman, J., Marchevsky, A.M. & Thornton, J. (1981). Quantitative Studies of APUD Cells in Airways of Rats. The effects of diethylnitrosamine and $NO_2$ *American Review of Respiratory Disease*, **124**, 458–62.

Lacy, E.R. & Ito, S. (1984). Rapid epithelial restitution of the rat gastric mucosa after ethanol injury. *Laboratory Investigation*, **51**, 573–83.

Lanzon-Miller, S., Pounder, R.E., Hamilton, M.R., Ball, S., Chronos, N.A.F., Raymond, F., Olausson, M. & Cederberg, C. (1987). Twenty-four-hour intragastric acidity and plasma gastrin concentration before and during treatment with either ranitidine or omeprazole. *Alimentary Pharmacology and Therapeutics*, **1**, 239–51.

Lauweryns, J.M., Cokelaere, M. & Theunynck, P. (1972). Neuro-epithelial bodies in the respiratory mucosa of various mammals. A light optical, histochemical and ultrastructural investigation. *Zeitschrift für Zellforschung*, **135**, 569–92.

Leslie, G.B., Noakes, D.N., Pollitt, F.D., Roe, F.J.C. & Walker, T.F. (1981). A two-year study with cimetidine in the rat: assessment for chronic toxicity and carcinogenicity. *Toxicology Applied Pharmacology*, **61**, 119–37.

Linnoila, R.I. (1982). Effects of diethylnitrosamine on lung neuroendocrine cells. *Experimental Lung Research*, **3**, 225–36.

Loser, C., Folsch, U.R., Mustroph, D., Cantor, P., Wunderlich, U. & Creutzfeldt, W. (1988). Pancreatic polyamine concentrations and cholecystokinin plasma levels in rats after feeding raw or heat-inactivated soyabean flour. *Pancreas*, **3**, 285–91.

Majke, J.A. & Sher, S. (1989). Spontaneous gastric carcinoid tumour in an aged Sprague-Dawley rat. *Veterinary Pathology*, **26**, 88–90.

Maton, P.N., Vinayek, R., Frucht, H., McArthur, K.A., Miller, L.S., Saeed, Z.A., Gardener, J.D. & Jensen, R.T. (1989). Long-term efficacy and safety of omeprazole in patients with Zollinger–Ellison syndrome: a prospective study. *Gastroenterology*, **97**, 827–36.

Mazzacca, G., Cascione, F., Budillon, G., D'Agostino, L., Cimino, L. & Femiano, C. (1978). Parietal cell hyperplasia induced by long-term administration of antacids to rats. *Gut*, **19**, 798–801.

McGuiness, E.E., Morgan, R.G.H. & Wormsley, K.G. (1984). Effects of soya bean flour on the pancreas of rats. *Environmental Health Perspectives*, **56**, 205–12.

Mignon, M., Lehy, T., Bonnefond, A., Ruszniewski, P., Labielle, D. & Bonfils, S. (1987). Development of gastric argyrophil carcinoid tumours in a case of Zollinger–Ellison syndrome with primary hyperparathyroidism during long-term antisecretory treatment. *Cancer*, **59**, 1959–62.

Moosavi, H., Smith, P. & Heath, D. (1973). The Feyrter cell in hypoxia. *Thorax*, **28**, 728–41.

Mori, T., Nagasawa, H., Namiki, H. & Niki, K. (1986). Development of pancreatic hyperplasia in female SHN mice receiving ectopic pituitary isografts. *Journal of the National Cancer Institute*, **76**, 1193–8.

Morton, D.M. (1987). Pharmacology and toxicology of nizatidine. *Scandinavian Journal Gastroenterology*, **22** (Suppl. 136), 1–8.

Moses, R.E., Frank, B.B., Leavitt, M. & Miller, R. (1986). The syndrome of type A chronic atrophic gastritis, pernicious anaemia, and multiple gastric carcinoids. *Journal Clinical Gastroenterology*, **8**, 61–5.

Naylor, D.C., Krinke, G.J. & Ruefenacht, H.J. (1988). Primary tumours of the thymus in the rat. *Journal of Comparative Pathology*, **99**, 187–203.

Pearse, A.G.E. (1968). Common cytochemical and ultrastructural characteristics of cells producing polypeptide hormones (the APUD series) and their relevance to thyroid and ultimobranchial C cells and calcitonin. *Proceedings of Royal Society B*, **170**, 71–80.

Penston, J. & Wormsley, K.G. (1987). Achlorhydria: hypergastrinaemia: carcinoids – a flawed hypothesis? *Gut*, **28**, 488–505.

Pour, P. M., Lawson, T., Helgeson, S., Donnelly, T. & Stepan, K. (1988). Effect of cholecystokinin on pancreatic carcinogenesis in the hamster model. *Carcinogenesis*, **9**, 597–601.

Poynter, D., Pick, C.R., Harcourt, R.A., Sutherland, M.F., Spurling, N. W., Alinge, G., Cook, J. & Gatehouse, D. (1982). Evaluation of ranitidine safety. In *Clinical use of Ranitidine: Proceedings of a Glaxo International Conference, London, 1981*, ed. J.J. Misiewicz, pp. 49–57. Oxford: Medical Educational Services.

Poynter, D., Pick, C.R., Harcourt, R.A., Selway, S.A.M., Ainge, G., Harman, I.W., Spurling, N.W., Fluck, P.A. & Cook, J.L. (1985). Association of long lasting unsurmountable histamine $H_2$-blockade and gastric carcinoid tumours in the rat. *Gut*, **26**, 1284–95.

Poynter, D., Selway, S.A.M., Papworth, S.A. & Riches, S.R. (1986).

Changes in the gastric mucosa of the mouse associated with long lasting unsurmountable histamine $H_2$ blockade. *Gut*, **27**, 1338–46.

Reeve, J.R., Dimaline, R., Shively, J.E., Hawke, D., Chew, P. & Walsh, J.H. (1981). Unique amino terminal structure of rat little gastrin. *Peptides*, **2**, 453–8.

Rehm, S., Sommer, R. & Deerberg, F. (1987). Spontaneous non-neoplastic gastric lesions in female Han: NMRI mice, and influence of food restriction throughout life. *Veterinary Pathology*, **24**, 216–25.

Roebuck, B.D., Longnecker, D.S., Baumgartner, K.J. & Thron, C.D. (1985). Carcinogen-induced lesions in the rat pancreas: effects of varying levels of essential fatty acid. *Cancer Research*, **45**, 5252–6.

Rode, J., Dhillon, A.P., Papadaki, L., Stockbrigger, R., Thompson, R.J., Moss, E. & Cotton, P.B. (1986). Pernicious anaemia and mucosal endocrine cell proliferation of the non-antral stomach. *Gut*, **27**, 789–98.

Rubin, W. (1969). Proliferation of endocrine-like (enterochromaffin) cells in atrophic gastric mucosa. *Gastroenterology*, **57**, 641–8.

Salyer, W.R., Salyer, D.C. & Eggleston, J.C. (1976). Carcinoid tumours of the thymus. *Cancer*, **37**, 958–73.

Seglen, P.O., Skomedal, H., Saeter, G., Schwarze, P.E. & Nesland, J.M. (1989). Neuroendocrine dysdifferentiation and bombesin production in carcinogen-induced hepatocellular rat tumours. *Carcinogenesis*, **10**, 21–5.

Scotti, T. (1973). Simian gastropathy with submucosal glands and cysts. *Archives of Pathology*, **96**, 403–8.

Simoens, C., Woudden-Colle, M.C. & Graef, . (1989). Effect of acute auppression of acid secretion by omeprazole on postprandial gastrin release in conscious dogs. *Gastroenterology*, **97**, 837–45.

Soga, J., Kohro, T., Tazawa, K., Kanahara, H., Sano, M., Sakashita, T., Tajima, K., Morooka, H. & Karaki, Y. (1975). Argyrophil cell microneoplasia in the Mastomys stomach – an observation on early carcinoid formation. *Journal of the National Cancer Institute*, **55**, 1001–6.

Solcia, E., Capella, C., Buffa, R., Fiocca, R., Frigerio, B. & Usellini, L. (1980). Identification, ultrastructure and classification of gut endocrine cells and related growths. *Investigative Cellular Pathology*, **3**, 37–49.

Solleveld, H.A. (1981). Praomys (Mastomys) natalensis *in aging research*. The Netherlands: Institute of Experimental Gerontology TNO.

Sorokin, S.P., Hoyt, R.F. & Pearsall, A.D. (1983). Comparative biology of small granule cells and neuroepithelial bodies in the respiratory system. *American Review of Respiratory Disease*, **128**, S26–S31.

Stewart, H.L. & Andervont, H.B. (1938). Pathologic observations on the adenomatous lesion of the stomach in mice of strain I. *Archives of Pathology*, **26**, 1009–22.

Sundaram, S. & Dayan, D. (1989). Inhibition of raw soya flour-induced pancreatic hyperplasia by a CCK Antagonist (L-364,718). *Proceedings of BTS/SDR Meeting 12–14/4/89.* Cambridge UK.

Streett, C.S., Robertson, J.L. & Crissman, J.W. (1988). Morphologic stomach findings in rats and mice treated with the $H_2$ receptor antagonists, ICI 125,211 and ICI 162,846. *Toxicologic Pathology,* **16,** 299–304.

Svendsen, L.B., Hansen, O.H., Larsen, J.K., Pedersen, T. & Johansen, A. (1986). Effect of cimetidine on gastric mucosal cell proliferation in man. *Scandinavian Journal of Gastroenterology,* **21,** 1271–4.

Tabassian, A.R., Nylen, E.S., Linnoila, R.I., Snider, R.H., Cassidy, M.M. & Becker, K.L. (1989). Stimulation of hamster pulmonary neuroendocrine cells and associated peptides by repeated exposure to cigarette smoke. *American Review of Respiratory Disease,* **140,** 436–40.

Tahara, E., Ito, H., Nakagami, K. & Shimamoto, F. (1981). Induction of carcinoids in the glandular stomach of rats by N-methyl-N'-nitro-N-nitrosoguanidine. *Journal of Cancer Research Clinical Oncology,* **100,** 1–12.

Tatsuta, M., Itoh, T., Okuda, S., Wada, A., Taniguchi, H., Tamura, H. & Yamamura, H. (1980). Effects gastrin and histamine on gastric carcinogenesis induced in rats by N-methyl-N'-nitro-N-nitrosoguanidine. *European Journal of Cancer,* **16,** 631–8.

Tatsuta, M., Yamamura, H., Taniguchi, H. & Tamura, H. (1982). Gastrin protection against chemically induced gastric adenocarcinomas in Wistar rats: histopathology of the glandular stomach and incidence of gastric adenocarcinoma. *Journal of the National Cancer Institute,* **69,** 59–66.

Van Zwieten, M.J., Burek, J.D., Zurcher, C. & Hollander, C.F. (1979). Aortic body tumours and hyperplasia in the rat. *Journal of Pathology,* **128,** 99–112.

Wick, M.R. & Scheithauer, B.W. (1984). Thymic carcinoid. A histological immunochemical, and ultrastructural Study of 12 Cases. *Cancer,* **53,** 475–84.

Willems, G., Galand, P., VanSteenkiste, Y. & Zeitoun, P. (1972). Cell population kinetics of zymogen and parietal cells in the stomach of mice. *Zeitschrift für Zellforschung,* **134,** 505–18.

Wisner, J.R., McLaughlin, R.E., Rich, K.A., Ozawa, S. & Renner, I.G. (1988). Effects of L-364,718, a new cholecystokinin receptor antagonist, on camostate-induced growth of the rat pancreas. *Gastroenterology,* **94,** 109–13.

Yasui, W. & Tahara, E. (1985). Effect of gastrin on gastric mucosal cyclic adenosine 3'5' monophosphate-dependent protein kinase activity in rat stomach carcinogenesis induced by N-methyl-N-nitro-N-nitrosoguanidine. *Cancer Research,* **45,** 4763–7.

# VII  Conclusion

# 13    The future: needs and opportunities

## Introduction

Two inter-related questions arise from the contents of the various chapters in this book. First, what place does endocrinology have in toxicology, and how can endocrinological effects be characterized and their importance assessed during the course of toxicological studies? Secondly, what is the importance of toxicology in endocrinology and what can toxic effects tell us about the control and responses of endocrine tissues and their targets under both normal and abnormal circumstances? The answer to these questions, which have importance not only for clinicians and toxicologists but also for basic researchers in the field of physiology, will eventually need to be expressed in terms of receptocytes, receptoactivation, signal transduction, mechanisms of hormone secretion, molecular biology, etc.

The endocrine system is heavily involved in homeostasis. In this context the distinction between endocrinology and the rapidly expanding knowledge of regulatory peptides is quite unclear. The term 'endocrine pathology' is seemingly limited to changes in the function and structure of classical endocrine glands and their more obvious targets. However, if its meaning were extended to embrace the effects of disturbance of regulatory peptide function, then it is likely to transpire that endocrine disturbance in this broader sense would be seen as being very widely implicated in toxicology.

There are four steps in the investigation of potential endocrine toxicity. First, appropriately sensitive clinical and pathological techniques for the detection of such toxicity need to be available and applied. Secondly, the evaluation, nature and magnitude of effects need to be measured. Thirdly, mechanisms need to be understood. And finally, the likely significance of an effect in terms of general health and wellbeing and of possible late effects on target organs needs to be assessed.

## Detection of endocrinological toxicity

As exemplified in almost every chapter in this book, effects of exposure to drugs, toxins, or other agents may be functional and/or structural in nature. Both functional and structural changes may lie within the range of normal physiological action and reaction (e.g. effects on oestrous cycling or a change in the circulating level of $T_4$ due to a rise in thyroxin binding globulin following exposure to an oestrogen). Alternatively, effects may be frankly abnormal (e.g. the sharp rise in circulating prolactin produced by a dopamine antagonist, or the reduction in circulating cortisol [or cortisone, depending on the species] caused by a dehydrogenase inhibitor). If the action of the toxicant is sufficiently prolonged and/or severe, then persistent morphological abnormalities are likely to develop in one or more organs of the endocrine orchestra or their target tissues. In these circumstances the histopathologist will report pathological change.

Effects on the endocrine system may be direct (e.g. the agent may have oestrogenic activity) or secondary to an effect on a target tissue for a hormone (e.g. destruction of the seminiferous tubules in the rat testis leads to the appearance of castration cells in the pituitary gland).

## The inadequacy of routine toxicological procedures with regard to the evaluation of effects on endocrine status

The usual first main purpose of toxicity tests is to detect and quantify adverse effects on behaviour, clinical appearances, bodily functions and the macroscopic and microscopic appearance of tissues. In many cases there is no *a priori* reason to expect any particular adverse effect, so that when an adverse effect is found at necropsy it may come as a surprise or, should we say, shock. Observations made during the in-life phase of studies may alert one to the probability of finding pathological changes in particular tissues. However, it is not at present usual practice routinely to measure the levels of circulating hormones. Consequently most toxicological effects on endocrine function and status are discovered for the first time at necropsy. There are, of course, notable exceptions to this. For instance, a high incidence of mammary tumours in female rats will lead one to expect to find a high incidence of prolactinomas of the pituitary gland at necropsy. Similarly, careful palpation of the testes of male rats may lead one to expect to find an increased incidence of interstitial (Leydig) cell tumours of that organ. Notwithstanding these exceptions, the majority of neoplasms and other lesions of the pituitary, thyroid follicular cells, thyroid C-cells, parathyroid gland, adrenal cortex, adrenal medulla, pancreatic islets, ovary and testis remain unsuspected until they are discovered at necropsy. Perhaps we should be asking ourselves, is this situation as it should be? Why have we not found fit to develop sensitive assay methods whereby we can detect in individual animals, lesions of endocrine glands as they develop? If we had such methods might we not have new and more sensitive tools for investigating the mechanisms of action of pharmaceutical agents, and the mechanisms responsible for the toxicity of environmental agents?

In reality, however, the situation is much worse than has been painted above. When rats and mice, and animals of other species, are killed at the termination of studies, they are subjected to a careful dissection and recording of macroscopic changes. However, whether abnormalities are seen or not, usual practice is simply to submit endocrine tissues like all other tissues to no other than routine fixation, embedding in paraffin wax, and preparation of sections stained only with haematoxylin and eosin. While this sequence of simple procedures will enable one to detect relatively major changes such as focal or generalized hyperplasia or the presence of neoplasms in endocrine tissues, it may be quite inadequate for the purposes of distinguishing between the different cell types that may be involved in these proliferative lesions. For this latter purpose it is sometimes possible by cutting further sections from formalin-fixed, paraffin wax embedded tissues, and applying special stains or immunochemical techniques to them to obtain the additional information one needs. However, in other cases the option to use optimal techniques may have been for ever forfeited by the routine approach to tissue processing.

Irrespective of what it is theoretically possible to do, the fact is that in most studies little or no attempt is made to distinguish the cell of origin of, for instance, pituitary or pancreatic islet cell tumours. In the case of rats it may well be that most tumours of the anterior pituitary consist mainly of prolactin-producing cells. However, eight other kinds of hormone are produced in the gland and it is clear from studies where special techniques have been used that areas of hyperplasia and neoplasia may consist of cells producing hormones other than prolactin or, not infrequently, of mixtures of cells. The question arises, therefore, should we not develop better and more precise techniques for processing and staining endocrine tissues, particularly in the case of the pituitary and pancreatic islets?

All these questions take on a special poignancy when we compare the kind of information about endocrinological disturbances we have for humans with the kind of information about such disturbances we have for animals in long-term toxicity tests. In the case of an individual human we may have, if we think we need it, detailed information on the level of virtually any circulating hormone, and may follow levels of each hormone of interest sequentially through hours, days, months or years. On the other hand, because necropsy rates are so low, we have very inadequate and inaccurate information about the incidences of neoplasms and foci of hyperplasia of endocrine tissues in humans.

By contrast in experimental animals – more often than not we have little or no information about circulating hormones during the in-life phase of tests and a super-abundance of necropsy data. If the object of toxicological tests is to determine toxicity for safety of test agents for man and to throw light on mechanisms of toxicity, and to alert physicians to potential toxicological – including endocrinological – problems, it really is difficult to imagine that the picture described above is optimal.

## Points to be borne in mind by the diagnostician in relation to endocrine toxicology

Many aspects of endocrine toxicology need to be borne in mind by the diagnostician. First, toxic effects on the endocrine system may involve more than one of the many endocrine organs or their target tissues. Secondly, the effects may be manifested as functional and/or structural (pathological) changes and both these kinds of effect may evolve with time. Obviously the diagnostician needs to take both sex and age into account since the sensitivity to toxicants and the manifestations of toxicity are likely to differ with age, and to be different between the sexes. Also, it should never be forgotten that response to endocrine toxicants can be crucially influenced by dietary ingredients (e.g. the iodine content of foodstuffs may modify response to otherwise marginal goitrogens).

In a conventional type of toxicity test, with its structured and relatively standardized set of observations, although the first hints of an effect on the endocrine system often come from treatment-related effects on organ size and weight or from differences in histological appearances of endocrine tissues or their targets, signals from general metabolic tests (e.g. changes in plasma electrolytes, lipid and triglyceride levels, metastatic calcification and cardiac function) should always be carefully considered since they can be indicative of, or associated with, endocrine dysfunction. Also, simple observations of behaviour, reflex responses, and especially of oestrous cycling and mating activity, can be powerful guides to endocrine effects, especially when viewed as part of a pattern.

Complex integrative processes are involved in maintaining homeostasis. When these become disordered as a result of toxicity a wide variety of patterns of disease and pathology may arise. Some signs of disturbed homeostasis are easier to detect than others and presenting signs in humans, who can describe their symptoms, may be different from those in animals who cannot do so. It is particularly important, therefore, in the evaluation of toxic responses to look for patterns rather than isolated effects, and also to take into account sequences of normal physiological responses. The value of this holistic approach is well illustrated by the consequences and causes of multi-site neoplasia in overfed rodents (e.g. overfeeding predisposes to ageing-related nephropathy which compromises calcium homeostasis and leads to parathyroid hyperplasia, and neoplasia and metastatic calcification).

In our view the most serious problem facing the investigator attempting to interpret observations in long-term toxicity studies in rodents is the need to consider whether an apparent toxic effect should be attributed to the substance being investigated, or whether it is or might be a non-specific consequence of ageing or of disturbance of physiological status. The next section discusses the need for such consideration with particular reference to the effects of overnutrition.

## Influence of ageing – particularly ageing secondary to overfeeding – on endocrine status

Before specified pathogen free (SPF) conditions became generally available for toxicological testing the duration of tests was curtailed by morbidity and mortality due to infectious diseases, and infestations by parasites. After the introduction of SPF conditions animals lived longer and the predominant pathology became one of age-related diseases, including, in the case of rats, a wide variety of endocrine disturbances. The spectrum of endocrine disturbances embraced high incidences of neoplasms of endocrine glands, and of hormone-responsive tissues, such as the mammary gland and uterus.

The incidences of endocrine tumours and of other endocrine changes among untreated control rats in carcinogenicity studies in SPF rats are now not frequently such that close to 100% of animals have one or more histologically-evident endocrine neoplasms. Control data reported by Kociba *et al*, (1979) from a two-year study illustrate the point in the case of *ad libitum*-fed Sprague-Dawley rats (see Table 13.1) and our own more recent data do so for *ad libitum*-fed Wistar rats (see Table 13.2).

Such data pose three series of questions. Firstly, does it make any sense to conduct general toxicological tests in animals which towards the end of studies are in such endocrinological disarray as the animals depicted in Tables 13.1 and 13.2? What does it mean if exposure to a test agent is associated with a significant increase or decrease in the incidence of a kind of endocrine tumour which is occurring in high incidence in the untreated control group? Would evidence of a treatment-related change

Table 13.1. *Endocrine tumour incidences in untreated Sprague-Dawley rats (Data from Kociba* et al., *1979)*

|  |  | Males | Females |
|---|---|---|---|
| Number of rats observed (%) |  | 86(100) | 86(100) |
| Number of rats with tumours of: |  |  |  |
| Adrenal | – cortex | 2 (2.3) | 6 (7.0) |
|  | – medulla | 44(51.2) | 7 (8.1) |
| Ovary | – granulosa cell | – | 4 (4.7) |
| Mammary | – fibroadenoma | 1 (1.2) | 65(75.6) |
|  | – cystfibroadenoma | – | 11(12.8) |
|  | – adenoma | – | 10(11.6) |
|  | – fibroma | – | 4 (4.7) |
|  | – adenocarcinoma | 2 (2.3) | 7 (8.1) |
| Pancreas | – islet cell | 14(16.3) | 8 (9.3) |
| Parathyroid |  | – | 1 (1.2) |
| Pituitary | – anterior lobe | 29(33.7) | 54(62.8) |
| Testis | – Leydig cell | 4 (4.7) | – |
| Thyroid | – C-cell | 7 (8.1) | 7 (8.1) |

in the incidence of a kind of endocrine tumour which is found in between 10 and 60% of untreated control animals have any toxicological significance for man? In circumstances where an endocrine tumour is occurring in high incidence in untreated control animals, should treatment-related changes in the incidence of tumours that fall into this category be used in the assessment of the test compound for carcinogenicity?

Secondly, can one assume that abnormality in endocrine status has no effect on the manifestation of other forms of toxicity? Many manifestations of toxicity in organs such as the liver and kidney differ in incidence and severity between males and females and are known to be influenced by castration and/or the administration of sex hormones.

Thirdly, although the more obvious disturbances of endocrine status in *ad libitum*-fed rats are most clearly seen at the termination of studies of two years or longer duration, it is clear that the beginnings of these changes take place much earlier in life. Foci of hyperplasia in the pituitary gland are already evident in *ad libitum*-fed rats of less than one year old, and prolactin levels well above the physiological range begin to be evident from the age of about six months onwards. In addition to this, irregularity of oestrus cycling is frequently rife in *ad libitum*-fed SPF female rats aged only about one year. Apart from its being obvious that rats showing such evidence of endocrine disturbance during middle life are not appropriate models for endocrinologically-normal humans, there

Table 13.2. *Percentage life-time incidence of certain endocrine tumours (benign and/or malignant) in* ad libitum-*fed Wistar rats in a study of 30-months duration*

| | Males | | Females | |
|---|---|---|---|---|
| | AL | 80% of AL[1] | AL | 80% of AL[1] |
| Number of rats | 100 | 100 | 100 | 100 |
| % rats with tumours of: | | | | |
| Adrenal | | | | |
| – cortex | 0 | 1 | 2 | 3 |
| – medulla | 3 | 4 | 3 | 1 |
| Ovary | – | – | 4 | 3 |
| Mammary | 0 | 0 | 37 | 9** |
| Pancreas | | | | |
| – islet cell | 10 | 1* | 2 | 1 |
| Parathyroid | 5 | 1 | 2 | 1 |
| Pituitary | | | | |
| – anterior lobe | 30 | 14** | 62 | 46* |
| – intermediate lobe | 13 | 9 | 6 | 0 |
| Testis | | | | |
| – Leydig cell | 23 | 30 | – | – |
| Thyroid | | | | |
| – Follicular | 1 | 1 | 2 | 0 |
| – C-cell | 2 | 2 | 8 | 4 |

AL = ad libitum; * = $p<0.01$; ** = $p<0.001$
[1]Survival was highly significantly better in the 80% of AL animals than in the AL animals hence the beneficial effects of diet restriction were actually greater than those shown and none of the apparently adverse effects are real.

is the fact that the manifestations of endocrine abnormality vary widely from rat to rat. And yet, as pointed out above, the design of studies is such that no attempt is made during the in-life phase of experiments to assess the endocrine status of individual animals.

There is abundant published evidence that, in rats, calorie-restriction prolongs life, and reduces the age-standardized incidences of many different ageing-related non-neoplastic and neoplastic diseases. Notable among the non-neoplastic conditions affected are chronic progressive nephropathy, polyarteritis, acute and chronic prostatitis, mammary gland hyperplasia, secretory activity and galactocoele formation, and a range of inflammatory conditions of the skin and subcutis. Severe chronic nephropathy impairs the maintenance of mineral balance with regard especially to calcium, magnesium and phosphate. A consequence of this impairment is hyperplasia and neoplasia of the parathyroid gland. A second consequence is an increased risk of hyperplasia and neoplasia of the adrenal medulla (Roe & Baer, 1985). Under conditions of slight dietary restriction, the incidence of parathyroid and adrenal medullary proliferative conditions tend to be significantly less. It is, however, not only the fact that overfeeding greatly increases the risk of development of ageing-related kidney disease which predisposes to parathyroid and adrenal disease, which gives cause for concern. There is also the fact that the effects vary widely from animal to animal and no attempt is being made during the in-life phase of studies to assess individual animals for the severity of nephropathy.

Obviously there exists a strong case for conducting all chronic toxicity and carcinogenicity experiments under conditions wherein premature ageing does not occur and does not introduce unwanted between-animal variation in endocrine status, and it is clear that one can partly achieve this by conducting tests under conditions of diet restriction. However, there are those who argue that dietary restriction does no more than postpone the evil day and that eventually, at an albeit later age, calorie-restricted rats end up with the same spectrum of ageing-related diseases, and in the same high incidence as *ad libitum*-fed rats. This is, in fact, not wholly true. The lifetime expectation of developing several conditions is in fact lower in calorie-restricted rats. Another commonly put forward argument is that carcinogenicity tests would have to be continued for longer than in *ad libitum*-fed animals. This, it is claimed, would simply increase the costs without any obvious benefit. We would argue, however, that experiments should not be continued after animals have begun to be in endocrinological disarray due to ageing. Experiments should be terminated while control rats are still in normal physiological status, that is, while it is still reasonable to claim that they are likely to be appropriate models for man.

The last point that we need to make here is that calorie-restriction is not a panacea for all the problems associated with the use of laboratory rats and mice in chronic toxicity and carcinogenicity tests. Although calorie restriction reduces the incidence of endocrine disturbances it by no means abolishes them. As illustrated in Table 13.2 tumours of the anterior lobe of the pituitary and of the testis may still be very high in calorie-restricted rats. This problem has been evident for years and yet no serious attempt has been made to overcome it. It is, of course, possible that genetic constitution is responsible for these unhuman-like character-istics. If so, then we need to be bold enough to abandon the strains we are using and start again to develop strains which are free from such genetic flaws. Alternatively, it is possible that the high incidences of endocrine changes which we are seeing, even in diet-restricted rats, are due to environmental factors which we as yet do not understand and cannot define. We would argue that complacency with regard to the adequacy of currently used animal models is misplaced and that there is an urgent need for fundamental research aimed at developing animal models that are more reliable, particularly from an endocrinological standpoint.

## Quantification of effects on endocrine status

When it is reasonably certain in a toxicological study that there has been an effect on endocrine status, it may be necessary to quantify it. If the mechanism involved is unclear further *in vivo* studies may be needed to elucidate it (e.g. further *in vivo* testing will be needed to explore hypo-thalamic-Leydig cell performance and adrenalcortico-steroids in a case presenting as simple virilization). On the other hand, if the mechanisms involved are known, quantification may sometimes be achieved by the use of well-established *in vitro* diagnostic and assay procedures (e.g. tissue culture methods are available for studying the effects of secretago-gues and membrane transport inhibitors of iodine uptake and metabolism by thyroid cells).

In no other area of toxicology is it more important than in endocrine toxicology to establish the specificity and sensitivity of methods used for measurement. The scientific literature is full of examples of erroneous conclusions being drawn in studies where non-specific and/or insufficiently sensitive methods have been used.

## Extrapolation from animals to man

The basic principles underlying the prediction from the findings in laboratory studies of risk for man (or for some other species in the case of veterinary products) are common to all areas of toxicology. They involve, *inter alia*, obtaining answers to four questions. First: 'Are the test species and man physiologically similar in relation to the function and activity of the endocrine gland(s) involved?' Secondly: 'Are the circumstances of exposure (i.e. dose and duration) to the test substance and its active metabolites, particularly at the target site(s), similar in man and the test species?' Thirdly: 'What is the mechanism of action in the test species: is it direct or indirect and would it be operative in man?' Lastly: 'If knowledge is lacking, is it possible, ethically, to determine whether the endocrine targets in the test animals are, in fact, targets in man?'

If the answers to all these questions are in the affirmative, the prediction of risk for humans may be straightforward. Often, however, variability of endocrine responses in different circumstances tends to engender uncertainty so that precise extrapolation is impossible and great caution is necessary.

Perhaps the most difficult areas in which to make a risk assessment are those in which the function and importance of a hormone and its consequential responses vary from one species to another (e.g. somatotrophin and prolactin in rodents versus humans), or in which the normal role of a hormone is uncertain (e.g. many neuropeptides in the gastrointestinal tract). Risk assessment is also difficult where it seems that the same hormone can have different effects at different sites (e.g. cholecystokinin and vasoactive intestinal peptide in the peripheral versus the central nervous systems), or where little or nothing is known of the mechanism of action of a hormone.

It may also be very difficult to evaluate properly the toxicological significance of tumours of the endocrine system that are endocrinologically silent (e.g. many chromophobe adenomas of the pituitary and adrenal cortical adenomas), or which do not appear to have been caused by conventional hormonal stimuli (e.g. adrenal medullary tumours secondary to disturbance of calcium homeostasis). Neoplasms of the diffuse neuroendocrine system are likely to fall into this class, at least until more is known about their pathogenesis and the physiological roles of their products.

## Future possibilities and uncertainties

Rapidly increasing knowledge in the fields of general receptorology, membrane receptors and channels, signal transduction mechanisms, and various areas of molecular biochemistry are impacting importantly on the understanding of mechanisms in endocrinology. These advances have been paralleled by greater understanding of the sources and nature of various dynamic integrative controlling systems. Even more exciting are recent discoveries of interactions between DNA and hormones and of how these may sometimes be subverted (e.g. the very recent identification of the possible receptor for peroxisome proliferation in the liver as a member of the oestrogen receptor super family). In this area, clearer understanding will surely lead to an ability to predict sites where xenobiotics may act to affect endocrine status.

At a different level, the discovery of endocrine, paracrine and autocrine controls on cell proliferation has not only enlightened our understanding of carcinogenesis, it has also brought the concepts of endocrinology into a broader area of pathology – i.e. neoplasia. That, in turn, emphasizes the importance of understanding of how normally responsive cells may become abnormal, insensitive, autochthonous tumour cells (e.g. the selective loss of control by insulin-like growth factor-1 in thyroid cells during at least one particular type of thyroid carcinogenesis).

Many uncertainties stem from the carrying out of very detailed and precise investigations on what are, in fact, nothing more than laboratory artefacts. Every investigator using model systems which are several stages away from real life should constantly be asking himself whether what he is observing relates to real life, or only to the model. If reliable micro methods requiring only very small samples of blood existed for the monitoring of circulating hormones in routine toxicity studies, they might be of great help in mapping out the pathogenesis of lesions which presently remain unsuspected until necropsy is carried out. At present, however, studies of endocrine effects is not an integral part of toxicological assessment, so that research on suspected endocrine effects has to be undertaken in separate and often quite costly studies. Clearly, careful thought combined with a full evaluation of chemical structure, known pharmacological activity, and the results of other toxicological studies, need to be given before special studies are contemplated.

An area that has not received much attention, and which merits further study, is the involvement of the endocrine system in toxicity. At a simple level, enzyme induction in the liver, which involves massive synthesis of proteins, requires normal somatotrophin, insulin and thyroxine levels for its full expression. How might it respond to limited abnormality of even just one of these factors? Similarly, renal clearance of many materials is sensitive to circulatory changes produced by a variety of peptide hormones. Other examples include the effect of androgens in inducing $2\mu$ globulin synthesis in the rat, and the partial permissive role of sex hormones in determining the response of sensitive epithelia to carcinogens, etc.

Overall, endocrinology seems well suited to toxicological experimentation, because its actions can be quantified and mechanisms can be explored, provided that a signal action is identifiable. An orderly progression of investigative studies can often be envisaged, extending from first detection of an effect in a simple experiment to precise mechanistic analysis at the molecular level. It has been argued that toxicology is no more than the flipside of pharmacology. What could be more satisfying to a toxicologist than to deduce from toxicological observations how a regulatory hormone works?

## References

Kociba, R.J., Keyes, D.G., Lisowe, R.W. *et al.* (1978). Results of a two-year chronic toxicity and oncogenicity study of 2, 3, 7, 8-tetrachlorodibenzo-p-dioxin in rats. *Toxicol. Appl. Pharmacol.*, **46**, 279–303.

Roe, F.J.C. & Baer, A. (1985). Enzootic and epizootic adrenal medullary proliferative disease of rats. *Human Toxicol.*, **4**, 27–52.

# Index